Amyotrophic Lateral Sclerosis

Amyotrophic Lateral Sclerosis
Understanding and Optimizing Quality of Life and Psychological Well-Being

Edited by

Francesco Pagnini
Department of Psychology
Università Cattolica del Sacro Cuor
Milan, Italy;
Department of Psychology
Harvard University
Cambridge, MA, USA

Zachary Simmons
Departments of Neurology and Humanities
Penn State Hershey Medical Center
Hershey, PA, USA

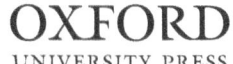

OXFORD
UNIVERSITY PRESS

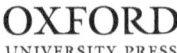
UNIVERSITY PRESS

Great Clarendon Street, Oxford, OX2 6DP,
United Kingdom

Oxford University Press is a department of the University of Oxford.
It furthers the University's objective of excellence in research, scholarship,
and education by publishing worldwide. Oxford is a registered trade mark of
Oxford University Press in the UK and in certain other countries

Published in the United States of America by Oxford University Press
198 Madison Avenue, New York, NY 10016, United States of America

British Library Cataloguing in Publication Data

Data available

Library of Congress Control Number: 2017955148

ISBN 978–0–19–875772–6

Printed in Great Britain by
Ashford Colour Press Ltd, Gosport, Hampshire

Foreword

Brian Dickie, PhD, Director of Research Development, Motor Neurone Disease Association

Over the past quarter-century we have seen ALS emerge from a relative backwater to the forefront of neurological science, with major advances in understanding disease pathogenesis, a much deeper insight into the clinical heterogeneity and syndromic nature of ALS, and of course, the welcome emergence of new treatment strategies. The signs are encouraging that this disease may not be as intractable as once believed.

It is often said that ALS is a disease of low prevalence, but high need. Certainly the wide diversity of symptoms—physical, cognitive, behavioural, and psychological—compounded by a relentless speed of progression, require a genuinely universal approach to management and support, not only for the patient, but also for their caregivers and family. The term 'holistic care' could have been coined specifically for ALS.

This book does not aim to follow the path of many predecessors by concentrating on the biological and clinical aspects of the disease, but instead seeks to complement the literature through a detailed evaluation of the complex psychosocial aspects of ALS that would, in the past, have probably been combined into a single final chapter. It does not shy away from difficult topics such as the relationship between 'quality of death' and 'quality of life'. It also recognizes that, in our modern information-driven society, patients and their families are increasingly well informed—and sometimes misinformed—creating novel challenges for health care professionals.

It is also said that if you can get the care right for ALS, you can get it right for any disease. This book will certainly be an asset to professionals with an interest in the former and make informative and insightful reading for others.

Foreword

Ammar Al-Chalabi, Professor of Neurology and Complex Disease Genetics

Francesco Pagnini is a psychologist and assistant professor at the Catholic University of the Sacred Heart in Milan, while Zachary Simmons is a neurologist and professor at Penn State Hershey Medical Center. This book, like its editors, is a fusion of the psychological with the neurological.

Like many others, my first contact with Francesco Pagnini, was on hearing him talk as recipient of the European Network to Cure ALS Young Investigator Award, where I was fortunate, as Chair of the Award Committee, to give him the international prize for outstanding and novel ALS research. I first met Zach Simmons during a meeting on ALS clinical trials, in which he was advocating a more holistic and patient-orientated approach to patient care, a direction he still follows passionately and very effectively. The two of them have worked as a formidable team, pulling together a superb collection of chapters written by the foremost figures and future leaders in quality of life and psychological well-being in ALS.

The book itself is like a welcoming silhouette, visible through blinding glare, the silhouette being the recognition of the role of the mind in ALS, and the glare being the overwhelming emphasis on physical symptoms. The most striking effect of ALS is physical weakness, manifesting not only as the main symptom, but also the most obvious finding on neurological examination; indeed, the other name for ALS, 'motor neuron disease', focuses our attention on the involvement of the motor system, while text books announce that it is a disease confined to the motor system. It is a welcome and timely contrast to this emphasis on the physical that we have, in one place, a set of accessible and relevant papers covering all aspects of the psychological. I was struck by how comprehensive the subjects covered are, from the internal reactions of people to the diagnosis and subsequent disability, to the external responses in engaging with conventional and alternative therapies; from the effect of ALS on sexuality and intimacy to the psychological support available from family, friends, professionals, and the virtual world; from the measurement of quality of life, to the most effective ways to improve it; from the effect of ALS on communication, cognition, and behaviour on the affected person, to the effects on caregivers.

I learned a huge amount reading this book. I am sure it will act as a landmark for the future in which we deeply understand the intertwining of the mind and body, the psychological, and the neurological, in ALS.

Contents

Contributors

Sharon Abrahams
Euan MacDonald Centre for Motor Neurone Disease Research, University of Edinburgh, UK; Human Cognitive Neuroscience Unit, School of Psychology, Philosophy, and Language Sciences, University of Edinburgh, UK

Paolo Banfi
Don Carlo Gnocchi Foundation, Milan, Italy

Tom Burke
Academic Unit of Neurology, Trinity College Dublin, Ireland; Beaumont Hospital, Dublin, Ireland

Jashelle Caga
Brain and Mind Centre, University of Sydney, Camperdown, NSW, Australia; Sydney Medical School, University of Sydney, Camperdown, NSW, Australia

Adriano Chiò
'Rita Levi Montalcini' Department of Neuroscience, University of Torino, Turin, Italy; Neuroscience Institute of Torino, Turin, Italy

Christopher Crockford
Euan MacDonald Centre for Motor Neurone Disease Research, University of Edinburgh, UK; Human Cognitive Neuroscience Unit, School of Psychology, Philosophy, and Language Sciences, University of Edinburgh, UK

Michelle L. Dube
Department of Psychology, Philadelphia College of Osteopathic Medicine, Philadelphia, PA, USA

Stephanie H. Felgoise
Department of Psychology, Philadelphia College of Osteopathic Medicine, Philadelphia, PA, USA

Miriam Galvin
Academic Unit of Neurology, Trinity College Dublin, Ireland

Chris Gibbons
Manchester Centre for Health Psychology, School of Psychological Sciences, University of Manchester, UK

Laura H. Goldstein
Institute of Psychiatry, Psychology and Neuroscience, King's College London, UK

Christopher D. Graham
Leeds Institute of Health Sciences, University of Leeds, UK; Department of Clinical Neuropsychology, St. James Hospital, Leeds, UK

Orla Hardiman
Academic Unit of Neurology, Trinity College Dublin, Ireland; Beaumont Hospital, Dublin, Ireland

Matthew C. Kiernan
Brain and Mind Centre, University of Sydney, Camperdown, NSW, Australia; Sydney Medical School, University of Sydney, Camperdown, NSW, Australia

Andrea Kübler
Institute of Psychology, University of Würzburg, Germany

Ellen Langer
Department of Psychology, Harvard University, Cambridge, MA, USA

Albert C. Ludolph
Department of Neurology, University of Ulm, Germany

Dorothée Lulé
Department of Neurology, University of Ulm, Germany

Sinead Maguire
Academic Unit of Neurology, Trinity College Dublin, Ireland; Beaumont Hospital, Dublin, Ireland

Anna Marconi
Neuromuscular Omnicentre (NEMO), Serena Onlus Foundation, Milan, Italy

David Oliver
Tizard Centre, University of Kent, Canterbury, UK

Francesco Pagnini
Department of Psychology, Università Cattolica del Sacro Cuore, Milan, Italy; Department of Psychology, Harvard University, Cambridge, MA, USA

Arianna Palmieri
Philosophy, Sociology, Education, and Applied Psychology Department, University of Padova, Italy; Padua Neuroscience Centre, University of Padova, Italy

Niall Pender
Academic Unit of Neurology, Trinity College Dublin, Ireland; Beaumont Hospital, Dublin, Ireland

Deborah Phillips
Department of Psychology, Harvard University, Cambridge, MA, USA

James A. Russell
Department of Neurology, Lahey Hospital and Medical Center, Burlington, MA, USA

Peggy Z. Shipley
Bloomsburg University Department of Nursing, Bloomsburg, PA, USA

Zachary Simmons
Departments of Neurology and Humanities, Penn State Hershey Medical Center, Hershey, PA, USA

Bryan J. Traynor
Neuromuscular Diseases Research Section, Laboratory of Neurogenetics, National Institute on Aging, National Institutes of Health, Bethesda, MD, USA; Brain Science Institute, Department of Neurology, Johns Hopkins University, Baltimore, MD, USA

Eleonora Volpato
Department of Psychology, Università Cattolica del Sacro Cuore, Milan, Italy; Don Carlo Gnocchi Foundation, Milan, Italy

Tamlyn J. Watermeyer
Centre for Dementia Prevention, University of Edinburgh, UK

Paul Wicks
PatientsLikeMe, Cambridge, MA, USA

Vincenzo Zaccheo
Department of Psychology, Philadelphia College of Osteopathic Medicine, Philadelphia, PA, USA

Chapter 1

Psychological research in amyotrophic lateral sclerosis: Past, present, and future

Tamlyn J. Watermeyer and Laura H. Goldstein

This chapter evaluates research that has investigated psychological interventions for optimizing well-being in people with amyotrophic lateral sclerosis (ALS) and their caregivers. It outlines earlier work that sought to identify correlates of reduced well-being and quality of life (QoL) in ALS, and delineates possible targets for intervention, such as hopelessness, depression, and anxiety. The chapter reviews current efforts to address the paucity of interventional research in ALS, focusing on five therapies that have so far been evaluated for treatment efficacy—hypnosis, mindfulness, cognitive behavioural therapy (CBT), expressive disclosure therapy, and dignity therapy. Positive effects for some therapies have been indicated, improving psychological and physical outcomes. However, caution in the interpretation of these findings is thought to be due to various methodological limitations present across these studies. Future research is needed to overcome these limitations and assess appropriate routes for implementation of these therapies in clinical settings.

Given the progressively debilitating and life-limiting nature of ALS, it is reasonable to expect that various psychological reactions might occur at different milestones over a patient's disease course. The study of these reactions enables greater insight into patients' psychological journeys through their illness. In turn, this information can better prepare clinical teams to support ALS patients and their families at varying stages of the disease. First, we will introduce early work that identified the psychological and psychosocial implications of the disease, and from which various targets for intervention were initially proposed. Following that, the main focus of this chapter is on current work investigating psychological interventions in ALS, with therapeutic paradigms examined in succession. Finally, we discuss future directions for this work and its implications for clinical practice.

Past

Historically, people with ALS were believed to remain 'stoic' in the face of their illness, experiencing little or no dysphoria (1). This viewpoint was then challenged by the variable prevalence rates reported for mood disorder within the disease (2–4) and the acknowledged limitations of using generic self-report outcome measures potentially confounded by somatically determined symptoms. Thus, debate persists as to whether psychological distress is an inevitable consequence as ALS progresses (see Chapter 3). Similarly, the assumption that compromised QoL accompanies patients' increasing debility appears to be mistaken. Several studies have shown that QoL is independent of physical impairment even in the late stages of disease (5–7). The noted paradox between physical impairment and well-being in ALS highlights the possible contributory role of psychological factors in patients' vulnerability (or resilience) to the development of distress. It has been suggested that patients undergo a 'response shift', whereby they maintain a sense of well-being through deriving more satisfaction from external factors, such as social networks and spirituality, in spite of the losses brought about by their unrelenting disability (6). Identifying personal characteristics or situational factors that may prevent or facilitate this 'shift' is pivotal to supporting patients' well-being (See Chapter 2).

Some premorbid traits, such as optimism, reflectiveness, and humour, have been shown to help sustain well-being in people with ALS (8, 9). Likewise, the role of pre-existing social relationships in determining QoL, mood, and self-esteem in ALS patients has been demonstrated through cross-sectional and longitudinal research (10–12). Patients' perceptions of the burden placed upon their caregiver are also correlated with their own level of depression (13, 14). These findings suggest that interventions might usefully aim to consolidate patients' social networks and interpersonal relationships, perhaps by incorporating support from and for patients' families and friends.

Spirituality and religiosity have also been shown to influence patients' perceived QoL and their attitudes towards dying (15, 16), possibly offering patients meaning and coherence in life-threatening crises (10). Indeed, patients' reflections on existential domains, such as death, freedom, and meaning, were the most important contributors to QoL scores in one study (16). Loss of meaning (purpose in life), together with an external locus of control, predicts a sense of hopelessness above and beyond the physical consequence of the disease (17). Hopelessness is mostly a future-orientated construct, defined as a system of cognitive schemas converging upon negative expectations about one's future and oneself (see Chapter 3). It is a common outcome for people with ALS (4) and a predictor of depression, low QoL, and suicidal ideation (3, 12, 18). Therefore, targeting hopelessness in ALS, through reorientating patients' thoughts to the present, as well as constructing an internal locus of control, and restoring purpose and meaning to their lives, might significantly alter patients' experiences of their illness.

Despite an established literature outlining the psychological and existential implications for those affected by ALS, efforts to address these consequences through targeted interventions are relatively recent. Pagnini and his colleagues were the first to appeal to the scientific community to address the paucity of studies evaluating the efficacy of psychological interventions for patients and their caregivers (19). Since then, various approaches have been evaluated for their efficacy, feasibility, and applicability for people with ALS. These approaches will be reviewed in the next section 'Present'. Additional details about study design and outcomes are provided in Table 1.1. An

Table 1.1 Summary of main findings for ALS psychological intervention studies

Authors	Therapeutic technique; study design	Participants	Main findings
Palmeri et al. (20)	Hypnosis intervention with autohypnosis training; Cohort study (pilot), pre-post-intervention assessments	Eight ALS patients; no control group; eight caregivers	Intervention effects for anxiety, depression, global QoL Subjective improvement in ALS symptoms Reduced anxiety and depression reported by caregivers
Kleinbub et al. (21)	Hypnosis intervention with autohypnosis training; pre-post-intervention assessments; follow-up assessments 3 and 6 months following treatment	15 ALS patients; 15 matched controls (from database); 15 caregivers	Intervention effects for anxiety, depression (patients and caregivers), QoL (patients) evident at post-treatment assessment Intervention effects for anxiety (patients and caregivers) and depression (caregiver) present at 3- and 6-month follow-ups. Patients and caregivers' defence style profiles showed an effect on these outcomes, independent of intervention effect Patients in intervention group showed slower disease progression than controls over observation period
Perez & Dapueto (27)	CBT and expressive-supportive models; case study	66-year-old female with ALS, study commenced 3 months after diagnosis until 3 years of disease	Patient reported reduced psychological distress, enhanced autonomy, dignity and self-esteem, better symptom control and communication with family and healthcare professionals
Diaz et al. (28)	CBT; non-randomized trial (allocation determined by participants' availability to complete sessions).	30 ALS patients; 30 controls	Patients showed reduced anxiety and depression symptoms; control participants showed opposite pattern of symptoms
van Groenestijn et al. (31)	CBT; TAU; RCT	15 ALS patients: 10 CBT arm; five TAU arm; 10 caregivers	Emotional functioning remained stable in CBT arm; declined in TAU arm Caregivers' burden remained stable in CBT arm; deteriorated in TAU arm Caregivers' QoL improved in the CBT arm; deteriorated in the TAU arm

(Continued)

Table 1.1 Continued

Authors	Therapeutic technique; study design	Participants	Main findings
Averill et al. (34)	Expressive disclosure; RCT	48 ALS patients: 24 treatment group (disclosure); 24 control group (no-disclosure)	Treatment group showed improvements in 'well-being composite' at 3-month post-intervention follow-up, with score reversing to baseline levels at 6-month follow-up. Control group showed reductions in 'wellbeing composite' at 3-month post-intervention, with scores improving to baseline levels at 6-month follow-up
Bentley et al. (41); Aoun et al. (42)*	Dignity therapy	29 ALS patients (Bentley et al., 2014)/27 ALS patients (Aoun et al., 2014)*	No intervention effects observed at the group level
Pagnini et al. (51)	Mindfulness; RCT	100 ALS patients: 50 treatment group (meditation training); 50 control group (usual care)	Treatment group showed improvement in quality of life, depression, and anxiety scores relative to the control group

* Aoun et al. 2014 sample only included participants recruited from MND Association for Western Australia who were registered members, while the Bentley et al. 2014 sample also comprised patients who were not registered with the organization; results were published separately.

RCT = randomized controlled trial; TAU = treatment as usual; CBT = cognitive behavioural therapy; QoL = quality of life.

overview of the strengths and limitations of these intervention studies will be presented in our discussion of future directions for work in this area.

Present

Hypnosis-based therapy

One of the first approaches to be evaluated for the treatment of psychological suffering in individuals with ALS was hypnosis. In a preliminary study, Palmieri et al. (20) recruited a pilot sample of eight patients to examine the possible effects of a 1-month hypnosis-based intervention and self-hypnosis training protocol on self-reported levels of depression, anxiety, and perceived QoL. Improvements, with large effect sizes, were observed on all the patients' outcome measures when comparing pre-treatment to post-treatment values. Patients also endorsed subjective improvements in symptoms of pain, emotional lability, and muscle fasciculations, attributing these improvements to the hypnosis intervention. Caregivers showed reduced anxiety and depression over the course of their partner's therapy, suggesting a possible indirect benefit for caregivers of ALS patients who engage in such therapeutic approaches. Following these encouraging results, the same research group investigated longer-term effects of hypnosis-based treatment on an ALS sample (21). Fifteen ALS patients received a 1-month hypnosis-based intervention and self-hypnosis training, similar to that described by Palmieri et al. (20). Psychological outcomes were measured at baseline, immediately after the treatment, and at 3 and 6 months after the end of treatment. In keeping with the preliminary evidence from the earlier study, patients and caregivers showed a reduction in anxiety and depression, while patients also reported higher QoL post-treatment. The improvements observed for patients' and caregivers' anxiety, as well as caregivers' depression scores persisted at the 3- and 6-month follow-ups. This study also assessed patient and caregivers' defensive styles (maladaptive, image-distorting, or adaptive) and defence mechanisms (e.g. passive aggression, fantasy, denial, affiliation, suppression). For both participant groups, defence style profiles impacted on mood scores over time, with higher scores for maladaptive defence styles associated with lower anxiety scores in patients, and lower anxiety and depression scores in caregivers. These effects were independent of the hypnosis treatment effects found for both groups, indicating that the effectiveness of the hypnosis treatment did not depend on the amount or type of defence styles employed by participants. The design and results of these two studies and the interpretations of their findings are discussed in more detail in Chapter 5.

Cognitive behavioural therapy

CBT is an intervention based on the premise that psychological distress is maintained through cognitive processes that affect emotion and behaviour. How a person thinks can affect how they behave and this in turn can affect how they think and feel. Maladaptive thoughts, which encourage dysfunctional behaviour, can be identified and challenged by examining the evidence for or against these cognitions, leading to their substitution with alternative more reality-orientated interpretations (22). The effectiveness of CBT for treating depression and anxiety, as well as reduced QoL, fatigue, and disability has been demonstrated for people with chronic neurological conditions such as multiple sclerosis (23, 24) and Parkinson's disease (25, 26).

Only three studies to date have considered the potential benefits of CBT for people with ALS. The first, a case study, adopted a psychotherapy based on a combination of CBT and expressive-supportive models (27). The therapy was eventually delivered using a computer-assisted language device to circumvent the patient's speech difficulties, which progressed over the course of treatment (from diagnosis to 3 years of disease). The intervention was deemed successful, with the patient, a 66-year-old woman, reporting a reduction in psychological distress, enhanced autonomy, dignity, and self-esteem, as well as improved symptom control and communication with family and healthcare professionals. As with all case-study designs, the generalizability of these results to the wider ALS population is limited, but exemplifies how CBT might be applied in the context of progressive disease severity.

In the same year, Diaz et al. (28) investigated the effects of CBT on symptoms of anxiety and depression in a group of 30 ALS patients. This sample was compared with a control group of 24 patients who had shown an interest in taking part in the CBT, but who could not participate due to the time or travel burden associated with the study. The frequency and number of CBT sessions offered to the intervention group varied according to individual need; patients were considered to have completed the intervention after four appointments. The sessions took place 15–25 days apart and varied in theme. An initial interview identified patients' thoughts and perceptions about their disease, evaluated their family relationships, and established the presence of coping styles or denial mechanisms. The remaining sessions focused on psychoeducation about ALS, CBT training (such as learning cognitive restructuring and emotional management tools), and addressing concerns regarding palliative aids and assisting the decision-making process surrounding these, as well as enhancing problem solving and self-esteem. While the intervention procedures followed a standardized delivery, each session was adjusted to accommodate the individual patient's requirements and characteristics. Results of the study showed that following the four treatment sessions, the intervention group showed a significant reduction in symptoms of anxiety and depression, while the control group showed the opposite pattern. It is possible that the intervention provided participants with adaptive coping mechanisms, which facilitated their emotional expression and regulation, thereby modifying their mood. However, the study did not incorporate a randomized design and it may be that more depressed, anxious, or motivated participants elected to complete the intervention. Indeed, the intervention group showed higher levels of anxiety than the control group at baseline. This group difference was not accounted for in the analyses and may have influenced the results obtained.

A randomized controlled trial (RCT), where participants are randomly assigned to treatment conditions following baseline assessment, but prior to the intervention delivery, is considered to be the gold-standard method for clinical research, as it mitigates the influence of selection bias and reduces the possibly of spurious causes for the observed effect. Van Groenetijn et al. (29) adopted this design to compare the efficacy of CBT, aerobic exercise therapy (AET), and treatment as usual (TAU, i.e. no additional intervention) on physical functioning and QoL in ALS patients. Participants in the CBT group were offered sessions, either individually or jointly with their caregiver, depending on the issue at hand. The authors intended to recruit 120 participants, using multicentre support. Participants were invited if they scored in the clinical range for anxiety or depression on the Hospital Anxiety and Depression Scale (30). Participation involved a 4-month intervention period, with follow-ups designated at 3 and 6 months from treatment allocation. Unfortunately, the trial concluded prematurely at 42 months due to poor recruitment ($n = 15$) and a lack of demand for joint patient-caregiver CBT sessions. The results were published as a study that compared CBT with TAU, since only three participants had been randomized to the AET condition at the termination of the trial (31). Ten participants received the CBT intervention, while five were allocated to the TAU condition. Participants in the CBT arm showed no change in scores on an index of emotional functioning, while the TAU participants' scores declined on the same measure. Similarly, levels of caregiver burden were maintained at a similar level in the CBT arm, but increased under the TAU condition. Finally, caregivers' scores on the Mental Component Summary (measuring mental health-related QoL from the Health Survey Short Form (SF-36)) (32), improved under the CBT intervention, but deteriorated under the TAU condition. While these results suggest some benefit of the CBT treatment over TAU for ALS patients and their caregivers, the small sample size and uneven distribution of participants between treatment conditions limits the generalizability of these findings.

Expressive-disclosure therapy

The disclosure of negative thoughts or traumatic events is commonplace in counselling and 'talking' therapies. Such disclosure may facilitate the cognitive re-appraisal of distressing thoughts and emotions surrounding the events and create more coherent narratives about the self, one's environment, and the events in question (33). The effects of expressive-disclosure therapy on the well-being of ALS patients were investigated in a study of 48 participants using an RCT design (34). Twenty-four participants were randomly assigned to a therapeutic condition in which they wrote or recorded (via voice recorder) their thoughts and feelings about their experiences of living with ALS for three 20-minute sessions over the course of one week. The remaining participants were assigned to the no-disclosure control condition, where, like the treatment group, they completed the study measures at baseline, and at 3 and 6 months post-intervention assessments, but were encouraged not to discuss emotional topics. The primary outcome measure, psychological well-being, was indexed by a composite score comprising measures of affect, QoL, and spirituality. At baseline, the study also measured participants' 'ambivalence over emotional expression' (the extent to which participants feel uncomfortable or regret expressing emotions), their tendencies for 'emotional coping' (the use of emotional processing strategies and freedom to express emotions), and their levels of perceived 'social constraints' (their perceived inadequacy of support from relatives or friends to express thoughts or feelings about ALS). Based on evidence from other medical populations (35, 36), these variables were considered as potential moderators for the effects of the intervention and were examined as such in the analyses.

The results of the trial revealed that participants allocated to the therapeutic intervention showed an improvement in the well-being composite scores from the baseline assessment to the 3-month follow-up, but that these scores returned to baseline levels at the 6-month follow-up. In contrast, the well-being composite scores for the control group decreased at the 3-month follow-up and then improved to baseline levels at the 6-month follow-up. These patterns across the groups might suggest that stressors, such as increasing disability, negatively affect well-being in both groups, but that disclosure therapy possesses a short-term (less than 6 months) buffering effect. However, this does not explain why the control group's scores improved back to baseline levels at the 6-month point. The authors suggest that the control participants may have actively inhibited negative thoughts and feelings following randomization which resulted in short-term (less than 3 months) negative effects on well-being. Nonetheless, without a measure of thought or emotion inhibition, the explanation for this observed pattern within the control group remains tentative. Notably, greater 'ambivalence over emotional expression' was related to a more robust intervention effect at the 3-month follow-up. This relationship suggests that people with ALS who are unable or feel more hesitant to express their emotions may benefit more from this type of intervention, in terms of well-being, than those who are already comfortable with expressive disclosure.

Dignity therapy

Dignity, as a construct, is not well-defined in ALS research, let alone in clinical practice, despite being an important existential issue for those affected by the illness (37). Its maintenance is a great challenge for palliative care, especially in the face of an increasingly debilitating disease course. Dignity therapy, an intervention based on empirical models of dignity at the end of life (38), offers patients an opportunity to address personally relevant issues and leave a legacy for their relatives, while also encouraging a sense of meaning and hope. The therapy is scheduled over several sessions, covering several themes, from the patients' sense of personhood to concerns over the implications of their death for their loved ones. Each session is transcribed and edited, with the aim of creating a physical document for the patient to bequeath to chosen individuals. Family-members can support the therapy during the interviewing and editing processes, and are often the intended recipients of the final document. Relative to standard and client-centred care practises, the intervention has been found to enhance dignity and improve QoL in patients with terminal illness (39). It has also been shown to moderate relatives' bereavement experiences 9 to 12 months following the patient's death (40).

An ALS study of dignity therapy in a cohort of 29 patients failed to find treatment effects on measured outcomes (41, 42). However, pre-intervention scores for hopefulness, spirituality, and dignity-related distress were high, moderate, and low, respectively. Thus, the benefits of the psychosocial intervention may not be as readily apparent in this small sample of patients. At the individual-level, four patients showed improvement in hopefulness, seven reported a deterioration, and 16 reported no change on this outcome. In line with evidence suggesting a relationship between spirituality and outcomes in ALS (10, 15, 16), those who showed an increase in hopefulness reported that they were both religious and spiritual, while 43% of patients whose hopefulness scores decreased reported that they were neither religious nor spiritual. Interestingly, two of the four patients with increased hopefulness scores had been diagnosed with ALS at least 4 years earlier, while 85% of the group whose scores declined had been diagnosed for 2 years or less (41). These results tentatively suggest that dignity therapy may be effective at increasing hopefulness in patients who are more spiritual and/or at the advanced stages of disease. Despite the lack of group effects, a large majority of patients deemed the intervention to be satisfactory and helpful to themselves and their families. Patients reported that the intervention assisted in supporting their unique identity, helped with their acceptance and concerns following their death, and aided their ability to find meaning and purpose. Endorsements such as these suggest that dignity therapy may influence other important aspects of patients' experiences, which might not have been captured by the primary outcome measures. The results of this study underscore the importance of participants' qualitative feedback as an adjunct to the quantitative measurement of study outcomes in the assessment of interventions for people with ALS.

Mindfulness-based therapies

There has been a recent resurgence of scientific interest in mindfulness techniques across academic disciplines (43). The positive effects of these therapies on physical and psychological health in medical and healthy populations have been indicated through meta-analyses (44, 45). In particular, the benefits of meditation training in the context of neurodegenerative disorders, such as multiple sclerosis (46) and Parkinson's disease (47) have been delineated. Mindfulness as a predictor of well-being has been indicated by two separate, but parallel studies of ALS patients ($n = 104$; 48) and ALS caregivers ($n = 55$; 49). In both studies, participants' levels of 'trait mindfulness' were assessed using the Langer Mindfulness Scale (LMS; 50), a measure that quantifies the person's tendency to seek new learning opportunities, have more awareness of their relationship with the environment, and apply new information to learn about their current experience. Patients scoring higher on this construct at baseline reported reduced depression and anxiety, and improved QoL at a 4-month follow-up (48). Similar results were revealed for the ALS caregivers with high LMS scores who reported reduced depression, anxiety, burden, and greater QoL over the same time-frame (49). Recently, an RCT design was used to investigate the physical and psychological implications of mindfulness meditation as an intervention for people affected by ALS (51). An impressive 100 people with ALS were recruited to the study and were randomized to receive either an 8-week meditation training, tailored to accommodate the ALS symptomatology, or to continue with their usual care (control group). Relative to the control group, patients receiving the meditation treatment reported improvements to their QoL as well as reduced anxiety and depression. Together, these findings suggest that mindfulness might serve as a protective factor against mood disorder and reduced QoL following disease onset. Furthermore, the caregiver study positions mindfulness as a potential cognitive strategy to reduce burden associated with caring for someone with the disease. The design and results of these studies and the interpretations of their findings are discussed in more detail in Chapter 4.

Future

The few studies to date evaluating psychological interventions for people with ALS provide some encouraging results. In particular, there is evidence that some therapies can improve patients' and caregivers' well-being in the short term (i.e. for less than 6 months), and might even influence disease progression or severity. Nonetheless, while progress in this area of ALS research is welcomed, there is still much work to be done before conclusions about the efficacy of these treatments in ALS can be reached.

The intervention studies reviewed in this chapter have employed varying therapeutic techniques, design, and patients samples. Due to some methodological issues, caution is warranted when interpreting the results of these studies (for a summary see 52). Most noticeably, the majority of sample sizes are small, lacking power to detect true effects. Furthermore, only one trial of CBT specified psychological morbidity as an inclusion criterion (31). Consequently, patients recruited to some of these studies were not necessarily experiencing significant psychological distress, possibly limiting demonstrable benefits of the applied therapies (41, 42).

Only two of the completed studies to date opted for a RCT design (34, 51), and many of the remaining studies did not include a control group (20, 41, 42). Where a control group was included (28), participants were not randomly assigned, but were instead allocated to the treatment condition on the basis of their availability for sessions, increasing the likelihood of self-selection bias. No study included an active control group and, thus, the presence of placebo effects for positive results cannot be excluded. Future studies should follow a RCT design and include an active control group to reduce the bias associated with participants' expectations about treatment outcomes, even though this will increase required sample sizes. In addition, while it is not always possible to blind participants to the therapeutic modality to which they are allocated, appropriate blinding methods for researchers assessing participants' outcomes should be applied. Piloting of trial procedures should be considered before an ambitious RCT project commences to ensure feasibility. For example, the main barrier to completion of Van Groenetjin et al.'s CBT trial was a poor recruitment rate. The intervention period for this study was prolonged (4 months) and patients and caregivers who already felt burdened due to ALS may have been unwilling to participate in an intervention of this length. Piloting might have highlighted patients' concerns regarding participation and informed the final study procedures.

Piloting is also useful for determining the most appropriate assessment measures. Caveats associated with the ascertainment of psychological distress and QoL in ALS will be discussed elsewhere in this book (See Chapters 2 and 3). The sensitivity of these measures to demonstrate change in outcomes over time is also pertinent, particularly for studies seeking to show prolonged effects of treatment. More research is required to determine which psychological measures are best suited for these purposes. Gaining qualitative information from participants, as an adjunct to quantitative measures, may further characterize their experiences of the treatments and barriers to participation, leading to interventions being more tailored to people with ALS in the future.

While tailoring therapeutic interventions to the disease is a key research objective, the individuality of the patient is paramount in a clinical situation. Characteristics such as cognitive status, personality traits, and behavioural styles, which may moderate changes in outcomes or at least how the therapy is delivered, deserve further investigation. One study found that defence mechanisms, such as 'denial', showed positive effects on mood, independent of the therapy's effect (21). Other studies suggest religiosity/spirituality may mediate perceived improvements (41, 42), while individuals who are less comfortable with emotional expression could benefit more from disclosure-type interventions (34). A therapist's knowledge of these factors in an individual patient might assist, complement, or modify on-going therapeutic treatments with that patient. Likewise, the therapist's experience in treating patients with ALS is an important component to a successful intervention as this can affect their own confidence in being able to support patients to express their fears regarding their illness, as well as help the therapist to identify non-physical impacts of the disease, such as cognitive or behavioural change (53).

Most studies excluded patients with cognitive impairment (although cognitive screens were either absent or limited to one measure). Therapies such as mindfulness, which require a level of focus and cognitive flexibility, may be more difficult for patients showing attentional and executive function deficits. Similarly, disclosure and dignity therapies rely heavily on abstraction, emotional regulation, and language functions, which have been shown to be compromised in some patients with ALS

(54). Future research should consider evaluation of whether psychological therapies are effective for, or can be modified to accommodate, individuals with cognitive impairment. Caregivers' burden is predicted not only by patients' disease variables, but also by their neuropsychiatric symptoms (55, 56), which in some cases may be more important (57, 58). Therefore, interventions that accommodate patients' cognitive and behavioural profiles could prove most useful to ALS couples who would otherwise be considered inappropriate for treatment. Most of the studies recognized the caregiver as a valuable enactor of patients' well-being, by inviting them to participate. Given the evidence for the relationship between patients' and caregivers' psychological status (10, 19, 55, 57) and reports that caregivers may show lower levels of QoL and greater depression than patients over time (59), it is important that interventions are offered to, and fit the needs of, both parties, either as a dyadic unit or as individuals.

A subsidiary question is how to adapt such therapies for the clinic environment where the patient's disease evolves over time. None of the intervention studies reviewed in this chapter examined outcomes beyond 6 months following the end of treatment, presumably to avoid high attrition due to illness progression. Inferences regarding the application of these therapies in advancing ALS are therefore restricted. Nonetheless, a case study did show that regular psychotherapy spanning a 3-year period from diagnosis could accommodate the patient's speech difficulties with the help of an alphabetic display and computer program (27). The use of communication aids or brain–computer interface technologies might circumvent some of the physical restrictions imposed by ALS, but the validity and convenience of their use in conjunction with the different therapies discussed here cannot be assumed. The economic costs associated with these devices may prevent treatment. An advantage of most of these psychological therapies is that they are relatively inexpensive, in some cases requiring only pen and paper (e.g. disclosure therapy). Some can be self-administered once a level of expertise is achieved (e.g. mindfulness, hypnosis), or managed via email or electronic portal (e.g. dignity therapy), but others such as CBT require the availability of trained therapists who can adapt the intervention to accommodate the physical (and potentially cognitive) impairments of the person with ALS. The evaluation of newer, third-wave CBT approaches such as acceptance and commitment therapy (ACT), which includes aspects of mindfulness, is also worthy of consideration for patients with ALS and already has an evidence base in life-limiting muscle disorders (60, 61). The cost-effectiveness of delivering these therapies within or alongside a multidisciplinary team will, however, need to be evaluated before they can become commonplace within ALS services.

Conclusions

Many studies have sought to understand the existential impacts of ALS on patients and their caregivers. There is now a move towards evaluating the applicability and effectiveness of various psychotherapeutic techniques to improve psychological outcomes in ALS. Positive effects for some therapies have been indicated, improving psychological and physical outcomes. However, the various methodological limitations present across intervention studies prevent robust conclusions regarding these treatments' effectiveness. How these therapies can be tailored to fit individual patients' needs, and their physical and cognitive limitations for the purposes of clinical management is a matter for future investigation.

References

1. Brown, W.A. and Mueller, P.S. (1970) Psychological function in individuals with amyotrophic lateral sclerosis (ALS). *Psychosomatic Medicine*, **32**(2), 141–52.
2. Taylor, L., Wicks, P., Leigh, P.N., and Goldstein, L.H. (2010) Prevalence of depression in amyotrophic lateral sclerosis and other motor disorders. *European Journal of Neurology*, **17**(8), 1047–53.
3. McLeod, J.E. and Clarke, D.M. (2007) A review of psychosocial aspects of motor neurone disease. *Journal of the Neurological Sciences*, **258**(1–2), 4–10.
4. Averill, A.J., Kasarskis, E.J., and Segerstrom, S.C. (2007) Psychological health in patients with amyotrophic lateral sclerosis. *Amyotrophic Lateral Sclerosis*, **8**(4), 243–54.
5. Simmons, Z., Bremer, B.A., Robbins, R.A., Walsh, S.M., and Fischer, S. (2000) Quality of life in ALS depends on factors other than strength and physical function. *Neurology*, **55**(3), 388–92.
6. Neudert, C., Wasner, M., and Borasio, G.D. (2004) Individual quality of life is not correlated with health-related quality of life or physical function in patients with amyotrophic lateral sclerosis. *Journal of Palliative Medicine*, **7**(4), 551–7.
7. Hardiman, O., Hickey, A., and O'Donerty, L.J. (2004) Physical decline and quality of life in amyotrophic lateral sclerosis. *Amyotrophic Lateral Sclerosis and Other Motor Neuron Disorders*, **5**(4), 230–4.
8. Nelson, N.D., Trail, M., Van, J.N., Appel, S.H., and Lai, E.C. (2003) Quality of life in patients with amyotrophic lateral sclerosis: perceptions, coping resources, and illness characteristics. *Journal of Palliative Medicine*, **6**(3), 417–24.
9. Young, J.M. and McNicoll, P. (1998) Against all odds: positive life experiences of people with advanced amyotrophic lateral sclerosis. *Health & Social Work*, **23**(1), 35–43.
10. Chiò, A., Gauthier, A., Montuschi, A., et al. (2004) A cross sectional study on determinants of quality of life in ALS. *Journal of Neurology, Neurosurgery & Psychiatry*, **75**(11), 1597–601.
11. Goldstein, L.H., Atkins, L., Landau, S., Brown, R., and Leigh, P.N. (2006) Predictors of psychological distress in carers of people with amyotrophic lateral sclerosis: a longitudinal study. *Psychological Medicine*, **36**(06), 865–75.
12. Matuz, T., Birbaumer, N., Hautzinger, M., and Kübler, A. (2010) Coping with amyotrophic lateral sclerosis: an integrative view. *Journal of Neurology, Neurosurgery & Psychiatry*, **81**(8), 893.
13. Rabkin, J.G., Wagner, G.J., and Del Bene, M. (2000) Resilience and distress among amyotrophic lateral sclerosis patients and caregivers. *Psychosomatic Medicine*, **62**(2), 271–9.
14. Gauthier, A., Vignola, A., Calvo, A., et al. (2007) A longitudinal study on quality of life and depression in ALS patient–caregiver couples. *Neurology*, **68**(12), 923–6.
15. Murphy, P.L., Albert, S.M., Weber, C.M., Del Bene, M.L., and Rowland, L.P. (2000) Impact of spirituality and religiousness on outcomes in patients with ALS. *Neurology*, **55**(10), 1581–4.
16. Roach, A.R., Averill, A.J., Segerstrom, S.C., and Kasarskis, E.J. (2009) The dynamics of quality of life in ALS patients and caregivers. *Annals of Behavioral Medicine*, **37**(2), 197–206.

17. **Plahuta, J.M., McCulloch, B.J., Kasarskis, E.J., Ross, M.A., Walter, R.A.,** and **McDonald, E.R.** (2002) Amyotrophic lateral sclerosis and hopelessness: psychosocial factors. *Social Science & Medicine*, **55**(12), 2131–40.

18. **Ganzini, L., Johnston, W.S.,** and **Hoffman, W.F.** (1999) Correlates of suffering in amyotrophic lateral sclerosis. *Neurology*, **52**(7), 1434–40.

19. **Pagnini, F., Simmons, Z., Corbo, M.,** and **Molinari E.** (2012) Amyotrophic lateral sclerosis: Time for research on psychological intervention? *Amyotrophic Lateral Sclerosis*, **13**(5), 416–17.

20. **Palmieri, A., Kleinbub, J.R., Calvo, V.,** et al. (2012) Efficacy of hypnosis-based treatment in amyotrophic lateral sclerosis: A pilot study. *Frontiers in Psychology*, **3**, 465.

21. **Kleinbub, J.R., Palmieri, A., Broggio, A.,** et al. (2015) Hypnosis-based psychodynamic treatment in ALS: a longitudinal study on patients and their caregivers. *Frontiers in Psychology*, **6**, 822.

22. **Beck, A.T., Rush, A.J., Shaw, B.F.,** and **Emery, G.** (1979) *Cognitive Theory of Depression*. New York: Guildford.

23. **Dennison, L.** and **Moss-Morris, R.** (2010) Cognitive–behavioral therapy: What benefits can it offer people with multiple sclerosis? *Expert Review of Neurotherapeutics*, **10**(9), 1383–90.

24. **Moss-Morris, R., Dennison, L., Landau, S., Yardley, L., Silber, E.,** and **Chalder, T.** (2013) A randomized controlled trial of cognitive behavioral therapy (CBT) for adjusting to multiple sclerosis (the saMS trial): Does CBT work and for whom does it work? *Journal of Consulting and Clinical Psychology*, **81**(2), 251–62.

25. **Dobkin, R.D., Menza, M., Allen, L.A.,** et al. (2011) Cognitive-behavioral therapy for depression in Parkinson's disease: A randomized, controlled trial. *American Journal of Psychiatry*, **168**(10), 1066–74.

26. **Feeney, F., Egan, S.,** and **Gasson, N.** (2005) Treatment of depression and anxiety in Parkinson's disease: A pilot study using group cognitive behavioural therapy. *Clinical Psychologist*, **9**(1), 31–8.

27. **Garcia Perez, A.I.** and **Dapueto, J.J.** (2014) Case report of a computer-assisted psychotherapy of a patient with ALS. *International Journal of Psychiatry in Medicine*, **48**(3), 229–33.

28. **Díaz, J.L., Sancho, J., Barreto, P., Bañuls, P., Renovell, M.,** and **Servera, E.** (2014) Effect of a short-term psychological intervention on the anxiety and depression of amyotrophic lateral sclerosis patients. *Journal of Health Psychology*, **21**(7), 1426–35.

29. **van Groenestijn, A.C., van de Port, I.G., Schröder, C.D.,** et al. (2011) Effects of aerobic exercise therapy and cognitive behavioural therapy on functioning and quality of life in amyotrophic lateral sclerosis: protocol of the FACTS-2-ALS trial. *BMC Neurology*, **11**(1), 1–11.

30. **Zigmond, A.S.** and **Snaith, R.P.** (1983) The hospital anxiety and depression scale. *Acta Psychiatrica Scandinavica*, **67**(6), 361–70.

31. **van Groenestijn, A.C., Schröder, C.D., Visser-Meily, J.M.A., Reenen, E.T.K-V., Veldink, J.H.,** and **van den Berg, L.H.** (2015) Cognitive behavioural therapy and quality of life in psychologically distressed patients with amyotrophic lateral sclerosis and their caregivers: Results of a prematurely stopped randomized controlled trial. *Amyotrophic Lateral Sclerosis and Frontotemporal Degeneration*, **16**(5–6), 309–15.

32. **Jenkinson, C., Hobart, J., Chandola, T., Fitzpatrick, R., Peto, V.,** and **Swash, M.** (2002) Use of the short form health survey (SF-36) in patients with amyotrophic lateral

sclerosis: tests of data quality, score reliability, response rate and scaling assumptions. *Journal of Neurology*, **249**(2), 178–83.

33. **Pennebaker, J.W.** and **Seagal, J.D.** (1999) Forming a story: The health benefits of narrative. *Journal of Clinical Psychology*, **55**(10), 1243–54.

34. **Averill, A.J., Kasarskis, E.J.,** and **Segerstrom, S.C.** (2013) Expressive disclosure to improve well-being in patients with amyotrophic lateral sclerosis: A randomised, controlled trial. *Psychology & Health*, **28**(6), 701–13.

35. **Lu, Q.** and **Stanton, A.L.** (2010) How benefits of expressive writing vary as a function of writing instructions, ethnicity and ambivalence over emotional expression. *Psychology & Health*, **25**(6), 669–84.

36. **Norman, S.A., Lumley, M.A., Dooley, J.A.,** and **Diamond, M.P.** (2004) For whom does it work? Moderators of the effects of written emotional disclosure in a randomized trial among women with chronic pelvic pain. *Psychosomatic Medicine*, **66**(2), 174–83.

37. **Bolmsjo, I.** (2001) Existential issues in palliative care: interviews of patients with amyotrophic lateral sclerosis. *Journal of Palliative Medicine*, **4**(4), 499–505.

38. **Chochinov, H.** (2002) Dignity-conserving care—a new model for palliative care: Helping the patient feel valued. *Journal of the American Medical Association*, **287**(17), 2253–60.

39. **Chochinov, H.M., Kristjanson, L.J., Breitbart, W.,** and et al. (2011) Effect of dignity therapy on distress and end-of-life experience in terminally ill patients: a randomised controlled trial. *Lancet Oncology*, **12**(8), 753–62.

40. **McClement, S., Chochinov, H.M., Hack, T., Hassard, T., Kristjanson, L.J.,** and **Harlos, M.** (2007) Dignity therapy: family member perspectives. *Journal of Palliative Medicine*, **10**(5), 1076–82.

41. **Bentley, B., O'Connor, M., Breen, L.J.,** and **Kane, R.** (2014) Feasibility, acceptability and potential effectiveness of dignity therapy for family carers of people with motor neurone disease. *BMC Palliative Care*, **13**(1), 1–9.

42. **Aoun, S.M., Chochinov, H.M.,** and **Kristjanson, L.J.** (2015) Dignity therapy for people with motor neuron disease and their family caregivers: A feasibility study. *Journal of Palliative Medicine*, **18**(1), 31–7.

43. **Pagnini, F.** and **Philips, D.** (2015) Being mindful about mindfulness. *Lancet Psychiatry*, **2**(4), 288–9.

44. **Khoury, B., Lecomte, T., Fortin, G.,** et al. (2013) Mindfulness-based therapy: A comprehensive meta-analysis. *Clinical Psychology Review*, **33**(6), 763–71.

45. **Khoury, B., Sharma, M., Rush, S.E.,** and **Fournier, C.** (2015) Mindfulness-based stress reduction for healthy individuals: A meta-analysis. *Journal of Psychosomatic Research*, **78**(6), 519–28.

46. **Simpson, R., Booth, J., Lawrence, M., Byrne, S., Mair, F.** and **Mercer, S.** (2014) Mindfulness based interventions in multiple sclerosis—a systematic review. *BMC Neurology*, **14**, 15.

47. **Pickut, B., Vanneste, S., Hirsch, M.A.,** et al. (2015) Mindfulness training among individuals with Parkinson's disease: Neurobehavioral effects. *Parkinson's Disease*, **2015**, 816404.

48. **Pagnini, F., Phillips, D., Bosma, C.M., Reece, A.,** and **Langer, E.** (2015) Mindfulness, physical impairment and psychological well-being in people with amyotrophic lateral sclerosis. *Psychological Health*, **30**(5), 503–17.

49. **Pagnini, F., Phillips, D., Bosma, C.M., Reece, A.,** and **Langer, E.** (2016) Mindfulness as a protective factor for the burden of caregivers of amyotrophic lateral sclerosis patients. *Journal of Clinical Psychology*, **72**(1), 101–11.

50. **Pirson, M., Langer, E.J., Bodner, T.,** and **Zilcha-Mano, S.** (2012) The development and validation of the Langer Mindfulness Scale-Enabling a socio-cognitive perspective of mindfulness in organizational contexts. *Fordham University Schools of Business Research Paper*.

51. **Pagnini, F., Marconi, A., Tagliaferri, A.,** et al. (2017) Meditation training for people with amyotrophic lateral sclerosis: A randomized clinical trial. *European Journal of Neurology*, **24**(4), 578–86.

52. **Gould, R.L., Coulson, M.C., Brown, R.G., Goldstein, L.H., Al-Chalabi, A.,** and **Howard, R.J.** (2015) Psychotherapy and pharmacotherapy interventions to reduce distress or improve well-being in people with amyotrophic lateral sclerosis: A systematic review. *Amyotrophic Lateral Sclerosis and Frontotemporal Degeneration*, **16**(5–6), 293–302.

53. **Rabbitte, M., Bates, U.,** and **Keane, M.** (2015) Psychological and psychotherapeutic approaches for people with motor neuron disease: A qualitative study. *Amyotrophic Lateral Sclerosis and Frontotemporal Degeneration*, **16**(5–6), 303–8.

54. **Goldstein, L.H.** and **Abrahams, S.** (2013) Changes in cognition and behaviour in amyotrophic lateral sclerosis: nature of impairment and implications for assessment. *Lancet Neurology*, **12**(4), 368–80.

55. **Chio, A., Gauthier, A., Calvo, A., Ghiglione, P.,** and **Mutani, R.** (2005) Caregiver burden and patients' perception of being a burden in ALS. *Neurology*, **64**(10), 1780–2.

56. **Watermeyer, T.J., Brown, R.G., Sidle, K.C.,** et al. (2015) Impact of disease, cognitive and behavioural factors on caregiver outcome in amyotrophic lateral sclerosis. *Amyotrophic Lateral Sclerosis and Frontotemporal Degeneration*, **16**(5–6), 316–23.

57. **Lillo, P., Mioshi, E.,** and **Hodges, J.R.** (2012) Caregiver burden in amyotrophic lateral sclerosis is more dependent on patients' behavioral changes than physical disability: a comparative study. *BMC Neurology*, **12**(1), 1–6.

58. **Chio, A., Vignola, A., Mastro, E.,** et al. (2010) Neurobehavioral symptoms in ALS are negatively related to caregivers' burden and quality of life. *European Journal of Neurology*, **17**(10), 1298–303.

59. **Gauthier, A., Vignola, A., Calvo, A.,** et al. (2007) A longitudinal study on quality of life and depression in ALS patient-caregiver couples. *Neurology*, **68**(12), 923–6.

60. **Graham, C.D., Gouick, J., Ferreira, N.,** and **Gillanders, D.** (2016) The influence of psychological flexibility on life satisfaction and mood in muscle disorders. *Rehabilitation Psychology*, **61**(2), 210–17.

61. **Graham, C.D., Rose, M.R., Hankins, M., Chalder, T.,** and **Weinman, J.** (2013) Separating emotions from consequences in muscle disease: comparing beneficial and unhelpful illness schemata to inform intervention development. *Journal of Psychosomatic Research*, **74**(4), 320–6.

Chapter 2

Quality of life in ALS: What is it and how do we measure it?

Vincenzo Zaccheo and Zachary Simmons

Defining quality of life

For physicians and other allied health professionals, the care of individuals with amyotrophic lateral sclerosis (ALS) typically involves efforts to maximize quality of life (QoL). This is driven by the reality that there is no medical treatment to cure, reverse, or stabilize this disease. However, to optimize QoL, one must first appreciate that QoL is a complex concept that may be defined and used in a variety of ways. One important distinction is that between health-related QoL (HRQOL) and global QoL.

HRQOL, also known as health status, pertains to an individual's perceived well-being related to their physical and mental functioning (1, 2). Global QoL, on the other hand, involves one's perceived well-being in the context of additional factors outside of medical issues, such as family, friends, finances, job, religion, and spirituality. According to the World Health Organization (3), global QoL is '... a broad-ranging concept affected in a complex way by the person's physical health, psychological state, level of independence, social relationships, personal belief and their relation to salient features of their environment.' Thus, QoL is a complex, multidimensional concept impacted by numerous factors.

Despite variations in the definition of QoL, a core concept is that it is a subjective reflection of the patient's perception of their well-being in various areas of their life. It has been consistently shown that QoL in patients with serious or life-threatening diseases is underestimated by others in comparison to the individual's self-report (4–8), and that this includes those closest to them such as caregivers, and those with professional health care training. This has specifically been demonstrated for those with ALS. In one study comparing self-ratings by those with ALS, of their energy and suffering, with the ratings of the patients provided by caregivers, those with ALS judged their energy to be greater and their suffering to be less (9). Those in good health judged depression to be more frequent, and the wish for euthanasia or suicide to be more common in patients with ALS than did those patients themselves (10). Family members in good health rated the perceived physical and psychological well-being of individuals with ALS as being lower than the self-ratings provided by the patients (11).

A possible explanation for the seemingly paradoxical high self-ratings of QoL by those with ALS is provided by the concept of 'response shift.' Also called 'frame shift,' and similar in concept to the 'well-being paradox,' response shift refers to an individual's psychological adjustment of their values and expectations in the face of chronic illness (12–14). It is tied to the concept that QoL is derived from a comparison of one's expectations with reality. Individuals with serious and debilitating illnesses often place greater importance on non-health-related, as opposed to health-related, areas as being significant contributors to their overall quality of life (15). Thus, for an individual with ALS, the initial diagnosis may lead to a discrepancy between expectations of finding meaning in activities requiring physical activity, which they can no longer perform, and the reality that meaning has not been found in the social supports or existential factors readily accessible by them. Over time, those who successfully maintain QoL or who experience a QoL improvement, recalibrate the factors that contribute to QoL so that these more closely reflect what is possible in the face of the individual's physical limitations. These individuals are able to preserve their QoL by placing greater importance on supports such as visits from family, conversations with friends, faith, and spirituality, and less emphasis on activities that rely on physical well-being, such as playing sports, doing yard work, travel, or workplace activities.

Understanding quality of life instruments

General concepts

Optimizing the QoL of the patient requires not only an understanding of the concept of QoL, but also an understanding of how QoL is measured, how the various aspects of QoL contribute to the whole, and the variety of QoL instruments that are available. QoL instruments usually are composed of specific areas, classified as domains, which are believed to contribute to QoL. These may include physical, psychological, existential, spiritual/religious, and social relationship domains. Domains generally contain questions to which the patient provides a scaled response (0–10, for example) in which the extremes of the scales are indicative of the best or worst possible perceptions of the quality of that person's life with respect to the item being questioned. Scores can then be summed within a domain or over the entire questionnaire to produce a domain-specific or overall QoL score.

Of course, assessing QOL could be simplified to a one-step process devoid of complexity. The clinician could simply ask the patient to assess his or her QOL. Indeed, there is excellent agreement between scores on the McGill single-item scale (a single question asking the person to assess overall QoL) and the 59-item, six-domain ALS Specific Quality of Life Instrument (ALSSQOL) (16). However, doing so robs the QoL assessment of much of its strength. At the level of clinical care, the domains of QoL instruments give the clinician valuable insights into aspects of the patient's life that can form the basis for care decisions. If completed with the clinician, the questionnaire may facilitate patients' insights and disclosures. Responses to specific questions within domains can be monitored over time, providing an understanding of the evolution of factors contributing to QoL and possibly of the efficacy of interventions. For researchers, QoL domains facilitate a more precise definition of QoL that permits comparisons across individuals and groups, knowing that the participants' understanding of the otherwise somewhat muddy construct of QoL should be similar in all participants.

Because there is no universally accepted definition of QoL, numerous instruments have been developed that vary with regard to the domains that are included and their relative importance. Navigating the variety of available instruments is challenging, but can be facilitated by some relatively simple dichotomous classifications. At the most basic level, QoL instruments can be divided into those that measure HRQOL (or health status) and those which provide a broader assessment of global QoL. A division into generic vs. disease-specific instruments is equally helpful. It is also valuable to consider instruments with patient-defined domains vs. ones with standardized domains

Health-related vs. global QoL instruments

HRQOL instruments solely assess physical and mental health. Examples of such measures include the Sickness Impact Profile (SIP) (17); the EuroQoL EQ-5D (18,19), and the Short Form Health Survey-36 (SF-36) (20). Early attempts to measure QoL in patients with ALS were of this type, with a clear weighting toward physical function. In particular, the SIP and a disease-specific 19-item version with items chosen by ALS experts as most relevant (SIP/AL-19) were identified as ALS QoL measures, and were shown to correlate well with measures of strength (17, 21, 22). While research demonstrating such a correlation is admirable, the outcome is that such instruments will inevitably show a decline in measured QoL over time, as individuals with ALS become physically weaker (23–25). Yet, individuals with life-threatening illnesses, as discussed earlier, often judge their QoL better than healthy individuals would expect and seemingly do not base their assessment on physical abilities alone. Thus, HRQOL measures capture health status, as would be expected, but fail to provide a broader assessment of QoL.

Global QoL measures, on the other hand, assess broader domains beyond health-related factors, such as existential factors, religion, spirituality, social relationships, employment, and finances. The World Health Organization Quality of Life questionnaire and its briefer version (WHOQOL-100 and WHOQOL-BREF) are examples of such measures (26–28). Each assesses an individual's self-perceived well-being in four domains: physical health, psychological health, social relationships, and environment. Both measures have been validated and demonstrate other strong psychometric properties. The McGill QoL Questionnaire (MQOL); (15, 29–31) is another example of a true global QoL instrument. It was developed in direct response to a concern about overemphasis on physical functioning in QoL measures at that time. It strongly emphasizes existential domains, such as meaning in life and perception of purpose, which are believed to be important for individuals with serious illnesses. The questionnaire consists of 16-items, and is divided into five subscales—physical symptoms, physical well-being, psychological symptoms, existential well-being, and support. Psychometric properties have been shown to be strong when assessing patients with a variety of life-threatening disorders and for the assessment of those in palliative care. Global QoL instruments are not without their shortcomings, however. Because these instruments place less emphasis on health-related factors, include many domains that change independently of medical interventions, and may be unrelated to disease course or treatment, they may be less useful for assessing whether medical care has affected an individual's self-perceived overall life quality.

Generic vs. disease-specific QoL instruments

Given the existence of validated global QoL instruments, why not simply use one or more of these as the standard for assessing QoL in patients with ALS? After all, the MQOL and the WHOQOL instruments have been rigorously tested on many patients with a variety of diseases. However, the weakness of these generic instruments is that they are not disease-specific. Disease-specific QoL instruments are able to address items unique to certain disease states and place less emphasis on items that are non-essential to the QoL for individuals within the disease state being assessed. Thus, an ALS-specific QoL instrument may inquire about bulbar function or sialorrhea, but not about adverse effects of therapy, such as chemotherapy-induced nausea, vomiting, and hair loss, which would be more appropriate for a cancer-specific QoL instrument.

An admirable attempt to address this need for a disease-specific global measure of QoL in the ALS population was the development of the 40-item ALS Assessment Questionnaire (ALSAQ-40) and its shorter version, the ALSAQ-5 (32–34). The ALSAQ-40 is comprised of five domains—physical mobility, activities of daily living and independence, eating and drinking, communication, and emotional reactions. It has been translated into and validated in several other languages, and is widely used (35–38). Nonetheless, it is still heavily weighted toward physical function, with 30 of the 40 questions specifically assessing limb or bulbar function, and is best considered a HRQOL measure, rather than a global QoL instrument.

The need for an ALS-specific, global QoL instrument led to the development of the 59-item ALS-Specific Quality of Life Instrument (ALSSQOL) (16) and its 46-item revised version, the ALSSQOL-R (39), both of which have been validated in large, multicentre studies. The development of the ALSSQOL was based on studies that utilized the MQOL and measures of religiosity to assess variables important to QoL for individuals with ALS (40). These studies subsequently demonstrated the importance of psychological and existential factors, and possibly of spirituality and support systems, in impacting on QoL. They also demonstrated the lack of correlation of QoL with physical function, thereby reinforcing the need to de-emphasize this variable in an ALS-specific QoL instrument. The ALSSQOL was developed through a multi-step process based on the MQOL questionnaire, additional items pertaining to religiosity and spirituality, and semi-structured interviews with ALS patients eliciting opinions about items perceived to be or not to be of importance in determining QoL. The resulting ALSSQOL and the ALSSQOL-R are each comprised of six domains—negative emotion, interaction with people and the environment, intimacy, religiosity, physical symptoms, and bulbar function. The specificity of these measures has allowed for more sensitive assessment of QoL for individuals with ALS. A shorter, 20-item version of this instrument, the ALSSQOL-20, has been developed and validated in a multi-centre study (unpublished data, Dr Zachary Simmons), and is available online (41).

Instruments with patient-defined domains vs. those with standardized domains

The Schedule for the Evaluation of Individual QoL (SEIQoL) and the Direct-Weighting version (SEIQoL-DW) are global QoL measures that deserve special consideration (42–51). These measures are based on the premise that an individual's QoL is individually determined, and thus the factors that make-up a person's QoL should be elicited on an individual basis. Both the SEIQoL and SEIQoL-DW use semi-structured interviews, wherein individuals are asked to identify the five most important areas contributing to their QoL, and subsequently rate the importance of these areas and their level of functioning in each area. This structure makes the SEIQoL and SEIQoL-DW inherently both global and disease-specific QoL instruments. The SEIQoL and SEIQoL-DW have been validated, and have been used to assess QoL in a variety of disorders. However, when used in ALS, the SEIQoL-DW was found to have great value in individuals but to have less suitability for assessing groups (52). This is simply a reflection of the use of non-standardized, individually defined domains. In contrast, instruments with standardized domains, which are comprised of specific items that have been identified through research and factor analysis, as being the primary contributors to a particular area, are suitable for assessing grouped data.

Mode of administration

Instruments may be self-administered or administered by trained staff. Advantages of self-administered measures, particularly for routine clinical (in contrast to research) use, are that trained staff are not required and individuals may complete measures at their own pace in places of their own choosing. The trade-off is a lack of control and standardization. For example, the clinician cannot be sure that the responses represent those of the individual in question, and that these were not influenced by a caregiver. This is of particular concern in patients with ALS who have severe physical or communication impairments. In addition, one cannot determine whether the environment in which the individual completed the measure was conducive to thoughtful contemplation, or whether it was noisy, hurried, stressful, or physically uncomfortable in such a way as to impact their responses. Beyond this, there is no way to ensure that the individual has understood the questions. Greater control is provided with interviewer-administered instruments, as these measures are usually completed within a structured outpatient setting by a health care professional, thus allowing for mitigation of the factors just described. The disadvantages for routine clinical use of such instruments are that they require trained staff, and may add both physical and mental burdens to an ALS clinic visit for a weak and fatigued patient. The implications of an administration format have been mixed, with some studies demonstrating that scores are impacted on by and administration format (53) and others finding no association (54,55). Thus, the choice between a self-administered or interviewer-administered measure is generally based on the other considerations discussed above.

General considerations of psychometric properties

A basic understanding of the psychometric properties of the available QoL instruments is vital for making appropriate choices between those instruments. All must possess validity, reliability, and sensitivity (56, 57). The validity of an instrument indicates the extent to which it measures the intended construct or variable. Reliability is an assessment of the ability of an instrument to produce consistent results across situations and time. Finally, sensitivity to changes that occur across various domains is essential if a QoL instrument is to be used to measure variations over time or to assess the meaningfulness of differences in scores between subjects. Instruments may also have cut-off scores that define specific classification groups, most commonly normal vs. abnormal. 'Ceiling' and 'floor' effects are important concepts, and are used to describe the maximum and minimum scores an individual can attain for the variable under investigation. For QoL instruments, it is important that an individual with a good QoL should not attain the highest score unless their QoL is truly exceptional. Similarly, only those individuals who view their QoL as truly terrible should attain the lowest score.

Quality of life in ALS: What has been found?

One of the earliest studies to demonstrate the lack of relationship between QoL and physical function suggested that psychological and existential factors were closely related to QoL, and that support systems and spirituality might play roles (40). Many other studies have failed to find a correlation between global QoL of individuals with ALS and physical function. Patients with ALS often rate their QoL on global QoL instruments as being quite good and as remaining so over time (23,40,52,58–63), despite increasing weakness. Consistent with this, QoL in ALS patients with tracheostomy and mechanical ventilation has been found to be similar to those not requiring ventilatory support (63,64). Recent studies of patients with ALS on tracheostomy and mechanical ventilation have found that most would choose this again if given the choice (65,66). The concept of response shift, discussed earlier (12–14), provides a useful framework for explaining why QoL is preserved in spite of physical decline, and highlights the need for adjustment and modification of expectations so that those factors contributing to QoL shift to ones that do not require intact physical function.

The relationship between bulbar function and QoL appears to be the exception to the pattern just described. A study using a dysphagia-specific, health-related QoL questionnaire, the SWAL-QoL, identified oropharyngeal dysphagia as directly impacting the mental health and social life of individuals with ALS, and as resulting in greater burden and fear (67–72). An even more recent study using an ALS-specific global QoL instrument demonstrated a poorer QoL in those with impaired verbal communication, particularly during the time of earliest speech impairment (73). This early period of impaired speech may represent an opportunity for intervention. Related to this, augmentative and alternative communication (AAC) devices, such as eye-tracking communication devices, have been consistently shown to have a beneficial impact on the QoL of individuals with ALS (74–76).

In contrast to physical function, there appears to be a clear relationship between psychological health and QoL. Depression is associated with a poor QoL (77–79), as are hopelessness (80) and anxiety (81,82), all of which appear to be higher among individuals with ALS than in the general population (2). Aside from the impact on QoL, psychological health can also impact physical health, and overall health outcomes and prognosis (83,84). Given these facts, it is imperative that psychological health be routinely assessed in individuals with ALS, in order to generate appropriate referrals to mental health providers and guide treatment. To aid in this regard, particular measures may prove useful. The ALS-Depression Inventory is a 12-item measure that assesses the presence of depressive symptomatology in individuals with ALS, and which has been validated (85). The Brief Symptom Inventory (BSI), which contains subscales for anxiety, depression, phobic anxiety, and somatization, has also been found to be helpful in identifying psychological distress in individuals with ALS (86). Additional discussion of psychological morbidity in ALS can be found in Chapter 3. A wide variety of other factors may impact QoL (2), and are discussed elsewhere in this book.

The ALS clinic itself deserves some consideration. Given the multitude of physical, psychological, and socioeconomic issues with which individuals with ALS must contend, virtually all of which have the potential to impact their QoL, multidisciplinary clinics (MDCs) have become the standard of care. Within such clinics, care is provided by a multidisciplinary team, usually consisting of a specialist physician, specialized nursing care, respiratory and nutritional management, speech therapy, physical therapy, occupational therapy, social work care, and mental health counselling. In addition to providing access to integrated, specialized care (87,88), MDCs have generally been associated with longer survival (89–92). Improved quality of life was found using the SF-36, a HRQOL instrument (93), but not using a global QoL instrument, the ALSSQOL-R (8). In view of the large number of variables that impact upon those with ALS, but are beyond the control of health care providers, such as interpersonal relationships, spirituality, and finances, it is clear not clear whether global QoL instruments are the best measures for assessing the potential benefits of the MDC. Alternatively, the lack of improvement in measured global QoL may simply reflect attendance at MDCs as a self-selecting process, whereby those who require MDCs to maintain their QoL attend them, and those who do not need these supports to maintain QoL avoid them (88).

Guidelines to choosing an ALS quality of life instrument

It is not uncommon for those of us who are familiar with QoL instruments to be asked to identify the 'best' QoL instrument. With the multitude of QoL measures that are available, it is not surprising that clinicians often feel overwhelmed and confused regarding what measures to select in particular situations. A good starting point is to determine into which of three primary categories the goal of the assessment falls:

- Facilitating best clinical care for the individual patient.
- Measuring research outcomes from a therapeutic intervention in one or more groups of patients.
- Measuring QoL in a group one time, or monitoring group changes over time.

A decision tree can be helpful, and will identify whether the best instrument is a HRQOL or global QoL instrument, and whether it should be disease-specific or generic (Fig. 2.1).

The use of a QoL instrument to facilitate clinical care for an individual can involve both baseline and serial assessments. The ideal instrument would be a global QoL questionnaire. If available and able to be administered in the available setting and time frame, a disease-specific instrument is preferred. Because large groups are not

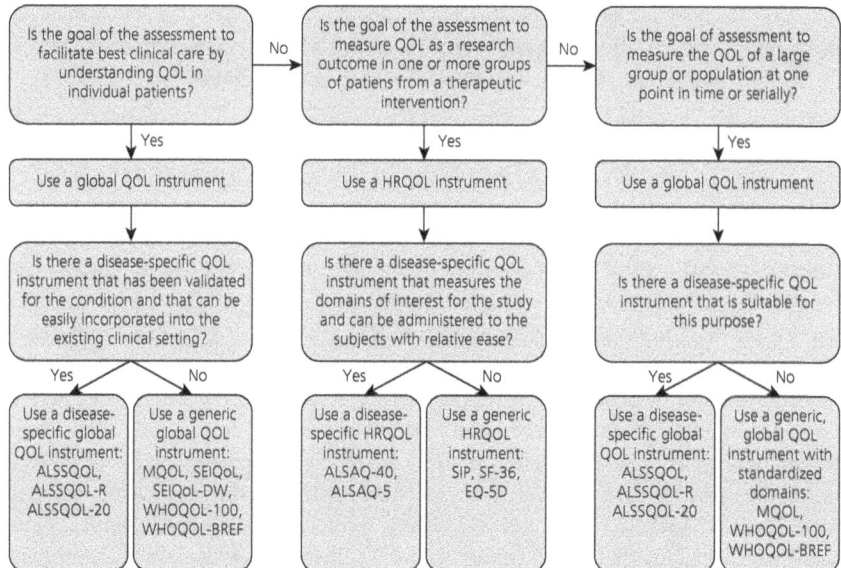

Fig. 2.1 Decision tree facilitating the choice of a quality of life instrument. ALSAQ-40 and ALSAQ-5: ALS Assessment Questionnaire, 40-item and five-item versions; ALSSQOL and ALSSQOL-R: ALS Specific Quality of Life Instrument and revised version; EQ-5D: EuroQoL 5D; MQOL: McGill Quality of Life Questionnaire; SEIQoL and SEIQoL-DW: Schedule for the Evaluation of Individual Quality of Life and direct-weighted version; SF-36: Short Form Health Survey-36; SIP: Sickness Impact Profile; WHOQOL-100 and WHOQOL-BREF: World Health Organization Quality of Life instrument and brief version.

being compared, instruments can be either those with standardized domains or those in the domains are patient-defined. In our multidisciplinary ALS clinic, the ALSSQOL-R is completed by each patient prior to each clinic visit, and is used by clinicians as part of the assessment when determining therapeutic interventions. Such information-sharing guides shared decision-making between patient, caregiver, and clinician. Scores in specific domains can guide the use of pharmacological and non-pharmacological interventions for symptom control, including sialorrhea, pain, sleep dysfunction, communication limitations, and swallowing difficulty. We have found the information to be particularly useful in assessing and managing psychological dysfunction such as depression and anxiety, both of which are assessed as part of the Negative Emotion subscale. Responses also can guide clinical decisions about assistive devices and durable medical equipment, and can lead to useful discussions about the need for help in the home, and methods to address social isolation, spiritual distress, and end-of-life counselling.

Assessing research outcomes from therapeutic interventions in groups of patients in clinical trials is best done currently with HRQOL instruments that assess the domains that contribute to study outcome measures. For example, if the primary outcome measure is an improvement in breathing, then there are HRQOL scales that focus primarily on respiratory symptoms that, if improved, result in a perception by the patient of an improved QoL. Such a measure might be a measure of sleep quality or of the impact on QoL of exertional dyspnoea. Global QoL instruments serve a more limited purpose in ALS trials in view of the modest efficacy of current therapeutics. Because ALS therapies slow progression, rather than leading to an improvement in strength, patients often will still experience response shifts that may stabilize QoL, while many other non-medical factors will continue to contribute disproportionately. If disease therapies evolve to the point of being able to stop or reverse disease progression, resulting in response shifts becoming more limited or absent, global QoL likely will improve as the patient experiences the effects of therapy, thereby making global QoL more suitable in such circumstances. The best instruments to use are disease-specific, but generic measures can be used if time or clinician training preclude use of these, or if a valid disease-specific instrument is not available for the condition being studied.

Finally, global QoL instruments in ALS are extremely useful for group analysis. If we wish to know how ALS patients rate their lives in general, and how this changes over time, then instruments such as the ALSSQOL can do this satisfactorily because they were designed precisely with this in mind. The defined domains permit comparisons of groups or populations over time. If a disease-specific instrument is not available for the disease being studied, or cannot be used because of limited time or training by clinicians, generic instruments can be used, but should have standardized domains if they are to be used in this manner.

As can be seen in Fig. 2.1, each path down the decision tree leads to a limited choice of instruments for patients with ALS. These are summarized in Box 2.1. All of the ones listed have good psychometric properties. Choices among those in any one category can then be made on the basis of operational criteria and available resources, such as time needed to complete the questionnaire, and whether or not it will be self-administered.

Conclusions

QoL is a complex, multidimensional concept that that has been defined, conceptualized, and used in numerous ways. It is a patient-derived concept, dependent on the judgment of the individual being assessed. A variety of generic and disease-specific instruments have been used to measure QoL, initially weighted toward physical function, but now much broader in scope. These have made it clear that QoL in those with ALS is not directly related to physical function (with the exception of bulbar functioning), but is dependent on a variety of psychological and existential factors. It is generally higher than judged by those around the affected individual and, on average, does not decline over time. The selection of the most suitable QoL instrument depends on the setting (clinical vs. research and individual vs. group) and on the question one is trying to answer. By thoughtful selection of the most appropriate measure, clinicians and researchers can help to provide consistent and well-defined information about a concept for which the literature is at times unclear, and to facilitate best clinical care and most accurate outcome measures for research.

Box 2.1 Quality of Life measures most commonly used in ALS

Health-related QOL

Generic

- Dysphagia-specific QoL Questionnaire (SWAL-QoL).
- EuroQol EQ-5D.
- Short Form-36 (SF-36).
- Sickness Impact Profile (SIP).
- SIP/ALS-19.

Disease-specific

ALS assessment Questionnaire (ALSAQ-40).

Global QoL

Generic

- World Health Organization WHOQOL-100 and WHOQOL-BREF.
- McGill QoL Questionnaire (MQOL).
- Schedule for the Evaluation of Individual QoL (SEIQoL and SEIQoL-DW).

Disease-specific

ALS-Specific Quality of Life Instrument (ALSSQOL and ALSSQOL-R).

References

1. **Burns, T.M., Graham, C.D., Rose, M.R., and Simmons, Z.** (2012) Quality of life and measures of quality of life in patients with neuromuscular disorders. *Muscle & Nerve*, **46**, 9–25.
2. **Simmons, Z.** (2014) Patient-perceived outcomes and quality of life in ALS. *Neurotherapeutics*, **12**, 394–402.
3. **World Health Organization, Division of Mental Health and Prevention of Substance Abuse.** (1997) *WHOQOL: Measuring Quality of Life*. Available at http://www.who.int/mental_health/media/68.pdf (accessed June 17, 2017).
4. **Kubler, A., Winter, A., Ludolph, A.C., Hautzinger, M., and Birbaumer, N.** (2005) Severity of depressive symptoms and quality of life in patients with amyotrophic lateral sclerosis. *Neurorehabilitation and Neural Repair*, **19**, 182–93.
5. **Slevin, M.L., Plant, H., Lynch, D., Drinkwater, J., and Gregory, W. M.** (1988) Who should measure the quality of life, the doctor or the patient? *British Journal of Cancer*, **57**, 109–12.
6. **Gerhart, K.A., Koziol-McLain, J., Lowenstein, S.R., and Whiteneck, G.G.** (1994) Quality of life following spinal cord injury: knowledge and attitudes of emergency care providers. *Annals of Emergency Medicine*, **23**, 807–12.

7. **Rothwell, P.M., McDowell, Z., Wong, C.K., and Dorman, P.J.** (1997) Doctors and patients don't agree: cross sectional study of patients' and doctors' perceptions and assessments of disability in multiple sclerosis. *British Medical Journal*, **314**, 1580–3.

8. **Trail, M., Nelson, N.D., Van, J.N., Appel, S.H., and Lai, E.C.** (2003) A study comparing patients with amyotrophic lateral sclerosis and their caregivers on measures of quality of life, depression, and their attitudes toward treatment options. *Journal of Neurological Sciences*, **209**, 79–85.

9. **Adelman, E.E., Albert, S.M., Rabkin, J.G., Del Bene, M.L., Tider, T., and O'Sullivan, I.** (2004) Disparities in perceptions of distress and burden in ALS patients and family caregivers. *Neurology*, **62**, 1766–70.

10. **Lule, D., Ehlich, B., Lang, D., et al.** (2013) Quality of life in fatal disease: the flawed judgement of the social environment. *Journal of Neurology*, **260**, 2836–43.

11. **Olsson, A.G., Markhede, I., Strang, S., and Persson, L.I.** (2010) Well-being in patients with amyotrophic lateral sclerosis and their next of kin over time. *Acta Neurologica Scandinavica*, **121**, 244–50.

12. **Schwartz, C.E. and Sprangers, M.A.** (1999) Methodological approaches for assessing response shift in longitudinal health-related quality of life research. *Social Science & Medicine*, **48**, 1531–48.

13. **Carr, A.J., Gibson, B., and Robinson, P.G.** (2001) Measuring quality of life: is quality of life determined by expectations or experience? *British Medical Journal*, **322**, 1240–3.

14. **Barclay, R. and Tate, R.B.** (2014) Response shift recalibration and reprioritization in health-related quality of life was identified prospectively in older men with and without stroke. *Journal of Clinical Epidemiology*, **67**, 500–7.

15. **Cohen, S.R., Mount, B.M., Bruera, E., Provost, M., Rowe, J., and Tong, K.** (1997) Validity of the McGill quality of life questionnaire in the palliative care setting: A multi-centre Canadian study demonstrating the importance of the existential domain. *Palliative Medicine*, **11**, 3–20.

16. **Simmon, Z., Felgoise, S,H., Bremer, B.A., et al.** (2006) The ALSSQOL: Balancing physical and nonphysical factors in assessing quality of life in ALS. *Neurology*, **67**, 1659–64.

17. **Bergner, M., Bobbitt, R.A., Carter, W.B., and Gilson, B.S.** (1981) The sickness impact profile: Development and final revision of a health status measure. *Medical Care*, **19**, 787–805.

18. **The EuroQol Group**. EuroQol—a new facility for the measurement of health related quality of life. *Health Policy*, **16**, 199–208.

19. **Brazier, J., Jones, N., and Kind, P.** (1993) Testing the validity of the EuroQoL and comparing it with the SF-36 health survey questionnaire. *Quality of Life Research*, **2**, 169–80.

20. **Ware, J.E. and Sherbourne, C.D.** (1992) The MOS 36-item short-form health survey (SF-36). I. Conceptual framework and item selection. *Medical Care*, **30**, 473–83.

21. **McGuire, D., Garrison, L., Armon, C., et al.** (1996) Relationship of the Tufts Quantitative Neuromuscular Exam (TQNE) and the Sickness Impact Profkle (SI) in measuring progression of ALS. Neurology, **46**, 1442–4.

22. **McGuire, D., Garrison, L., Armon, C., et al.** (1997) A brief quality-of-life measure for ALS clinical trials based on a subset of items from the sickness impact profile. *Journal of Neurological Sciences*, **152**(Suppl.), S18–S22.

23. **Neudert, C., Wasner, M., and Borasio, G.D.** (2004) Individual quality of life is not correlated with health related quality of life or physical function in patients with amyotrophic lateral sclerosis. *Journal of Palliative Medicine*, **7**, 551–7.

24. **Kiebert, G.M., Green, C., Murphy, C.,** et al. (2001) Patients' health-related quality of life and utilities associated with different stages of amyotrophic lateral sclerosis. *Journal of Neurological Sciences*, **191**, 87–93.

25. **Green, C., Kiebert, G., Murphy, C.,** et al. (2003) Patients' health-related quality of life and health state values for motor neurone disease/amyotrophic lateral sclerosis. *Quality of Life Research*, **12**, 565–74.

26. **The WHOQOL Group.** (1998) The World Health Organization Quality of Life Assessment (WHOQOL): development and general psychometric properties. Social Science & Medicine, **46**, 1569–85.

27. **The WHOQOL Group.** (1998) Development of the World Health Organization WHOQOL-BREF quality of life assessment. *Psychological Medicine*, **28**, 551–8.

28. **Skevington, S.M.** and **O'Connell, K.A.** (2004) The World Health Organization's WHOQOL-BREF quality of life assessment: psychometric properties and results of the international field trial. A report from the QHOQOL group. *Quality of Life Research*, **13**, 299–310.

29. **Cohen, S.R., Mount, B.M., Strobel, M.G.,** and **Bui, F.** (1995) The McGill quality of life questionnaire: a measure of quality of life appropriate for people with advanced disease. A preliminary study of validity and acceptability. *Palliative Medicine*, **9**, 207–19.

30. **Cohen, S.R., Hassan, S.A., Lapointe, B.J.,** and **Mount, B.M.** (1996) Quality of life in HIV disease as measured by the McGill Quality of Life Questionnaire. *AIDS*, **10**, 1421–27.

31. **Cohen, S.R., Mount, B.M., Tomas, J.J.,** and **Mount, L.F.** (1996) Existential well-being is an important determinant of quality of life. *Cancer*, **77**, 576–86.

32. **Jenkinson, C., Fitzpatrick, R., Brennan, C.,** and **Swash, M.** (1998) Evidence for the validity and reliability of the ALS assessment questionnaire: The ALSAQ-40. *Amyotrophic Lateral Sclerosis and Other Motor Neuron Disorders*, **1**, 33–40.

33. **Jenkinson, C., Fitzpatrick, R., Brennan, C., Bromberg, M.,** and **Swash, M.** (1999) Development and validation of a short measure of health status for individuals with amyotrophic lateral sclerosis/motor neurone disease: The ALSAQ-40. *Journal of Neurology*, **246**(Suppl. 3), 11116–21.

34. **Jenkinson, C., Levvy, G., Fitzpatrick, R.,** and **Garratt, A.** (2000) The amyotrophic lateral sclerosis assessment questionnaire (ALSAQ-40): Tests of data quality, score reliability and response rate in a survey of patients. *Journal of Neurological Sciences*, **180**, 94–100.

35. **Yamaguchi, T., Ohbu, S., Saito, M.,** et al. (2004) Validity and clinical applicability of the Japanese version of Amyotrophic Lateral Sclerosis—Assessment Questionnaire-40 (ALSAQ-40). *No To Shinkei*, **56**, 483–94.

36. **Maessen, M., Post, M.W., Maille, R.,** et al. (2007) Validity of the Dutch version of the Amyotrophic Lateral Sclerosis Assessment Questionnaire, ALSAQ-40, ALSAQ-5. *Amyotrophic Lateral Sclerosis*, **8**, 96–100.

37. **Salas, T., Mora, J., Esteban, J., Rodriguez, F., Diaz-Lobato, S.,** and **Fajardo, M.** (2008) Spanish adaptation of the Amyotrophic Lateral Sclerosis Questionnaire ALSAQ-40 for ALS patients. *Amyotrophic Lateral Sclerosis*, **9**, 168–72.

38. **Palmieri, A., Soraru, G., Lombardi, L.,** et al. (2010) Quality of life and motor impairment in ALS: Italian validation of ALSAQ. *Neurological Research*, **32**, 32–40.

39. **Felgoise, S.H., Walsh, S.M., Stephens, H.E., Brothers, A.,** and **Simmons, Z.** (2011) The ALS Specific Quality of Life-Revised (ALSSQOL-R) User's Guide. Available at: http://www.pennstatehershey.org/c/document_library/get_file?uuid=b9de0a6a-9c1d-4f77-bdf0-5c6c846e018e&groupId=22147 (accessed June 17, 2016).

40. **Simmons, Z., Bremmer, B.A., Robbins, R.A., Walsh, S.M.,** and **Fischer, S.** (2000) Quality of life in ALS depends on factors other than strength and physical function. *Neurology*, **55**, 388–92.

41. **ALS Specific Quality of Life Questionnaire—Brief Form (ALSSQOL-20).** (2015) Available at: http://www.pennstatehershey.org/documents/22147/375615/ALSSQOL-20+Form+with+Logo/fd2bde44-6008-43b6-b191-766c5a2c9918 (accessed June 17, 2016).

42. **McGee, H.M., O'Boyle, C.A., Hickey, A., Joyce, C.R.B.,** and **O'Malley, K.** (1991) Assessing the quality of life of the individual: the SEIQoL with a healthy and a gastroenterology unit population. *Psychological Medicine*, **21**, 749–59.

43. **O'Boyle, C., McGee, H., Hickey, A., O'Malley, K.,** and **Joyce, C.R.B.** (1992) Individual quality of life in patients undergoing hip replacement. *Lancet*, **339**, 1088–91.

44. **O'Boyle, C.A.** (1994) The schedule for the evaluation of individual quality of life. *International Journal of Mental Health*, **23**, 3–23.

45. **Hickey, A.M., Bury, G., O'Boyle, C.A., Bradley, F., O'Reilly, F.,** and **Shannon, W.** (1996) A new short form individual quality of life measure (SEIQoL-DW): application in a cohort of individuals with HIV/AIDS. *British Medical Journal*, **313**, 29–33.

46. **Browne, J.P., O'Boyle, C.A., McGee, H.M., McDonald, N.J.,** and **Joyce, C.R.B.** (1997) Development of a direct weighting procedure for quality of life domains. *Quality of Life Research*, **6**, 301–9.

47. **Hickey, A., O'Boyle, C.A., McGee, H.M.,** and **Joyce, C.R.B.** (1999) The schedule for the evaluation of individual quality of life. In: Joyce, C.R.B., McGee, H.M., and O'Boyle, C.A. (eds). *Individual Quality of Life: Approaches to Conceptualization and Assessment*, pp. 119–33. Amsterdam: Harwood.

48. **Campbell, S.** and **Whyte, F.** (1999) The quality of life in cancer patients participating in phase I clinical trials using SEIQoL-DW. *Journal of Advanced Nursing*, **30**, 335–43.

49. **Waldron, D., O'Boyle, C.A., Kearny, M., Moriarty, M.,** and **Carney, D.** (1999) Quality of-life measurement in advanced cancer: assessing the individual. *Journal of Clinical Oncology*, **17**, 3603–11.

50. **Prince, P.N.** and **Gerber, G.J.** (2001) Measuring subjective quality of life in people with serious mental illness using the SEIQoL-DW. *Quality of Life Research*, **10**, 117–22.

51. **Lintern, T.C., Beaumont, J.G., Kenealy, P.M.,** and **Murrell, R.C.** (2001) Quality of life (QoL) in severely disabled multiple sclerosis patients: comparison of three QoL measures using multidimensional scaling. *Quality of Life Research*, **10**, 371–8.

52. **Felgoise, S.H., Stewart, J.L., Bremer, B.A., Walsh, S.M., Bromberg, M.B.,** and **Simmons, Z.** (2009) The SEIQoL-DW for assessing quality of life in ALS: strengths and limitations. *Amyotrophic Lateral Sclerosis*, **10**, 456–62.

53. **Cheung, Y.B., Goh, C., Thumboo, J., Khoo, K.S.,** and **Wee, J.** (2006) Quality of life scores differed according to mode of administration in a review of three major oncology questionnaires. *Journal of Clinical Epidemiology*, **59**, 185–91.

54. **Puhan, M.A., Ahuja, A., Van Natta, M.L., Ackatz, L.E.,** and **Meinert, C.** (2011) Interviewer versus self-administered health-related quality of life questionnaires-does it matter? *Health & Quality of Life Outcomes*, **9**, 30.

55. **Lopes, A.D., Furtado, R.D.V.E., Silva, C.A., Yi, L.C., Malfatti, C.A.,** and **Araujo, S.D.** (2009) Comparison of self-report and interview administration methods based on the Brazilian versions of the western Ontario rotator cuff index and disabilities of the arm,

shoulder and hand questionnaire in patients with rotator cuff disorders. *Clinics (Sao Paulo)*, **64**, 121–25.

56. **Groth-Marnat, G.** (2009) *Introduction. Handbook of Psychological Assessment*, 5th edn. Hoboken, NJ: John Wiley & Sons, Inc.

57. **Kazdin, A.E.** (2003) *Assessment methods and strategies. Research Design in Clinical Psychology*, 4th edn. Boston, MA: Allyn & Bacon.

58. **Robbins RA, Simmons Z, Bremer BA, Walsh SM, Fischer S.** (2001) Quality of Life in ALS is maintained as physical function declines. *Neurology*, **56**, 442–4.

59. **Neudert, C., Wasner, M.,** and **Borasio, G.D.** (2001) Patients' assessment of quality of life instruments: a randomized study of SIP, SF-36 and SEIQoL-DW in patients with amyotrophic lateral sclerosis. *Journal of Neurological Sciences*, **191**, 103–9.

60. **Bromberg, M.B.** and **Forshew, D.A.** (2002) Comparison of instruments addressing quality of life in patients with ALS and their caregivers. *Neurology*, **58**, 320–2.

61. **Goldstein, L.H., Atkins, L.,** and **Leigh, P.N.** (2002) Correlates of quality of life in people with motor neuron disease (MND). *Amyotrophic Lateral Sclerosis and Other Motor Neuron Disorders*, **3**, 123–9.

62. **Carlson, D.** (1995) Speaking from experience: ALS patients can lead happy lives. *Registered Nurse*, **58**, 10.

63. **Abramson, N.** (2000) Quality of life: who can make the judgment? *American Journal of Medicine*, **100**, 365–6.

64. **McDonald, E.R., Hillel, A.,** and **Wiedenfeld, S.A.** (1996) Evaluation of the psychological status of ventilator-supported patients with ALS/MND. *Palliative Medicine*, **10**, 35–41.

65. **Rousseau MC, Pietra S, Blaya J, Catala A.** (2011) Quality of life of ALS and LIS patients with and without invasive mechanical ventilation. *Journal of Neurology*, **258**, 1801–4.

66. **Vianello, A., Arcaro, G., Palmieri, A.,** et al. (2011) Survival and quality of life after tracheostomy for acute respiratory failure in patients with amyotrophic lateral sclerosis. *Journal of Critical Care*, **26**, 329.e7–14.

67. **McHorney, C.A., Bricker, D.E., Kramer, A.E.,** et al. (2000) The SWAL-QOL outcomes tool for oropharyngeal dysphagia in adults: I. conceptual foundation and item development. *Dysphagia*, **15**, 115–21.

68. **McHorney, C., Bricker, D., Robbins, J., Kramer, A., Rosenbek, J.,** and **Chignell, K.** (2000) The SWAL-QOL outcomes tool for oropharyngeal dysphagia in adults: II. Item reduction and preliminary scaling. *Dysphagia*, **15**, 122–33.

69. **McHorney, C., Robbins, J., Lomax, K.,** et al. (2002) The SWAL-QOL and SWAL-CARE outcomes tool for oropharyngeal dysphagia in adults: III. Documentation of reliability and validity. *Dysphagia*, **17**, 97–114

70. **McHorney, C.A., Martin-Harris, B., Robbins, J.,** and **Rosenbek, J.** (2006) Clinical validity of the SWAL-QOL and SQAL-CARE outcome tools with respect to bolus flow measures. *Dysphagia*, **21**, 141–8.

71. **Tabor L, Gaziano J, Watts S, Robison R, Plowman EK.** (2016) Defining swallowing-related quality of life profiles in individuals with amyotrophic lateral sclerosis. *Dysphagia*, **31**, 376–82.

72. **Paris G, Martinaud O, Petit A,** et al. (2013) Oropharyngeal dysphagia in amyotrophic lateral sclerosis alters quality of life. *Journal of Oral Rehabilitation*, **40**, 199–204.

73. **Felgoise, S.H., Zaccheo, V., Duff, J.,** and **Simmons, Z.** (2016) Verbal communication impacts quality of life in patients with amyotrophic lateral sclerosis. *Amyotrophic Lateral Sclerosis and Frontotemporal Degeneration*, **17**, 179–83.

74. **Caligari M, Godi M, Guglielmetti S, Franchignoni F,** and **Nardone A.** (2013) Eye tracking communication devices in amyotrophic lateral sclerosis: Impact on disability and quality of life. *Amyotrophic Lateral Sclerosis and Frontotemporal Degeneration*, **14**, 546–52.

75. **Korner, S., Siniawski, M., Kollewe, K.,** et al. (2012) Speech therapy and communication device: Impact on quality of life and mood in patients with amyotrophic lateral sclerosis. *Amyotrophic Lateral Sclerosis and Frontotemporal Degeneration*, **14**, 20–5.

76. **Hwang, C.S., Weng, H.H., Wang, L.F., Tsai, C.H.,** and **Chang, H.T.** (2014) An eye-tracking assistive device improves the quality of life for ALS patients and reduces the caregivers' burden. *Journal of Motor Behaviour*, **46**, 233–8.

77. **Lou, J.S., Reeves, A., Benice, T.,** and **Sexton, G.** (2003) Fatigue and depression are associated with poor quality of life in ALS. *Neurology*, **60**, 122–3.

78. **Korner, S., Kollewe, K., Abdulla, S., Sapf, A., Dengler, R.,** and **Petri, S.** (2015) Interaction of physical function, quality of life, and depression for amyotrophic lateral sclerosis: characterization of a large patient cohort. *BMC Neurology*, **15**, 84.

79. **Pizzimenti A, Aragona M, Onesti E, Inghilleri M.** (2013) Depression, pain and quality of life in patients with amyotrophic lateral sclerosis: a cross-sectional study. *Functional Neurology*, **28**, 115–9.

80. **Ganzini, L., Johnston, W.S.,** and **Hoffman, W.F.** (1999) Correlates of suffering in amyotrophic lateral sclerosis. *Neurology*, **52**, 1434–40.

81. **Vignola, A., Guzzo, A., Calvo, A.,** et al. (2008) Anxiety undermines quality of life in ALS patients and caregivers. *European Journal of Neurology*, **15**, 1231–6.

82. **Diener, E., Emmons, R.A., Larsen, R.J.,** and **Griffin, S.** (1985) The satisfaction with life scale. *Journal of Personal Assessment*, **49**, 71–5.

83. **Larson, S.L., Owens, P.L., Ford, D.,** and **Eaton, W.** (2001) Depressive disorder, dysthymia, and risk of stroke: Thirteen-year follow-up from the Baltimore epidemiological catchment area study. *Stroke*, **32**, 1979–83.

84. **May M, McCarron P, Stansfeld S,** et al. (2002) Does psychological distress predict the risk of ischemic stroke and transient ischemic attack? The Caerphilly study. *Stroke*, **33**, 7–12.

85. **Hammer EM, Hacker S, Hautzinger M, Meyer TD, Kubler A.** (2008) Validity of the ALS-Depression-Inventory (ADI-12)—a new screening instrument for depressive disorders in patients with amyotrophic lateral sclerosis. *Journal of Affective Disorders*, **109**, 213–19.

86. **Felgoise, S.H., Chakraborty, B.H., Bond, E.,** et al. (2010) Psychological morbidity in ALS: The importance of psychological assessment beyond depression alone. *Amyotrophic Lateral Sclerosis*, **11**, 351–8.

87. **Stephens, H.E., Young, J., Felgoise, S.H.,** and **Simmons, Z.** (2015) A qualitative study of multidisciplinary ALS clinic use in the United States. *Amyotrophic Lateral Sclerosis and Frontotemporal Degeneration*, **17**, 55–61.

88. **Stephens, H.E., Felgoise, S., Young, J.,** and **Simmons, Z.** (2015) Multidisciplinary ALS clinics in the USA: a comparison of those who attend and those who do not. *Amyotrophic Lateral Sclerosis and Frontotemporal Degeneration*, **16**, 196–201.

89. **Traynor, B.J., Alexander, M., Corr, B., Frost, E.,** and **Hardiman, O.** (2003) Effect of a multidisciplinary amyotrophic lateral sclerosis (ALS) clinic on ALS survival: a population based study, 1996–2000. *Journal of Neurology and Neurosurgical Psychiatry*, **74**, 1258–61.

90. **Chio, A., Bottacchi, E., Buffa, C., Mutani, R.,** and **Mora, G.** (2006) Positive effects of tertiary centres for amyotrophic lateral sclerosis on outcome and use of hospital facilities. *Journal of Neurology and Neurosurgical Psychiatry*, **77**, 948–50.

91. **Rooney, J., Byrne, S., Heverin, M.,** et al. (2015) A multidisciplinary clinic approach improves survival in ALS: a comparative study of ALS in Ireland and Northern Ireland. *Journal of Neurology and Neurosurgical Psychiatry,* **86,** 496–501.

92. **Aridegbe, T., Kandler, R., Walters, S.J., Walsh, T., Shaw, P.J.,** and **McDermott, C.J.** (2013) The natural history of motor neuron disease: assessing the impact of specialist care. *Amyotrophic Lateral Sclerosis and Frontotemporal Degeneration,* **14,** 13–19.

93. **Van Den Berg, J.P., Kalmijn, S., Lindeman, E.,** et al. (2005) Multidisciplinary ALS care improves quality of life in patients with ALS. *Neurology,* **65,** 1264–7.

Chapter 3

Psychological morbidity in amyotrophic lateral sclerosis: Depression, anxiety, hopelessness

Dorothée Lulé, Albert C. Ludolph, and Andrea Kübler

Psychological well-being in amyotrophic lateral sclerosis

The well-being of a person according to the World Health Organization (WHO) includes at minimum physical (individuals' perception of their physical state), psychological (individuals' perception of their cognitive and affective state), and social (individuals' perception of their interpersonal relationships and social roles in their lives) dimensions. It is therefore not simply a state of physical integrity (1). One way of defining well-being is to use the concept of quality of life as detailed in Chapter 2. Psychological well-being indicated by affective state is another indicator of psychosocial adaptation to chronic illness and disability(2), and is increasingly recognized as an objective clinical or biological measure to evaluate health care provision and interventions in research and clinical trials (3).

The diagnosis of amyotrophic lateral sclerosis (ALS) is a major stressful event for patients and their families. It threatens hope and expectations for the future, forcing patients and their significant others to rewrite their life plans and change dreams (4). Despite the devastating diagnosis, observations concerning psychological well-being in serious chronic illnesses, such as ALS are often counter-intuitive. Deterioration of physical strength and function does not necessarily parallel a decline in perceived well-being(5). Accordingly, ALS patients may experience a surprisingly moderately altered affective state compared with healthy subjects of the same age and educational status (6–14). The lack of association of severity of illness and psychological well-being has been shown for several diseases and is referred to as the 'well-being- paradox' (15). Psychological well-being in serious illness is highly dependent on several intrinsic and extrinsic factors, which we will discuss in the current chapter.

Indicators of altered affective state: Depression, anxiety, and hopelessness

Affective state of a person as an indicator of psychological well-being addresses emotions, feelings, and moods. Altered affective state may present as depression, anxiety, and hopelessness. Depression, anxiety, and hopelessness may evolve independently of any lifetime event or may occur when an individual is discouraged by severely distressing or negative life events, such as the diagnosis of ALS. Depression and anxiety are psychiatric disorders, whereas hopelessness is a symptom that may occur in association with a variety of mental health conditions. Depression is a state of low mood that can affect a person's thoughts, behaviour, and feelings, whereas anxiety is a state of inner turmoil, often accompanied by restless behaviour. Hopelessness is defined by negative thoughts about the future or a negative view of oneself, associated with inhibited motivation and a lack of interest.

The prevalence of anxiety and depression in patients with ALS varies widely, estimated as between 0 and 30% for anxiety, and between 0 and 50% for depression, and numbers change with the assessment methods (16–18). Hopelessness is the most common marker of psychological morbidity in ALS and it is a key determinant of psychological well-being (19).

When reporting on affective state in ALS, the transient feeling of sadness and grief for losing the 'healthy self' (20) must be distinguished from clinically relevant depression, a mental disease that is conceptualized as a mood that is pervasive and non-responsive to environmental changes (21). As defined by Diagnostic and Statistical Manual of Mental Disorders (DSM-V)(22) criteria, major depression and generalized anxiety disorders are rather rare events in ALS, ranging in frequency between 2% and 11% for depression(6,17,23,24), and up to 20% for anxiety disorders (17,18). Patients with clinical depression in the course of ALS are often those with at least one prior episode of depression (6). Although the prevalence of depression is higher for those with ALS than for healthy adults in the same age group (6,23,24), it is not increased when compared with that of other patients with more benign disorders and better outcomes, such as patients with irritable bowel syndrome and chronic gastric ulcer (6).

The reasons for depression in ALS are heterogeneous and vary between patients despite the evidence that the incidence of depression is closely related to breaking the news of the fatal diagnosis. Roos and colleagues demonstrated in a nested population based study in Sweden that patients in the first year after diagnosis are most vulnerable to depression (25). In some cases, it might even be a prodromal symptom of ALS (25). Following first symptoms and before the final diagnosis is made, depression might be a results of psychological distress due to uncertainty (26). Following diagnosis, patients face a fatal diagnosis without any (current) medical cure. They are also confronted with a decreasing ability to perform activities of daily living, resulting in the need for help from others, which threatens their feeling of autonomy (27). Accordingly, early in the course of the disease, affective state is at risk and may decline (18,28). This may be regarded as part of the normal grieving process that accompanies a terminal diagnosis and may be diagnosed as 'adjustment disorder with depressive mood', rather than a depressive disorder as defined by DSM- V (20,22). With time, patients may adapt to the altered circumstances and experience an improved affective state (29,30). There are several factors determining the course and occurrence of depression in ALS. One of them is the time available to adapt. Accordingly, if disease progression is very rapid, patients are more likely to be depressed (31). In the terminal phase of the disease,

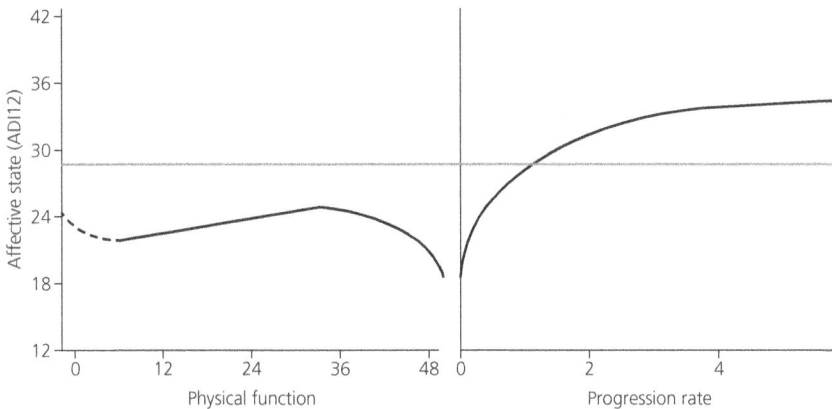

Fig. 3.1 (Left) Model of psychosocial adjustment and psychological morbidity in ALS (based on clinical experience and unpublished data by Lulé). Association of affective state as measured with the ADI-12 (ALS depression inventory 12 items; scores range 12–48, where increased scores indicate increased depressive mood; cut-off for clinically relevant depression >30 as indicated by the red line; [35]) and physical function as measured with the ALSFRS-R is depicted (ALS functional rating scale; scores range 0–48, lower scores indicating poorer physical function). On average, patients' depression scores increase with increasing physical dysfunction (represented by a decline in ALS-FRS) in the first year after diagnosis and then decrease when psychosocial adaptation is successful. In the terminal phase (e.g. ALSFRS<5) it might increase in some patients (end-of-life despair) but not in others (dashed blue line). (Right) Association of affective state and progression rate (maximum ALS-FRS-R (48) minus current ALS-FRS-R score divided by disease duration). A loss of more than 1.4 points per month on the ALS-FRS impairs successful psychosocial adjustment as indicated by clinically significant depression (above threshold of ADI-12 > 30 indicated by red line).

patients may experience end-of-life despair and depressive symptoms might increase again (Fig. 3.1). However, Rabkin and colleagues (32) showed that depression does not necessarily increase in the terminal phase, despite increased anxiety in the last days and hours before death as reported retrospectively by caregivers(33,34).

Non-disease associated characteristics such as demographics and educational status are critical factors also influencing psychological well-being in ALS, e.g. higher education was associated with better well-being, probably due to higher psychological capacity for adaptation and coping, and greater financial resources for care, in a German sample (6). In a Chinese study, higher education and female gender were associated with increased depression and anxiety(36).

Well-being among ALS patients also depends on pre-existing individual differences(37). These differences are personality dependent, but also triggered by external factors such as family. The choice and application of coping strategies are a key factor for psychological well-being(38). Perceived social support, the appraisal of one's own coping potential, avoidance, and search for support and information were found to be negatively linked with depression(9). These variables explained 47% of the variance of psychological well-being at the second measurement 3–6 months later(30). For many patients, coping strategies showed some variance during disease progression(39). In the early phase, 'avoidance' predicted good well-being in some patients but in the long run, coping strategies such as 'searching for information and support' were most effective strategies for psychological well-being in ALS(9,30).

Self-efficacy(40), self-perception of health (41) and trust in one's own coping potential (30) also appeared to impact psychological well-being. Thinking about the past, but not about the present and future, is linked to poor well-being, and this is mediated by rumination(42). Many years of research about adapting to and living with chronic diseases suggest that mindfulness in the sense of accepting the circumstances that cannot be changed (43) reduces the negative psychological impact of the illness(44,45). Accordingly, those patients focusing on abilities and qualities that are lost in the course of ALS, such as mobility and physical health, experience a reduced well-being, whereas those who focus on intrinsic factors such as spirituality report a better psychosocial adaptation(6,46). Accordingly, loss of hope(19,47), which refers to lack of meaning in life and inability of living in the moment is associated with low psychological well-being(42,46,48).

Other successful mechanisms to ensure well-being are intellectual stimulation, the development of wisdom, and interpersonal relationships(49). Meaning in life is highly interrelated with psychological well-being and this meaning may be provided in several ways(50). Spirituality and religiousness may provide a source of comfort for patients(41,50,51), but the degree to which spirituality is used as a strategy may be highly culturally specific, and so may vary greatly between countries(38). In the course of the disease, hope can be positively affected by spiritual beliefs (50) and hopelessness, similar to anxiety and depression, is often reduced in spiritual patients(52), but this is not true for all patient samples(32). Importantly, spirituality and psychological well-being may drive medical interventions(53–55).

In conclusion, continuous evaluation of psychological well-being as measured by symptoms of depression, anxiety, and hopelessness is mandatory and, if such symptoms are present, support must be provided.

Diagnosis and symptom management

Psychological well-being may interact with many fields of medical care (e.g. choice of medical care(56); disease state and progression) (57). Therefore, timely standard screening for psychological well-being in ALS and support within multidisciplinary professional teams (39) are important cornerstones of medical care. The most valid attempt to determine depression and anxiety is a clinical diagnosis according to DSM-V (22) criteria by a specialist. However, there is evidence that screening instruments might provide a fast and easy means to determine major changes in psychological well-being in ALS(58). In ALS, the focus has been mostly on anxiety, depression, and hopelessness, although others have suggested using broader concepts of psychological well-being, because a substantial number of individuals with ALS experience psychological distress of various types(59). The most commonly used measures to screen for anxiety in ALS are the Hamilton rating scale for anxiety (HAM-A) (60), the subscale anxiety of the Hospital Anxiety and Depression Scale (HADS (61); modified version by Gibbons et al.) (62) and the State and Trait Anxiety Inventory (STAI) (63). Depression can be estimated with the Beck's depression inventory (64), the Hamilton rating scale (65), the depression part of the HADS and the Zung depression scale(66). Hopelessness is often determined with the Beck's Hopelessness Scale (67).

There are limitations that impact upon the assessment of depression, anxiety, hopelessness, and other measures of psychological well-being in patients with ALS. Most of the scales mentioned are self-rating scales and patients with severe physical symptoms might experience difficulty filling them out. Furthermore, the scales are not specific for ALS and some physical symptoms specific for ALS might interfere with these items. Such instruments may overestimate depression and anxiety in these patients. Examples of such items are loss of energy, appetite, and body weight (as symptoms of depression in the Beck's depression inventory) as these are findings associated with progressive weakness or severe bulbar symptoms; cramps preventing the ability to relax might be misclassified as a symptom of anxiety (17,23,68). Finally, being faced by a threatening disease without cure provides no comfort and hope to the patient, leading to feeling of hopelessness. Therefore, based on the BDI, the ALS depression inventory was developed (the scale is available for request at andrea.kuebler@uni-wuerzburg.de); it is specifically designed for ALS patients, and thus does not include questions whose answers would be impacted by physical symptoms associated with disease progression (35). For other aspects of psychological well-being, there are no scales designed for ALS, with the possible exclusion of some ALSSQoL-R subscales (69).

Discrepancies in frequency of depression, anxiety, and hopelessness in studies might be due to different methods and instruments used to detect psychological morbidity in ALS. Furthermore, selection bias in studies may explain the high variance in findings of psychological morbidity in ALS. Sampling methods that enrol patients at their initial visit in multicenter trials may lead to a larger variance in psychological well-being because it may disproportionately include patients in whom the disease is progressing rapidly or who are early in their disease course. In contrast, longitudinal studies are skewed toward patients with longer survival, allowing them to adapt to the changing circumstances of life with ALS (9,30).

With regards to management, there is sparse literature on how to improve psychological well-being in ALS patients. The primary goal of clinical intervention is physical symptom management. However, psychological intervention may not only impact psychological well-being (70), but may have a significant impact on physical symptoms and lifespan. For example, early depressive symptoms have negative predictive value for survival (71,72). Even in a devastating condition such as ALS, there is evidence that psychological intervention might have positive impact on psychological well-being by leading to a sense of reduced depression and anxiety (73–75). Mindfulness seems to be a promising approach in managing psychological morbidity in ALS (see Chapter 4) (44,74). Additionally, approaches such as expressive disclosure, cognitive behavioural therapy, and hypnosis might provide important support for the patients to improve psychological well-being, at least in the short term (see also Chapter 5) (74). Whether these strategies have a long-term effect on psychological well-being is currently unknown. Long-term randomized controlled trials for management and intervention of psychological well-being are needed. The understanding of the need for psychosocial intervention in ALS in clinical care is evolving.

Extrinsic determinants of psychological well-being: Physical condition

External factors such as lack of effective medical treatment and fatality of the diagnosis are features impacting well-being in ALS (36). Some studies suggest a negative association between loss of physical function and both psychological well-being (76,77) and satisfaction with life (32). Physical function explained up to 25% of psychological well-being in a Spanish study with decreasing impact as the disease progressed (19). However, other studies provided evidence that depression is not necessarily associated with loss of physical function in patients with ALS (71,78) and physical parameters (the ALSFRS score and time since diagnosis) were not predictive for severity of depressive symptoms (30). Accordingly, mental health can be preserved despite declining physical function (79) and the relation between the two may be indirect and more complex (Fig. 3.1) (6,14,18,31). For example, the specific body area affected by loss of physical function, rather than general loss of strength, influences psychological well-being; swallowing and respiratory dysfunction are more troubling for patients and are, thus, more closely associated with affective state than loss of limb function (28,80). In line with these results, Mora and colleagues provided evidence that communication abilities had the highest impact on psychological well-being (19). The use of non-invasive ventilation has no negative impact (23,32,81,82), but rather a beneficial effect, on psychological well-being in ALS (6,83,84).

In cross-sectional analyses, rate of progression seems to be critical. If physical function and strength are lost rapidly, patients have insufficient time to cope (29,56). Patients with fast progression, as indicated by a loss of physical function of more than 1.4 points per month on the ALS Functional Rating Scale (ALSFRS), had a significantly increased risk of depressiveness (31). The rapid changes do not permit the patients to adapt to medical interventions, such as artificial ventilation or a wheelchair (29). Diagnostic uncertainty also plays an important role. Caga and colleagues (20) analysed factors of depression in a sample of 27 ALS patients of whom 10 had depressive symptoms. For every additional month between symptom onset and the diagnosis of ALS, patients were 1.12 times more likely to report symptoms of depression. During the diagnostic phase, patients with suspected ALS are particularly likely to experience marked distress (18). Thus, patients with rapidly progressive disease or those with a long period of diagnostic uncertainty require particular attention to their mental health.

Extrinsic determinants of psychological well-being: Family and primary caregivers

Caregivers are often patients' relatives and family members, most commonly spouses. Caregivers and patients often have very close relationships, and thus, the patients' QoL is affected by the well-being of the caregivers and vice versa (see also Chapter 16)

(8,23,85,86). Some studies provide evidence that the caregivers' affective state (50,85) is in the range of that of the patient. Other studies suggest that caregivers of ALS patients may have increased levels of depression and anxiety (87) and Lo Coco (50) provided evidence that despite some similarities, patients and caregivers do not necessarily represent a unified psychological entity. Caregivers have to face the burden of watching the physical decline of the patient and the future loss of a loved one (88). The physical and psychological burden on primary caregivers is high (16,89,90). This is especially true for caregivers of patients in advanced stages of the disease (89,91). However, Lo Coco (50) reported that caregivers who present with lower psychological well-being are not always those who look after the most physically impaired patients. What seems to be even more burdensome than physical state per se is patients' cognitive and behavioural status (87,92–95). Specifically, behavioural changes such as disinhibition and impulsivity affect the well-being of the caregiver (95,96). Furthermore, the degree of burden is not necessarily determined by objective parameters of caregiving, but rather by intrinsic strategies of finding positive meaning in caregiving (23). Finally, the worse the affective state of caregivers the more burdensome they experienced the daily task of providing care (85).

Caregivers often experience severe restrictions in their personal life. Rabkin (85) demonstrated that the stronger these restrictions and the less likely the caregiver is to 'have a plan of action' or 'pay attention to good areas of life', the higher the degree of depression. Other factors such as age, gender, education, income, relationship with the patient, and marital status were unrelated to caregiver depression. Similarly, caregiver depression was not correlated with access to resources, as measured by hospice enrolment or weekly hours of paid help. In contrast to other studies, 'health care context' (including access to services and information) was an essential aspect of caregivers' well-being in the study of Cipolletta and Amicucci (97). Passive coping styles of caregivers are negative prognostic factors for psychological well-being, whereas actual (98) and perceived social support and (family) relationships (97) have a positive impact (99). Accordingly, support by multidisciplinary caregiver teams, including psychological intervention, is beneficial for the psychological well-being of family caregivers (59). Furthermore, spirituality—and religiousness are positively associated with psychological well-being in caregivers (100). In in-depth interviews with caregivers, Cipolletta and Amicucci (97) found 'meaning of ALS', including the peculiarity of ALS and its comparison with other illnesses, to be the most essential aspect of living with an ALS patient until death. Overall, caregivers have similar determinants of psychosocial adaptation to the disease as patients, e.g. active coping, social support and spiritual well-being.

Family members, who are the primary caregivers and usually spend many hours of time with the patient every day, are unable to correctly anticipate the patient's well-being. Specifically, caregivers often overestimate patients' psychological morbidity (14,31,85,101,102). The more depressed the caregivers, the more they overrated depression in the respective patient (31,85). This may be regarded as a psychological defence mechanism of healthy persons (103). As psychosocial adaptation is a gradual process (104), healthy persons are poor at imagining a patient's internal process of adaptation. Healthy persons generalize from their own perspective and thus, judge life with severe physical impairment not worth living (6,105). Even patients shortly after diagnosis cannot imagine adjusting to a life with ALS

(29). Against all odds, many patients psychologically adapt during the course of the disease (29,106). Interestingly, physicians' ability to correctly evaluate patients' well-being increased with professional experience: The more ALS patients a physician has encountered over the years, the better he or she estimated the actual level of patients' well-being (107).

The heavy burden on primary caregivers, the close interrelation of patients' and caregivers' well-being, and the caregivers' inability to correctly anticipate the patients' psychological well-being has major implications. Caregivers need to be closely integrated into the patient-centred concept of care and support. Multidisciplinary teams should also be attentive to the caregivers' and families' well-being. Because patients' and caregivers' emotional states are highly interrelated, support of caregivers will have positive effect on patients (23). As caregivers affect patient's decisions to opt for specific therapeutic treatments (29,44,53), support, and positive intervention concerning caregiver's psychological well-being might finally even interfere with clinical management and survival of ALS patients.

Models of psychosocial adjustment in ALS

The interaction of intrinsic and extrinsic determinants of psychological well-being may explain the broad variance of psychological adaptation seen in ALS. Pakenham adapted the stress-coping model of Lazarus and Folkman (108) to chronic disease (109,110). According to this stress model, the stressor itself—receiving the diagnosis itself is a very stressful moment for the patient (111)—might be similar for all patients—reduced survival, progressive immobility, and loss of verbal communication (Fig. 3.2) (109). However, patients may identify, evaluate, and respond to different aspects of the same stressor. Consequently, patients mobilize their personal resources individually and selectively. The more limited the personal resources, the more a patient experiences stress. Coping strategies, which may be either problem- or emotion-focused, can be used to adapt to the situation (see Chapter 7) (57). Different coping strategies explain much of the variance in psychological well-being in ALS (9).

Reappraisal and reframing help the patient to adjust to the devastating conditions of ALS (Fig. 3.2)(109, 112) and are used by ALS patients with good psychosocial adaptation (38,48). Levels of functioning in and importance of specified life areas and/or changes in the life areas themselves explain dynamics in psychological well-being over time (5). Social and medical support and well-being of significant others contribute to the ability to cope with the disease. Reframing is an important process for adjusting human behaviour in the context of a given situation according to the TOTE (Test-Operate-Test-Exit) model (113). In that model, in the test phase, an actual value (necessity of living with ALS) is compared with the desired target value (being healthy, having a long life) and if those do not match, an operant phase is entered to adjust the expectations. For successful psychosocial adaptation, this procedure is repeated in a feedback loop until the expectations and the outcomes match. In ALS, extrinsic factors (physical dysfunction and fatal diagnosis) cannot be changed, requiring an adaptation of the desired target value. If the process of adaptation, also referred to as response shift (105), is successful, ALS patients may experience a good psychological well-being (29).

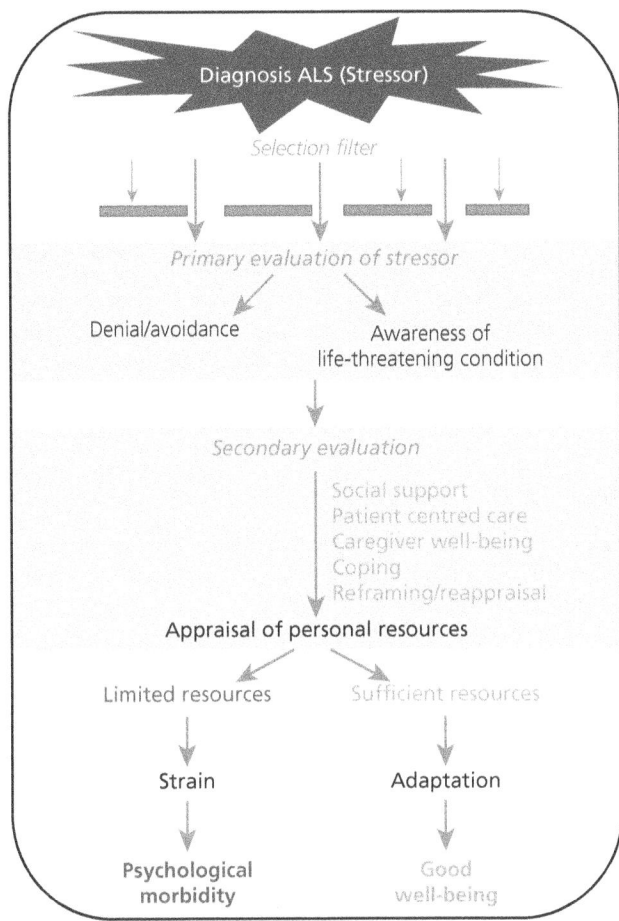

Fig. 3.2 Process model of psychological well-being with the life threatening stressor ALS. Source: data from Lazarus RS, Emotion and Adaptation, Copyright (1991), Oxford University Press.

Conclusion

Living with a fatal disease creates a crisis loaded environment and psychological well-being is at stake following first symptoms and diagnosis (114). There is not yet a cure for ALS, but there is evidence that extensive medical and psychosocial support positively impact upon psychological well-being (43). Following physical decline, psychological well-being is a hazard, especially if bulbar function and communication is impaired. Poor psychological well-being might shorten survival time and impact upon medical treatment in the terminal phase. Patients' preferences for or against treatments and the wish for a hastened death are biased by patients' depression, anxiety and hopelessness (29,44,55). The primary pathology in ALS is biologically driven. However, psychological morbidity strongly influences physical parameters. Patients' adaptation to the disease is a psychological process that is influenced by intrinsic and extrinsic factors. A holistic view of the patient responded to by a multidisciplinary team positively impacts psychosocial adaptation which ultimately determines psychological well-being in ALS (75).

Funding

This is an EU Joint Programme—Neurodegenerative Disease Research (JPND "NEEDSinALS" www.NEEDSinALS, 01ED1405) project. The project is supported through the following organizations under the aegis of JPND—www.jpnd.eu, e.g. Germany, Bundesministerium für Bildung und Forschung (BMBF, FKZ), Sweden, Vetenskapr å det Sverige, and Poland, Narodowe Centrum Bad á n i Rozwoju (NCBR). This work was supported by the Deutsche Forschungsgemeinschaft and the Bundesministerium für Bildung und Forschung (BMBF MND-Net 01GM1103A).

References

1. **World Health Organization.** (1995) The World Health Organization Quality of Life assessment (WHOQOL): position paper from the World Health Organization. *Social Science & Medicine*, **41**(10), 1403–9.

2. **Livneh, H.** (2001) Psychosocial adaptation to chronic illness and disability: A conceptual framework. *Rehabilitation Counseling Bulletin*, **44**(3), 151.

3. **Carr, A.J.** and **Higginson, I.J.** (2001) Are quality of life measures patient centred? *British Medical Journal*, **322**, 1357–60.

4. **McLeod, J.E.** and **Clarke, D.M.** (2007) A review of psychosocial aspects of motor neurone disease. *Journal of the Neurological Sciences*, **258**, 4–10.

5. **Joyce, C.R.**, **Hickey, A.**, **McGee, H.M.**, and **O'Boyle, C.A.** (2003) A theory-based method for the evaluation of individual quality of life: the SEIQoL. *Quality of Life Research*, **12**(3), 275–80.

6. **Lulé, D.**, **Häcker, S.**, **Ludolph, A.**, **Birbaumer, N.**, and **Kübler, A.** (2008) Depression and quality of life in patients with amyotrophic lateral sclerosis, **105**(23), 397–403.

7. **Lulé, D.**, **Pauli, S.**, **Altintas, E.**, et al. (2012) Emotional adjustment in amyotrophic lateral sclerosis (ALS). *Journal of Neurology*, **259**(2), 334–41.

8. **Chiò, A.**, **Gauthier, A.**, **Montuschi, A.**, et al. (2004) A cross sectional study on determinants of quality of life in ALS. *Journal of Neurology, Neurosurgery and Psychiatry*, **75**(11), 1597–601.

9. **Matuz, T.**, **Birbaumer, N.**, **Hautzinger, M.**, and **Kübler, A.** (2010) Coping with amyotrophic lateral sclerosis: an integrative view. *Journal of Neurology, Neurosurgery and Psychiatry*, **81**(8), 893–8.

10. **Cupp, J.**, **Simmons, Z.**, **Berg, A.**, **Felgoise, S.H.**, **Walsh, S.M.**, and **Stephens, H.E.** (2011) Psychological health in patients with ALS is maintained as physical function declines. *Amyotrophic Lateral Sclerosis*, **12**(4), 290–6.

11. **Hardiman, O.**, **Hickey, A.**, and **O'Donerty, L.J.** (2004) Physical decline and quality of life in amyotrophic lateral sclerosis. *Amyotrophic Lateral Sclerosis and Other Motor Neuron Disorders*, **5**(4), 230–4.

12. **Simmons, Z.**, **Bremer, B.A.**, **Robbins, R.A.**, **Walsh, S.M.**, and **Fischer, S.** (2000) Quality of life in ALS depends on factors other than strength and physical function. *Neurology*, **55**(3), 388–92.

13. **Neudert, C., Wasner, M.,** and **Borasio, G.D.** (2004) Individual quality of life is not correlated with health-related quality of life or physical function in patients with amyotrophic lateral sclerosis. *Journal of Palliative Medicine*, **7**(4), 551–7.

14. **Grehl, T., Rupp, M., Budde, P., Tegenthoff, M.,** and **Fangerau, H.** (2011) Depression and QOL in patients with ALS: How do self-ratings and ratings by relatives differ? Quality of Life Research, **20**(4), 569–74.

15. **Herschbach, P.** (2002) The Well-Being Paradox in Quality-of-Life Research—On what does our sense of well-being depend? *Psychotherapy and Psychosomatic Medicine*, **52**, 141–50.

16. **Pagnini, F., Rossi, G., Lunetta, C.,** et al. (2010) Burden, depression, and anxiety in caregivers of people with amyotrophic lateral sclerosis. *Psychology, Health & Medicine*, **15**(6), 685–93.

17. **Kurt, A., Nijboer, F., Matuz, T.,** and **Kübler, A.** (2010) Depression and anxiety in individuals with amyotrophic lateral sclerosis: epidemiology and management. *CNS Drugs*, **21**(4), 279–91.

18. **Vignola, A., Guzzo, A., Calvo, A.,** et al. (2008) Anxiety undermines quality of life in ALS patients and caregivers. *European Journal of Neurology*, **15**(11), 1231–6.

19. **Mora, J.S., Salas, T., Fajardo, M.L., Iváñez, L.,** and **Rodríguez-Santos, F.** (2013) Self perceived emotional functioning of Spanish patients with amyotrophic lateral sclerosis: a longitudinal study. *Frontiers in Psychology*, **3**, 609.

20. **Caga, J., Ramsey, E., Hogden, A., Mioshi, E.,** and **Kiernan, M.C.** (2015) A longer diagnostic interval is a risk for depression in amyotrophic lateral sclerosis. *Palliative Support Care*, **13**(4), 1019–24.

21. **Norris, L., Que, G.,** and **Bayat, E.** (2010) Psychiatric aspects of amyotrophic lateral sclerosis (ALS). *Current Psychiatry Reports*, **12**(3), 239–45.

22. **American Psychiatric Association.** (2013) *Diagnostic and Statistical Manual of Mental Disorders* (5th edn). Arlington, VA: American Psychiatric Publishing.

23. **Rabkin, J.G., Wagner, G. J.,** and **Del Bene, M.** (2000) Resilience and distress among amyotrophic lateral sclerosis patients and caregivers. *Psychosomatic Medicine*, **62**(2), 271–9.

24. **Ganzini, L., Johnston, W.S., McFarland, B.H., Tolle, S.W.,** and **Lee, M.A.** (1998) Attitudes of patients with amyotrophic lateral sclerosis and their care givers toward assisted suicide. *New England Journal of Medicine*, **339**(14), 967–73.

25. **Roos E, Mariosa D, Ingre C,** et al. (2016) Depression in amyotrophic lateral sclerosis. *Neurology*, **86**, 2271–7.

26. **Cragg, J.J., Seals, R., Cashman, N.,** and **Weisskopf, M.G.** (2016) Journal Club: Depression before and after diagnosis with amyotrophic lateral sclerosis. *Neurology*, **87**(21), e257–9.

27. **Connolly, S., Galvin, M.,** and **Hardiman, O.** (2015) End-of-life management in patients with amyotrophic lateral sclerosis. *Lancet Neurology*, **14**(4), 435–42.

28. **Hillemacher, T., Grässel, E., Tigges, S.,** et al. (2004) Depression and bulbar involvement in amyotrophic lateral sclerosis. *Amyotrophic Lateral Sclerosis and Other Motor Neuron Disorders*, **5**(4), 245–9.

29. **Lulé, D., Nonnenmacher, S., Sorg, S.,** et al. (2014) Live and let die: Existential decision processes in a fatal disease. *Journal of Neurology*, **261**(3), 518–25.

30. **Matuz, T., Birbaumer, N., Hautzinger, M.,** and **Kübler, A.** (2015) Psychosocial adjustment to ALS: A longitudinal study. *Frontiers in Psychology*, **6**, 1197.

31. **Lulé, D., Ehlich, B., Lang, D.,** et al. (2013) Quality of life in fatal disease: The flawed judgement of the social environment. *Journal of Neurology*, **260**(11), 2836–43.

32. **Rabkin, J.G., Albert, S.M., Del Bene, M.L.,** et al. (2005) Prevalence of depressive disorders and change over time in late-stage ALS. *Neurology*, **65**(1), 62–7.

33. **Neudert, C., Oliver, D., Wasner, M.,** and **Borasio, G.D.** (2001) The course of the terminal phase in patients with amyotrophic lateral sclerosis. *Journal of Neurology*, **248**(7), 612–16.

34. **Ganzini, L., Johnston, W.S.,** and **Silveira, M.J.** (2002) The final month of life in patients with ALS. *Neurology*, **59**(3), 428–31.

35. **Hammer, E.M., Häcker, S., Hautzinger, M., Meyer, T.D.,** and **Kübler, A.** (2008) Validity of the ALS-Depression-Inventory (ADI-12)—a new screening instrument for depressive disorders in patients with amyotrophic lateral sclerosis. *Journal of Affective Disorders*, **109**(1–2), 213–19.

36. **Cui, F., Zhu, W., Zhou, Z.,** et al. (2015) Frequency and risk factor analysis of cognitive and anxiety-depressive disorders in patients with amyotrophic lateral sclerosis/motor neuron disease. *Neuropsychiatric Disease and Treatment*, **11**, 2847–54.

37. **Roach, A.R., Averill, A.J., Segerstrom, S.C.,** and **Kasarskis, E.J.** (2009) The dynamics of quality of life in ALS patients and caregivers. *Annals of Behavioural Medicine*, **37**(2), 197–206.

38. **Montel, S., Albertini, L.,** and **Spitz, E.** (2012) Coping strategies in relation to quality of life in amyotrophic lateral sclerosis. *Muscle & Nerve*, **45**(1), 131–4.

39. **Jakobsson Larsson, B., Nordin, K.,** and **Nygren, I.** (2016) Coping with amyotrophic lateral sclerosis; from diagnosis and during disease progression. Journal of Neurological Sciences, **361**, 235–42.

40. **Stephens, H.E., Lehman, E., Raheja, D., Yang, C., Walsh, S.,** and **Simmons, Z.** (2016) The role of mental health and self-efficacy in the pain experience of patients with amyotrophic lateral sclerosis. *Amyotrophic Lateral Sclerosis and Frontotemporal Degeneration*, **17**(3–4), 1–7.

41. **Bremer, B.A., Simone, A.L., Walsh, S., Simmons, Z.,** and **Felgoise, S.H.** (2004) Factors supporting quality of life over time for individuals with amyotrophic lateral sclerosis: The role of positive self-perception and religiosity. *Annals of Behavioural Medicine*, **28**(2), 119–25.

42. **Real, R.G., Dickhaus, T., Ludolph, A., Hautzinger, M.,** and **Kübler, A.** (2014) Well-being in amyotrophic lateral sclerosis: a pilot experience sampling study. *Frontiers in Psychology*, **5**, 704.

43. **Langer, E.** (1989) *Mindfulness*. Reading, MA: Addison-Wesley.

44. **Pagnini, F., Phillips, D.,** and **Langer, E.** (2014) A mindful approach with end-of-life thoughts. *Frontiers in Psychology*, **5**, 138.

45. **Pagnini F, Phillips D, Bosma CM, Reece A, Langer E.** (2015) Mindfulness, physical impairment and psychological well-being in people with amyotrophic lateral sclerosis. *Psychology & Health*, **30**(5), 503–17.

46. **Plahuta, J.M., McCulloch, B.J., Kasarskis, E.J., Ross, M.A., Walter, R.A.,** and **McDonald, E.R.** (2002) Amyotrophic lateral sclerosis and hopelessness: psychosocial factors. *Social Science and Medicine*, **55**(12), 2131–40.

47. **Ganzini, L., Johnston, W.S.,** and **Hoffman, W.F.** (1999) Correlates of suffering in amyotrophic lateral sclerosis. *Neurology*, **52**(7), 1434–40.

48. **Fanos, J.H., Gelinas, D.F., Foster, R.S., Postone, N.,** and **Miller, R.G.** (2008) Hope in palliative care: From narcissism to self-transcendence in amyotrophic lateral sclerosis. *Journal of Palliative Medicine*, **11**, 470–5.

49. **Young, J.M.** and **McNicoll, P.** (1998) Against all odds: positive life experiences of people with advanced amyotrophic lateral sclerosis. *Health & Social Work*, **23**(1), 35–43.

50. **Walsh, S.M., Bremer, B.A., Felgoise, S.H.,** and **Simmons, Z.** (2003) Religiousness is related to quality of life in patients with ALS. *Neurology*, **60**, 1527–9.

51. **Lo Coco, G., Lo Coco, D., Cicero, V.,** et al. (2005) Individual and health-related quality of life assessment in amyotrophic lateral sclerosis patients and their caregivers. *Journal of Neurological Sciences*, **238**(1–2), 11–17.

52. **Pagnini, F., Lunetta, C., Rossi, G.,** et al. (2011) Existential well-being and spirituality of individuals with amyotrophic lateral sclerosis is related to psychological well-being of their caregivers. *Amyotrophic Lateral Sclerosis*, **12**(2), 105–8.

53. **Murphy, P.L., Albert, S.M., Weber, C.M., Del Bene, M.L.,** and **Rowland, L.P.** (2000) Impact of spirituality and religiousness on outcomes in patients with ALS. *Neurology*, **55**, 1581–4.

54. **Boehm, S., Ludolph, A.C.,** and **Lulé, D.** (2015) Lebensverlängernde oder –verkürzende Maßnahmen bei ALS-Patienten. *Neurotransmitter*, **26**, 38–41.

55. **Ganzini, L., Silveira, M.J.,** and **Johnston, W.S.** (2002) Predictors and correlates of interest in assisted suicide in the final month of life among ALS patients in Oregon and Washington. *Journal of Pain and Symptom Management*, **24**(3), 312–17.

56. **Ganzini, L., Goy, E.R.,** and **Dobscha, S.K.** (2008) Prevalence of depression and anxiety in patients requesting physicians' aid in dying: cross sectional survey. *British Medical Journal*, **337**, a1682.

57. **Jelsone-Swain, L., Persad, C., Votruba, K.L.,** et al. (2012) The relationship between depressive symptoms, disease state, and cognition in amyotrophic lateral sclerosis. *Frontiers in Psychology*, **3**, 542.

58. **van Groenestijn, A.C., Schröder, C.D., Visser-Meily, J.M., Reenen, E.T., Veldink, J.H.,** and **van den Berg, L.H.** (2015) Cognitive behavioural therapy and quality of life in psychologically distressed patients with amyotrophic lateral sclerosis and their caregivers: Results of a prematurely stopped randomized controlled trial. *Amyotrophic Lateral Sclerosis and Frontotemporal Degeneration*, **16**(5–6), 309–15.

59. **Felgoise, S.H., Chakraborty, B.H., Bond, E.,** et al. (2010) Psychological morbidity in ALS: The importance of psychological assessment beyond depression alone. *Amyotrophic Lateral Sclerosis*, **11**(4), 351–8.

60. **Hamilton, M.** (1959) The assessment of anxiety states by rating. *British Journal of Medical Psychology*, **32**, 50–5.

61. **Zigmond, A.S.** and **Snaith, R.P.** (1983) The hospital anxiety and depression scale. *Acta Psychiatrica Scandinavica*, **67**, 361–70.

62. **Gibbons, C.J., Mills, R.J., Thornton, E.W.,** et al. (2011) Rasch analysis of the hospital anxiety and depression scale (HADS) for use in motor neurone disease. *Health & Quality of Life Outcomes*, **9**, 82.

63. **Spielberger, C.D., Gorsuch, R.L., Lushene, P.R., Vagg, P.R.,** and **Jacobs, A.G.** (1968) *Spielberger State-Trait Anxiety Inventory*. Menlo Park, CA: Mind Garden.

64. **Beck, A.T., Ward, C.H., Mendelson, M., Mock, J.,** and **Erbaugh, J.** (1961) An inventory for measuring depression. *Archives of General Psychiatry*, **4**, 561–71.

65. **Hamilton, M.** (1960) A rating scale for depression. *Journal of Neurology and Neurosurgerical Psychiatry*, **23**, 56–62.

66. **Zung, W.W.** (1965) A self-rating depression scale. *Archives of General Psychiatry*, **12**, 63–70.

67. **Beck, A.T.** (1988). Beck Hopelessness Scale. New York, NY: The Psychological Corporation.

68. Ferentinos, P., Paparrigopoulos, T., Rentzos, M., Zouvelou, V., Alexakis, T., and Evdokimidis, I. (2011) Prevalence of major depression in ALS: comparison of a semi-structured interview and four self-report measures. *Amyotrophic Lateral Sclerosis*, **12**(4), 297–302.

69. Simmons, Z., Felgoise, S.H., Bremer, B.A., et al. (2006) The ALSSQOL balancing physical and nonphysical factors in assessing quality of life in ALS. *Neurology*, **67**(9), 1659–64.

70. Palmieri, A., Kleinbub, J.R., Calvo, V., et al. (2012) Efficacy of hypnosis-based treatment in amyotrophic lateral sclerosis: a pilot study. *Frontiers in Psychology*, **3**, 465.

71. Thakore, N.J. and Pioro, E.P. (2016) Depression in ALS in a large self-reporting cohort. *Neurology*, **86**(11), 1031–8.

72. McDonald, E.R., Wiedenfeld, S., Hillel, A., Carpenter, C., and Walter, R. (1994) Survival in amyotrophic lateral sclerosis: the role of psychological factors. *Archives of Neurology*, **51**, 17–23.

73. Díaz, J.L., Sancho, J., Barreto, P., Bañuls, P., Renovell, M., and Servera, E. (2016) Effect of a short-term psychological intervention on the anxiety and depression of amyotrophic lateral sclerosis patients. *Journal of Health & Psychology*, **21**(7), 1426–35.

74. Pagnini, F., Simmons, Z., Corbo, M., and Molinari, E. (2012) Amyotrophic lateral sclerosis: time for research on psychological intervention? *Amyotrophic Lateral Sclerosis*, **13**(5), 416–17.

75. Gould, R.L., Coulson, M.C., Brown, R.G., Goldstein, L.H., Al-Chalabi, A., and Howard, R.J. (2015) Psychotherapy and pharmacotherapy interventions to reduce distress or improve well-being in people with amyotrophic lateral sclerosis: A systematic review. *Amyotrophic Lateral Sclerosis and Frontotemporal Degeneration*, **16**(5–6), 293–302.

76. Körner, S., Kollewe, K., Abdulla, S., Zapf, A., Dengler, R., and Petri, S. (2015) Interaction of physical function, quality of life and depression in Amyotrophic lateral sclerosis: Characterization of a large patient cohort. *BMC Neurology*, **15**, 84.

77. Oh, H., Sin, M.K., Schepp, K.G., and Choi-Kwon, S. (2012) Depressive symptoms and functional impairment among amyotrophic lateral sclerosis patients in South Korea. *Rehabilitation Nursing*, **37**:136–44.

78. McElhiney, M.C., Rabkin, J.G., Gordon, P.H., Goetz, R., and Mitsumoto, H. (2009) Prevalence of fatigue and depression in ALS patients and change over time. *Journal of Neurology and Neurosurgical Psychiatry*, **80**(10), 1146–9.

79. De Groot, I.J., Post, M.W., van Heuveln, T., Van den Berg, L.H., and Lindeman, E. (2007) Cross-sectional and longitudinal correlations between disease progression and different health-related quality of life domains in persons with amyotrophic lateral sclerosis. *Amyotrophic Lateral Sclerosis*, **8**(6), 356–61.

80. Tabor, L., Gaziano, J., Watts, S., Robison, R., and Plowman, E.K. (2016) Defining swallowing-related quality of life profiles in individuals with amyotrophic lateral sclerosis. *Dysphagia*, **31**(3), 376–82. (Epub ahead of print)

81. Zamietra, K., Lehman, E.B., Felgoise, S.H., Walsh, S.M., Stephens, H.E., and Simmons Z. (2012) Non-invasive ventilation and gastrostomy may not impact overall quality of life in patients with ALS. *Amyotrophic Lateral Sclerosis*, **13**(1), 55–8.

82. Gelinas DF, O'Connor P, Miller RG. (1998) Quality of life for ventilator-dependent ALS patients and their caregivers. *Journal of Neurological Sciences*, **160** (1), 134–6.

83. Butz, M., Wollinsky, K.H., Wiedemuth-Catrinescu, U., et al. (2003) Longitudinal effects of noninvasive positive-pressure ventilation in patients with amyotrophic lateral sclerosis. *American Journal of Physical and Medical Rehabilitation*, **82**(8), 597–604.

84. **Piepers, S., van den Berg, J.P., Kalmijn, S.**, et al. (2006) Effect of non-invasive ventilation on survival, quality of life, respiratory function and cognition: A review of the literature. *Amyotrophic Lateral Sclerosis*, **7**(4), 195–200.

85. **Rabkin, J.G., Albert, S.M., Rowland, L.P.**, and **Mitsumoto, H.** (2009) How common is depression among ALS caregivers? A longitudinal study. *Amyotrophic Lateral Sclerosis*, **10**(5–6), 448–55.

86. **Mockford, C., Jenkinson, C.**, and **Fitzpatrick, R.** (2006) A review: Carers, MND and service provision. *Amyotrophic Lateral Sclerosis*, **7**, 132–41.

87. **Gauthier, A., Vignola, A., Calvo, A.**, et al. (2007) A longitudinal study on quality of life and depression in ALS patient–caregiver couples. *Neurology*, **68**, 923–6.

88. **Boerner, K.** and **Mock, S.E.** (2012) Impact of patient suffering on caregiver well-being: the case of amyotrophic lateral sclerosis patients and their caregivers. *Psychology & Health Medicine*, **17**(4), 457–66.

89. **Chio, A., Gauthier, A., Calvo, A., Ghiglione, P.**, and **Mutani, R.** (2016) Caregiver burden and patients' perception of being a burden in ALS. *Neurology*, **64**, 1780–2

90. **Mitsumoto, H.** (2002) Caregiver assessment: Summary. *Amyotrophic Lateral Sclerosis*, **3**(1), 31–4.

91. **Bruletti, G., Comini, L., Scalvini, S.**, et al. (2015) A two-year longitudinal study on strain and needs in caregivers of advanced ALS patients. *Amyotrophic Lateral Sclerosis and Frontotemporal Degeneration*, **16**(3–4), 187–95.

92. **Burke, T., Elamin, M., Galvin, M., Hardiman, O.**, and **Pender, N.** (2015) Caregiver burden in amyotrophic lateral sclerosis: a cross-sectional investigation of predictors. *Journal of Neurology*, **262**(6), 1526–32.

93. **Mioshi, E., McKinnon, C., Savage, S., O'Connor, C.M.**, and **Hodges, J.R.** (2013) Improving burden and coping skills in frontotemporal dementia caregivers: a pilot study. *Alzheimer Disease and Associated Disorders*, **27**, 84–86.

94. **Elamin, M., Bede, P., Byrne, S.**, et al. (2013) Cognitive changes predict functional decline in ALS: a population-based longitudinal study. *Neurology*, **80**, 1–8.

95. **Tremolizzo, L., Pellegrini, A., Susani, E.**, et al. Behavioural but not cognitive impairment is a determinant of caregiver burden in amyotrophic lateral sclerosis. *European Neurology*, **75**(3–4), 191–4.

96. **Lillo, P., Mioshi, E.**, and **Hodges, J.R.** (2012) Caregiver burden in amyotrophic lateral sclerosis is more dependent on patients' behavioral changes than physical disability: a comparative study. *BMC Neurology*, **12**, 156.

97. **Cipolletta, S.** and **Amicucci, L.** (2015) The family experience of living with a person with amyotrophic lateral sclerosis: a qualitative study. *International Journal of Psychology*, **50**(4), 288–94.

98. **Qutub, K., Lacomis, D., Albert, S.M.**, and **Feingold, E.** (2014) Life factors affecting depression and burden in amyotrophic lateral sclerosis caregivers. *Amyotrophic Lateral Sclerosis and Frontotemporal Degeneration*, **15**(3–4), 292–7.

99. **O'Connor, E.J., McCabe, M.P.**, and **Firth, L.** (2008) The impact of neurological illness on marital relationships. *Journal of Sex & Marital Therapy*, **34**, 115–32.

100. **Calvo, A., Moglia, C., Ilardi, A.**, et al. (2011) Religiousness is positively associated with quality of life of ALS caregivers. *Amyotrophic Lateral Sclerosis*, **12**(3), 168–71.

101. **Kübler, A., Winter, S., Ludolph, A.C., Hautzinger, M.**, and **Birbaumer, N.** (2005) Severity of depressive symptoms and quality of life in patients with amyotrophic lateral sclerosis. *Neurorehabilitation and Neural Repair*, **19**(3), 182–93.

102. **Olsson, A.G., Markhede, I., Strang, S.,** and **Persson, L.I.** (2010) Differences in quality of life modalities give rise to needs of individual support in patients with ALS and their next of kin. *Palliative Support & Care,* **8**(1), 75–82.

103. **Ganzini, L.** and **Block, S.** (2002) Physician-assisted death—a last resort? *New England Journal of Medicine,* **346,** 1663–5.

104. **Schwartz, C.E.** (2010) Applications of response shift theory and methods to participation measurement: a brief history of a young field. *Archives of Physical and Medical Rehabilitation,* **91**(9), 38–43.

105. **Moss, A.H., Casey, P., Stocking, C.B., Roos, R.P., Brooks, B.R.,** and **Siegler, M.** (1993) Home ventilation for amyotrophic lateral sclerosis patients: Outcomes, costs, and patient, family, and physician attitudes. *Neurology,* **43**(2), 438–43.

106. **Lemoignan, J.** and **Ells, C.** (2010) Amyotrophic lateral sclerosis and assisted ventilation: How patients decide. *Palliative Support & Care,* **8**(2), 207–13.

107. **Aho-Özhan, H.E., Böhm, S., Keller, J.,** et al. (2017) Experience matters: Neurologists' perspectives on ALS patients' well-being. *Journal of Neurology,* **264**(4), 639–46.

108. **Lazarus, R.S.** and **Folkman, S.** (1984) *Stress, Appraisal and Coping.* New York, NY: Springer.

109. **Pakenham, K.I.** (1999) Adjustment to multiple sclerosis: application of a stress and coping model. *Health & Psychology,* **18,** 383e92.

110. **Pakenham, K.I., Dadds, M.R.,** and **Terry, D.J.** (1994) Relationships between adjustment to HIV and both social support and coping. *Journal of Consulting Clinic Psychology,* **62,** 1194e203.

111. **Seeber, A.A., Pols, A.J., Hijdra, A., Grupstra, H.F., Willems, D.L.,** and **de Visser, M.** (2016) Experiences and reflections of patients with motor neuron disease on breaking the news in a two-tiered appointment: a qualitative study. *British Medical Journal of Support and Palliative Care.* Published Online First: 02 February 2016. doi:10.1136/bmjspcare-2015-000977.

112. **Lazarus, R.S.** (1991) *Emotion and Adaptation.* New York, NY: Oxford University Press.

113. **Miller, G.A., Galanter, E.,** and **Pribram, K.A.** (1960) *Plans and the Structure of Behavior.* New York, NY: Holt, Rhinehart, & Winston.

114. **Oliver, D.J.** and **Turner, M.R.** (2010) Some difficult decisions in ALS/MND. *Amyotrophic Lateral Sclerosis,* **11**(4), 339–43.

Chapter 4

Mindfulness and mindlessness and ALS

Francesco Pagnini, Deborah Phillips, Eleonora Volpato, Paolo Banfi, and Ellen Langer

Mindfulness and mindlessness

Mindfulness is a complex and multifaceted psychological construct that has been a topic of investigation for over 40 years, with the number of research papers increasing exponentially (1). As a simple comparison, a Pubmed search for the term 'mindfulness' between 2000 and 2005 yielded 124 results, while the same search conducted between 2010 and 2015 resulted in 2452 results. Despite the increased interest in mindfulness however, we believe that its construct is often misunderstood (1,2).

It is not our intention to define this concept in an absolute way, as being mindful is a subtle non-verbal experience (3). Two broad approaches characterize the general construct and investigations. The first approach is rooted in Buddhism and brought into the scientific and clinical contexts by Jon Kabat-Zinn. It defines mindfulness as remembering to pay attention, on purpose, in the present moment and non-judgmentally (4). It generally involves meditation as the key to developing mindfulness. The Western perspective derives from social and clinical psychological research conducted since the mid-1970s using the framework developed by Ellen Langer (5). In this approach, mindfulness is simply defined as the process of actively drawing novel distinctions, regardless of importance, as long as they are new to the viewer (6). In this chapter we refer to 'Langerian mindfulness' as the primary construct[1].

The epistemological background of mindfulness is that the world is in a state of constant change, that is, nothing endures in a static state (6). Langerian mindfulness is the act of noticing both obvious and subtle changes in the situational context and within oneself. One is able to create new ways of seeing and understanding, rather than remaining stuck in previous categories. Mindfulness is being aware that everything can be perceived from different perspectives, thereby rejecting a concept of absolute (e.g. 'right' or 'wrong'). This framework has as its basis the construct of absoluteness only in the uncertainty of things and from that we can derive an understanding that uncertainty is the basis for change, which opens up possibilities. In other words, that

---

[1] For more information about mindfulness and meditation, see Chapter 5.

things are *indeterminate* rather than *uncontrollable* (5), meaning that we don't know and, therefore, that we can create possibility.

This awareness of multiple perspectives promotes open-mindedness, reducing the need for using previously established categories. Some of the most common such categories deal with judgment; for example, the concepts of 'good' and 'bad' (or 'positive' and 'negative'). A mindful outlook is the recognition that an event is not 'good' or 'bad' in itself, but depends on the point of view being considered, which itself can be changed depending upon the situation.

The opposite of mindfulness is mindlessness, a construct rooted in its reliance on previously established categories that define what we mean by good, bad, wealth, health, and well-being (7). When mindless, a person relies upon distinctions and categories drawn from the past experience (of oneself or others) without the awareness of other possible points of view, and without incorporating the novelties and changes of the current context. Mindlessness is operating on 'autopilot,' as when a person drives somewhere and upon arrival cannnot recall how he/she got there (8).

Although we say that people are either being mindful or mindless, we need to be careful about making such a rigid distinction that would itself not be mindful. The distinctions between mindfulness and mindlessness can be perceived at the levels of both trait and state. Some people have a more mindful disposition than others. At the same time, mindfulness (as with everything) changes with time. For example, when noticing new stimuli, as when visiting a new place, people tend to be more mindful. It is theoretically easier to be mindless in an environment that is not new as one assumes there is no novelty in a previously-experienced situation. Such false knowledge produces behavioural responses that can be harmful or not, depending upon how the context has changed.

Mindfulness is a trending topic in clinical and health psychology, with psychological interventions that promote quality of life referring to this construct (1). An increasing number of studies associate a mindful disposition with positive well-being, life satisfaction, high self-esteem, and good quality of life (9,10). Furthermore, in the general population mindfulness appears strongly associated with lower anxiety, depression, and distress (11). As mindfulness is a complex construct, it is strongly related to several other psychological constructs, including flexibility, openness, awareness, reappraisal, and creativity, all of which have been considered positively related to resilience and well-being. A flexible (mindful) person can manage in situations that are uncertain or unpredictable, and thus require adaptation to novelty and unexpected events (12). On the other hand, a lack of flexibility (rigidity) may result in psychological morbidity (13) or in a reduction of the quality of life. Openness is one the *big five* factors of personality (14); it describes individuals who tend to be receptive to experience, curious, imaginative, and broad-minded (15) and it is a predictor of positive affect (16). Noticing that the world is constantly changing allows people to be aware of the present moment, which is a way to cultivate well-being in both minds and bodies (17). What has been termed reappraisal, the insight that things may be different than they were initially perceived, is actually a form of mindfulness (18). The Langerian mindfulness construct incorporates the view that there are always different available points of view of the same event, and it is possible to focus on one that we perceive to be less stressful. A curious attitude promotes attention to novelty and openness to new experiences (19), resulting in positive feelings related to this exploration process, and also operating as a countermeasure to the attempt to avoid difficult situations, thoughts or feelings (20).

Mindlessness, mindfulness, and chronic diseases

Examples of mindlessness can be found in everyday-life events, for example:

* buying a product simply because of adherence to a habitual brand;
* crossing the street without noticing that the light is red;
* dividing people by in-group/out-group stereotypes (e.g. all Asian people are similar);

thinking that 'a diagnosis of a chronic disease is a death sentence or a life of pain and accompanying misery' (8). A diagnosis of a severe chronic disorder, such as ALS, can be psychologically devastating (21). Together with the need to cope with worries and concerns, there are risks for a mindless processing of the diagnostic information. In fact, the risk of a diagnosis mindlessly perceived is the 'embodiment' of the diagnosis, with may become the most defining aspect of a person's identity.

Mindfulness is an important concept in ALS care. A longitudinal study (22,23) suggested that mindfulness predicts higher quality of life, lower depression and anxiety, and slower progression of the disease in people with ALS. Specifically, mindful individuals, as assessed using the Langer Mindfulness Scale (LMS) (24), reported higher psychological well-being when compared with less mindful people. Mindfulness was able to predict different trends in quality of life, anxiety, and depression after 4 months: people who scored higher on the LMS reported higher levels of quality of life (QoL), and lower levels of anxiety and depression (see Fig. 4.1–4.3).

Interestingly, the degree of mindfulness may be correlated with the course of the disease. Despite a decline in physical function with disease progression (23), patients who scored higher in mindfulness reported less severe decrement in functioning as measured by the ALS Functional Rating Scale (ALSFRS). As the rate of change in the ALSFRS is highly predictive of survival rates (25), this preliminary finding suggests

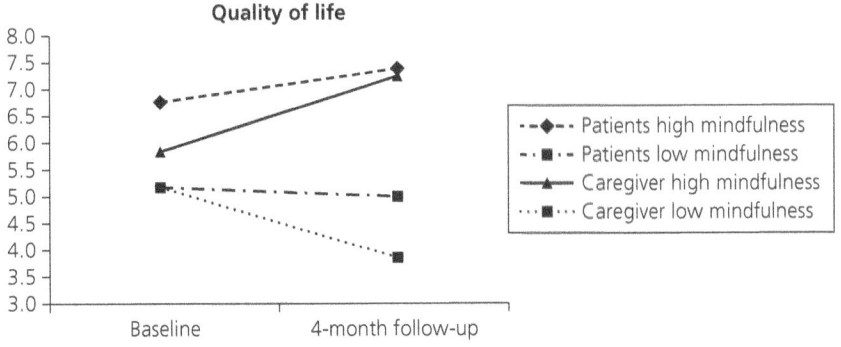

Fig. 4.1 Quality of life and mindfulness.

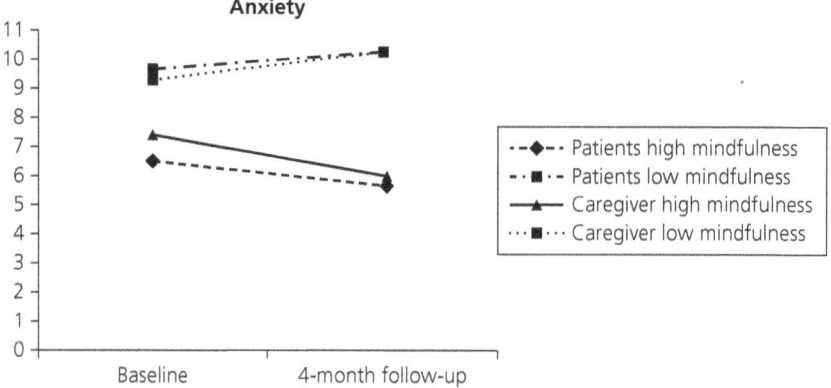

Fig. 4.2 Anxiety and mindfulness.

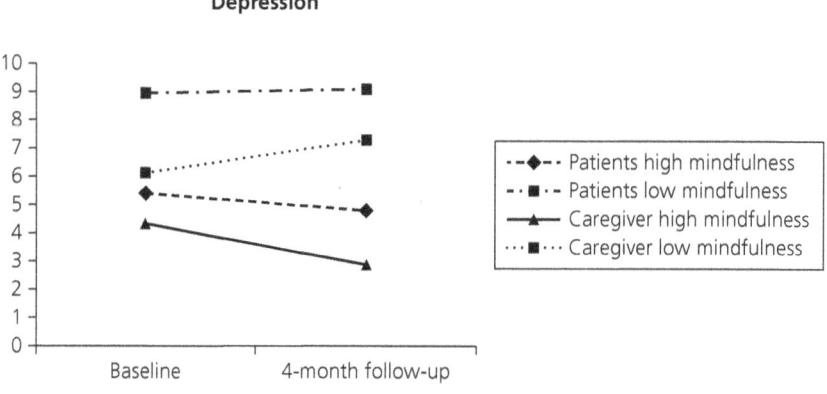

Fig. 4.3 Depression and mindfulness.

that mindful individuals with ALS may experience longer survival and a slower decline in physical functioning over the same period than others who are less mindful (Fig. 4.4). Interestingly, no correlation was found between physical function and QoL, suggesting that the mechanisms by which mindfulness is associated with these two outcomes may be different from one another.

Being mindful about the diagnosis: Mindfulness and quality of life

There is a vast amount of literature reporting similar results in different chronic popu-lations (26), suggesting an intuitive association between mindfulness, psychological well-being, and QOL. This is in line with previous findings (11), suggesting that a mindful attitude towards life, the self, and others promotes a higher degree of satisfac-tion and a lower risk of mood disturbances. In chronic disorders, the ability to perceive

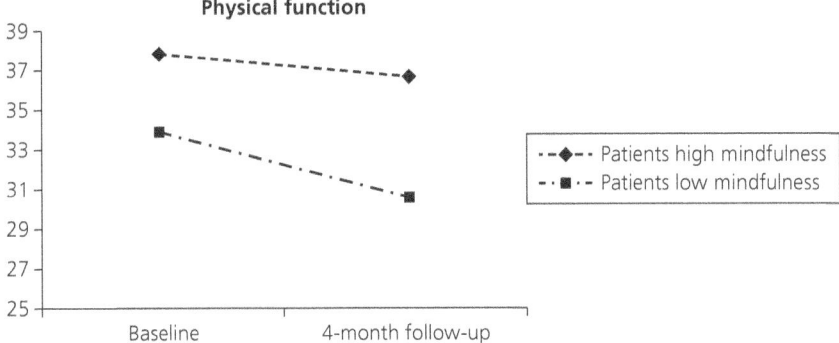

Fig. 4.4 Physical function and mindfulness.

stressful events from multiple perspectives allows one to better cope with them (27). Mindful individuals may be aware that, no matter how severe the disorder is, there are aspects of the self that are not involved. In other words, a more mindful outlook can promote a less narrow view of the self in which one identifies either exclusively or predominantly with the disease (28). That, in turn, can provide greater ease in accepting the illness as it is at any point in time, and in realizing the potential to create positive connections at any stage of the illness. An individual who is unable to move his/her arms can appreciate watching a sporting match or enjoying family love, no matter how severe their disability. This is an example of accepting the state of the illness and seeing that there is much potential to appreciate things in life in spite of what cannot be done to improve the person's physical strength and function. Multiple perspectives promote a point of view in which the value of 'negative' and 'positive' judgments is not absolute. Previous studies (29,30) suggest that people are able to envision and experience positive aspects of having a chronic disease, for example by reporting higher tolerance or being able to better understand people (31). There is a generally accepted principle in clinical psychology and in Langerian mindfulness, that stress is not caused by the event itself, but by the perception, interpretation, and the judgment that the person applies to the event (32). Being mindful allows one to be flexible, creative, and less judgmental when looking at a source of distress, such as the diagnosis and even the symptoms.

How can mindsets influence the course of ALS?

We suggest two ways by which mindfulness can influence the course of the disease, one of which is direct and one indirect. The former may include a mechanism similar to the placebo/nocebo effect (33) in which a person who adheres to the stereotypical course of the disease can create a self-fulfilling prophecy (34), exacerbating the severity of neurological symptoms. In other words, the expectation that symptoms will worsen can promote deterioration, acting as a nocebo. In other areas investigated by clinical psychologists(35), this effect happens in particular when the person's identity is exclusively attached to the diagnostic label (i.e. 'John' becomes 'John the

ALS patient'). This mindless assumption may lead to indirect effects as well, through behavioural changes such as reducing physical activity directly following the diagnosis even prior to symptoms that would require such reductions, resulting in a psychologically induced physiological deterioration (e.g. 'why should I exercise, I have ALS!'). In the Langerian mind/body unity theory, a more mindful person would understand that the fluctuations in symptoms act as a mechanism that varies the ability to use muscles that can thereby maintain movement and delay the onset of other symptoms (8).

Importance of mindfulness and caregivers

We collected data from the caregivers as (22) through use of a similar online survey and including a 4-month follow-up. Together with mindfulness, we assessed burden, quality of life, anxiety, and depression. Again, mindfulness was associated with higher quality of life, and lower anxiety and depression (see Fig. 4.1–4.3). We also found that mindfulness was a predictor of low levels of burden, with mindfulness acting as a protective factor for burden in ALS caregivers (Fig. 4.5). Similar to the considerations for stress reduction in people with ALS, caregivers may benefit from a high degree of openness, flexibility, and the ability to shift between multiple perspectives. For example, being mindful reduces the risk of identifying exclusively with the caregiving role, forgetting the rest of the self. One of the reasons that caregivers often report high levels of stress is the identity change process, from the original familial role (husband, wife, son, daughter) to simply 'caregiver' (36). A mindful outlook towards the care process allows one to integrate new aspects of the identity with the old one, without narrowing the perspective to one of solely being a caregiver. Furthermore, when mindful, people engage in activities exerting a protective effect against depressive reactions that are often characterized by withdrawal from life experiences (37).

Interestingly, while data from both ALS patients and caregivers show positive effects on mindfulness, their scores on the LMS are significantly different. On average, patients' mindfulness was higher than that of their caregivers, a finding that is in line with differences found in quality of life scores (38). While this result is not simple to interpret, it is possible that the diagnosis itself helps to encourage the patient to change perspectives, paying more attention to the variability of symptoms, and trying to adapt and cope

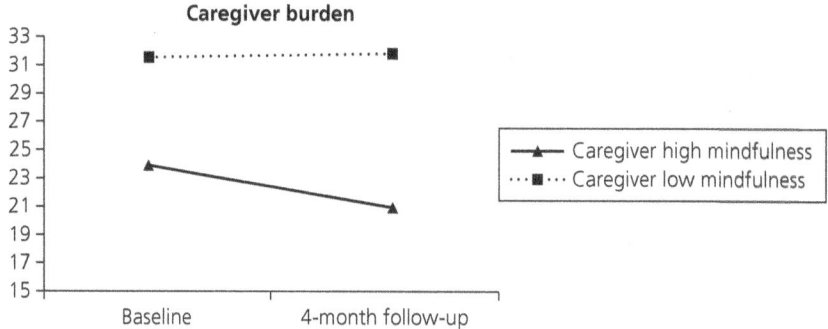

Fig. 4.5 Caregiver burden and mindfulness.

with the negative perception of the illness (8). By contrast, caregivers, facing challenges that reduce their QOL, such as being overwhelmed by the diagnosis and implications for patient care, and the future trajectory of the disease, may view caregiving solely or predominantly as a burden. This would theoretically result in less focus on any positive aspects (e.g. the relationship with the patient). If one is able to take a different, potentially positive view, the benefit could be a sense of meaning and more positive emotions.

Mindlessness in people with ALS also correlated with psychological symptoms, such as anxiety, depression, and burden experienced by their caregivers. Therefore, increasing mindfulness of people with who have been diagnosed with ALS may have a positive impact on both the patient and the caregiver.

Developing mindfulness

As mindfulness is a multifaceted concept, there are multiple ways to increase people's disposition towards it. While a large part of the literature focuses on meditation as a way to improve in mindfulness (2), a recent review showed that no more than 10% of people report having meditated during their lives (39). Therefore, while meditation represents an effective way to improve QoL (see Chapter 5), we believe physicians, psychologists, and other health care professionals should be aware that it is not the only choice for increasing mindfulness (1). Moreover, becoming more mindful can be easier than it may seem when looking at the structure of formal meditation protocols. Simply stated, the essence of mindfulness is paying attention to variability in the current environment, situation, or broadly speaking, the current context—both in other people and within oneself. Mindful people are aware of the existence of multiple perspectives and have a high level of flexibility. Therefore, to become mindful, people can learn to conceptualize their experiences in different ways, by changing their prior perspective about the course of the disease, as well as drawing distinctions between one's own experiences of the illness and one's self-identity. This can be achieved with a focus on simple everyday life awareness or relatively simple cognitive reframing exercises, such as the following:

Pay attention to variability

The key concept is that the world around us, and each one of us, is always changing. Many people have the mindless tendency to hold things as if they are unchanging, despite the changing environment (6). When things perceived as unchanging are also perceived as negative, they may lead to severe distress. For example, ALS symptoms may be considered as stable or, even more stressful, in a 'stable' sort of degeneration. This outlook is in line with the statistical consideration that physical functions are gradually decreasing due to disease progression. A person, however, is not a statistic, and available data are hardly able to describe idiographic changes, as they derive from aggregated analyses (40). In fact, plateaus and small reversals are quite common, in particular over brief intervals (41). If people are able to notice subtle changes in their symptoms or in how they can limit them, they may be able to appreciate that the illness is not as stable as presented. That helps to detach the illness-related identity (e.g. I am a patient) from the personal one (e.g. I am John). For example, when a person is watching a movie with family members or friends, the effects of ALS symptoms on that experience may be minimal or even irrelevant. Simple mental exercises can promote this attention to variability. The person can pay attention to subtle differences between two situations that may seem exactly the same at a first glance. For example, one can ask the patient to 'identify five ways in which you look different from the way you looked yesterday' or to 'think about how you felt after waking up in the morning on the weekend last week and this week—how are they different?' Similar exercises can be very helpful in reducing the perception that symptoms are unchanging, and can lead to the realization that they are not always worse: 'Think about discomforts or pains you are having today. Think about how they feel different from an hour ago, or from yesterday, or from the last time these feelings really bothered you.'

Seek and produce novelty

The attitude of paying attention to new elements is related to an open and curious orientation towards the world and oneself. An individual who has an inclination towards novelty-seeking shows high levels of adaptation, as he/she can be open to feedback and information from the environment that were not present before, resulting in responsive adaptations to one's thinking and behaviour. People who have a propensity for novelty-producing show an active attendance to changes, from both the external and the internal worlds. These individuals tend to create new categories, rather than relying on previous distinctions, which is the essence of mindfulness. This concept is otherwise known as 'creativity'. These two attitudes are highly related and can be taught and improved upon, resulting in higher mindfulness. Novelty seeking and novelty producing can be implemented by trying to consider different perspectives, no matter how unusual they may seem at a first glance. Simple cognitive exercises that can promote these attitudes are 'Imagine taking a new route to get from your house to any place to which you go very regularly. What new reactions occur to you?', or 'What are five ways you could change your bathroom—even slightly—in order to make it easier for you to get in and out of the shower?' People with ALS may find this attitude particularly useful, as it helps create positive ways to compensate for loss of function: 'Imagine a friend whose arms are paralysed. Suggest a new way that he can brush his/her teeth.' Any form of creativity could be encouraged, as it benefits mindfulness, but it also allows the person to express a part of himself/herself. Arts and crafts are ways to improve mindfulness and self-expression (42). This self-expression is always possible, no matter how severe the person's physical impairment, and it is not even hindered by the presence of frontotemporal dementia (43).

Understand that 'positive' and 'negative' depend on our view of events, and not to the events themselves. We generally act as if events, people, and situations are intrinsically either positive or negative, rather than understanding that such assessments are based on individual judgments of external events, and that there is no 'bad' or 'good' in any absolute or total sense. For example, the same event can be considered as either 'positive' or 'negative', on the basis of our perspective, and can be seen as either or both simultaneously. That is, something can be seen as both good and bad at the same time depending upon perspective. A simple example is that the end of a football match can be considered positive from the winner's perspective and negative from that of the loser. The losing team, however, can find some positive aspect of loss such as a previously unexplored defence move that could be helpful in the future, or the resilience of the team, or the enjoyment experienced by the fans. If we change our point of view then our perception about what we were certain is a negative event can, from that different perspective, be viewed as positive. That is, we can reframe a negative perception of an event by answering a simple question: 'In what ways might this be good for me?' Or 'What about this situation could be seen as good?'. With a disorder such as ALS, we can be aware of pain and suffering, and simultaneously try to find a different perspective about the illness. We see that our experience of the illness is a reflection of the view we take, rather than of the illness itself. This may seem counterintuitive at first, but we can find many individuals who are able to reframe their experiences of their own illnesses by including views that express the positive experiences or opportunities the illness has brought to their lives (e.g. a focus on the important things they missed, whether it be family or philanthropy or art) (31). This perspective shifting is a very mindful exercise and a very valuable coping resource. Examples of exercises could be 'Let's say that you miss a bus to meet an important person in your life. Try to find 5 ways in which that could be a positive event' or 'If you have difficulty speaking or raising your arm or leg, think of three new opportunities that this difficulty provides.'

Accepting and playing with unpredictability

As reality is in constant change, we cannot 'know' the future with certainty. Furthermore, since uncertainty is often associated with loss of control and considered a key stressor in chronic disease (44) it benefits us to view it as a resource that can reduce distress and lead to an increase of perceived control. One way to understand this concept is to see that just as the future is ultimately unpredictable, so is the course of the disease, regardless of statistical probabilities. That opens up different possibilities for the future than those perceived by individuals who rely on aggregated statistics. Accepting unpredictability and using it as a resource to be grounded in the present, reminding ourselves that we do not know with certainty what is going to happen, is also a good strategy for paying attention to changes and novelties. One example of an exercise that can help develop comfort with uncertainty in a mindful way is the following: 'Find 3 possible reasons that explain why you are certain that an event might occur, and then propose 3 reasons that it might not. For each of those reasons, describe the way in which it is both positive and negative.'

Making sense of symptoms

Illness and symptoms tend to be perceived as unchanging (i.e. I *have* ALS, or I *am* an ALS patient) and the course of the disease as progressively worsening. However, it is unlikely that all symptoms are always present at the same intensity or always produce the same level of impairment. Reflecting about symptoms allows one to understand and experience their variability, and making sense of this can help one understand that there are reasons for their variability. Once we can identify even a few reasons, feelings of increased control and awareness follow. We may or may not be able to make changes at the symptomatic level, but we may be able to exert control on the functional level of the impact that a possible impairment can have on us. One example of this is: 'Is today a better day than yesterday? What about compared with last week? In what ways is it better and worse? Can you think of three reasons why or how?'.

Add humour

Humour is a form of mindfulness. It forces the person to see another side of the situation, in an unexpected mode of thinking and behaviour, releasing stress and negative beliefs. Humour can be an ally in going beyond the rigidity of thinking that often accompanies depressive thoughts. Noticing humorous aspects of the self or being able to see funny sides of something previously judged as negative, helps people become more accepting and less worried (9). Humour can be cultivated in several ways, and receiving a diagnosis of ALS does not prevent people from laughing at their own behaviours and beliefs, or inserting silliness in their lives. It can be both refreshing and comforting, particularly in such circumstances.

Conclusions

As stated earlier, the epistemological background of mindfulness is that the world's constant state of change brings with it possibilities, and that Langerian mindfulness is very simply the acknowledgment of these possibilities through uncertainty, and through the act of noticing both obvious and subtle changes in one's situation, and in oneself. With the ability to create new ways of seeing and understanding, and not being committed to prior categories or labels, one opens up the possibility of creating new and different perceptions of the world and one's personal situation. We believe that people can become more mindful by learning to conceptualize their experiences in different ways, by changing rooted perspectives about the course of the disease, and by distinguishing between the experience of the illness and the identification of that with the self. This process of mind-openness can be achieved with cognitive reframing exercises, often quite simple, such as those described above. For both the person with ALS and that person's caregiver, the ability to see positives in a situation, even when experiencing severe negative sensations or thoughts, should help to improve quality of life and possibly to slow disease progression.

References

1. **Pagnini, F.** and **Phillips, D.** (2015) Being mindful about mindfulness. *Lancet Psychiatry*, **2**(4), 288–9.
2. **Hart, R., Ivtzan, I.,** and **Hart, D.** (2013) Mind the gap in mindfulness research: A comparative account of the leading schools of thought. *Review of General Psychology*, **17**(4), 453.
3. **Germer, C.** (2004) What is mindfulness. *Insight Journal*, **22**, 24–9.
4. **Kabat-Zinn J.** (1990) *Full Catastrophe Living: Using the Wisdom of your Body and Mind to Face Stress, Pain, and Illness*. New York, NY: Delacorte.
5. **Langer, E.** (1989) *Mindfulness*. Boston, MA: Addison-Wesley/Addison Wesley Longman.
6. **Langer, E.** and **Moldoveanu, M.** (2000) The construct of mindfulness. *Journal of Social Issues*, **56**(1),1–9.
7. **Langer, E.** (1992) Matters of mind: Mindfulness/mindlessness in perspective. *Consciousness and Cognition*, **1**(3), 289–305.

8. **Phillips, D.** and **Pagnini, F.** (2014) A mindful approach to chronic illness. In: Le, A., Ngnoumen, C.T., and Langer, E. (eds) *The Wiley-Blackwell Handbook of Mindfulness*, pp. 852–63. London: Wiley-Blackwell.

9. **Carson, S.H.** and **Langer, E.J.** (2006) Mindfulness and self-acceptance. *Journal of Rational-emotive and Cognitive-behavior Therapy*, **24**(1), 29–43.

10. **Langer E.** (2005) Well-being. In: Snyder, C.R. and Lopez, L.S. (eds) *The Handbook of Positive Psychology*, pp. 214–30. Oxford: Oxford University Press.

11. **Brown, K.W.** and **Ryan, R.M.** (2003) The benefits of being present: mindfulness and its role in psychological well-being. *Journal of Personality and Social Psychology*, **84**(4), 822.

12. **Kashdan, T.B.** and **Rottenberg, J.** (2010) Psychological flexibility as a fundamental aspect of health. *Clinical Psychology Review*, **30**(7), 865–78.

13. **Greenberg, J., Reiner, K.,** and **Meiran, N.** (2012) 'Mind the trap': Mindfulness practice reduces cognitive rigidity. *PloS One*, **7**(5), e36206.

14. **Goldberg, L.R.** (1990) An alternative 'description of personality': the big-five factor structure. *Journal of Personality and Social Psychology*, **59**(6), 1216.

15. **Giluk, T.L.** (2009) Mindfulness, Big Five personality, and affect: A meta-analysis. *Personality and Individual Differences*, **47**(8), 805–11.

16. **Gutiérrez, J.L.G., Jiménez, B.M., Hernández, E.G.,** and **Pcn, C.** (2005) Personality and subjective well-being: Big five correlates and demographic variables. *Personality and Individual Differences*, **38**(7), 1561–9.

17. **Siegel, D.J.** (2007) Mindfulness training and neural integration: differentiation of distinct streams of awareness and the cultivation of well-being. *Social Cognitive and Affective Neuroscience*, **2**(4), 259–63.

18. **Pagnini, F.** and **Langer, E.** (2015) Mindful reappraisal: Comment on 'Mindfulness broadens awareness and builds eudaimonic meaning: A process model of mindful positive emotion regulation'. *Psychological Inquiry*, **26**(4), 365–7.

19. **Kashdan, T.B., Rose, P.,** and **Fincham, F.D.** (2004) Curiosity and exploration: Facilitating positive subjective experiences and personal growth opportunities. *Journal of Personality Assessment*, **82**(3), 291–305.

20. **Kashdan, T.B., Afram, A., Brown, K.W., Birnbeck, M.,** and **Drvoshanov, M.** (2011) Curiosity enhances the role of mindfulness in reducing defensive responses to existential threat. *Personality and Individual Differences*, **50**(8), 1227–32.

21. **Pagnini, F.** (2013) Psychological wellbeing and quality of life in amyotrophic lateral sclerosis: A review. *International Journal of Psychology*, **48**(3), 194–205.

22. **Pagnini, F., Bosma, C., Phillips, D., Reece, A.,** and **Langer, E.** (2016) Mindfulness as a protective factor for the burden of caregivers of amyotrophic lateral sclerosis patients. *Journal of Clinical Psychology*, **72**(1), 101–11.

23. **Pagnini, F., Phillips, D., Bosma, C., Reece, A.,** and **Langer, E.** (2015) Mindfulness, physical impairment and psychological well-being in people with amyotrophic lateral sclerosis. *Psychology & Health*, **30**(5), 503–17.

24. **Pirson, M., Langer, E.J., Bodner, T.,** and **Zilcha, S.** (2012) The development and validation of the Langer mindfulness scale-enabling a socio-cognitive perspective of mindfulness in organizational contexts. Available at SSRN: https://ssrn.com/abstract=2158921 or http://dx.doi.org/10.2139/ssrn.2158921 (accessed 18 July 2017).

25. **Kimura, F., Fujimura, C., Ishida, S.,** et al. (2006) Progression rate of ALSFRS-R at time of diagnosis predicts survival time in ALS. *Neurology*, **66**(2), 265–7.

26. **Bohlmeijer, E., Prenger, R., Taal, E.,** and **Cuijpers, P.** (2010) The effects of mindfulness-based stress reduction therapy on mental health of adults with a chronic medical disease: a meta-analysis. *Journal of Psychosomatic Research,* **68**(6), 539–44.

27. **Carson, S.L.** and **Langer, E.J.** (2004) Mindful practice for clinicians and patients. In: Haas, L. (ed.) *Handbook of Primary Care Psychology,* pp. 173–86. New York, NY: Oxford University Press.

28. **Aujoulat, I., Luminet, O.,** and **Deccache, A.** (2007) The perspective of patients on their experience of powerlessness. *Qualitative Health Research,* **17**(6), 772–85.

29. **de Ridder, D., Geenen, R., Kuijer, R.,** and **van Middendorp, H.** (2008) Psychological adjustment to chronic disease. *Lancet,* **372**(9634), 246–55.

30. **McDonald, E.R., Wiedenfeld, S.A., Hillel, A., Carpenter, C.L.,** and **Walter, R.A.** (1994) Survival in amyotrophic lateral sclerosis: the role of psychological factors. *Archives of Neurology,* **51**(1), 17–23.

31. **Young, J.M.** and **McNicoll, P.** (1998) Against all odds: positive life experiences of people with advanced amyotrophic lateral sclerosis. *Health & Social Work,* **23**(1), 35–43.

32. **Lazarus, R.S.** and **Folkman, S.** (1984) *Stress, Appraisal, and Coping.* Berlin: Springer Publishing Company.

33. **Benedetti, F., Pollo, A., Lopiano, L., Lanotte, M., Vighetti, S.,** and **Rainero, I.** (2003) Conscious expectation and unconscious conditioning in analgesic, motor, and hormonal placebo/nocebo responses. *Journal of Neuroscience,* **23**(10), 4315–23.

34. **Robertson DA, Savva GM, King-Kallimanis BL, Kenny RA.** (2015) Negative perceptions of aging and decline in walking speed: A self-fulfilling prophecy. *PloS One,* **10**(4), e0123260.

35. **Khoury, B., Langer, E.J.,** and **Pagnini, F.** (2014) The DSM: mindful science or mindless power? A critical review. *Frontiers in Psychology,* **5**, 602.

36. **Montgomery, R.** and **Kosloski, K.** (2009) Caregiving as a process of changing identity: Implications for caregiver support. *Generations,* **33**(1), 47–52.

37. **Mausbach, B.T., Coon, D.W., Patterson, T.L.,** and **Grant, I.** (2008) Engagement in activities is associated with affective arousal in Alzheimer's caregivers: A preliminary examination of the temporal relations between activity and affect. *Behavior Therapy,* **39**(4), 366–74.

38. **Gauthier, A., Vignola, A., Calvo, A.,** et al. (2007) A longitudinal study on quality of life and depression in ALS patient–caregiver couples. *Neurology,* **68**(12), 923–6.

39. **Clarke, T.C., Black, L.I., Stussman, B.J., Barnes, P.M.,** and **Nahin, R.L.** (2015) Trends in the use of complementary health approaches among adults: United States, 2002–2012. *National Health Statistics Reports,* **2015**(79), 1.

40. **Pagnini, F., Gibbons, C.J.,** and **Castelnuovo, G.** (2012) The importance of an idiographic approach for the severe chronic disorders-the case of the amyotrophic lateral sclerosis patient. *Frontiers in Psychology,* **3**, 509.

41. **Bedlack, R.S., Vaughan, T., Wicks, P.,** et al. (2015) How common are ALS plateaus and reversals? *Neurology,* **86**(9), 808–12.

42. **Langer EJ.** (2007) *On Becoming an Artist: Reinventing Yourself Through Mindful Creativity.* New York, NY: Ballantine Books.

43. **Liu, A., Werner, K., Roy, S.,** et al. (2009) A case study of an emerging visual artist with fronto-temporal lobar degeneration and amyotrophic lateral sclerosis. *Neurocase,* **15**(3), 235–47.

44. **McCormick, K.M.** (2002) A concept analysis of uncertainty in illness. *Journal of Nursing Scholarship,* **34**(2), 127–31.

Chapter 5

Complementary and alternative medicines and ALS

Arianna Palmieri, Francesco Pagnini, and Chris Gibbons

Complementary and alternative medicine (CAMs) refers to a broad range of medical therapies that are neither taught widely in medical schools nor available as part of conventional medical practice (1). CAMs are used in conjunction with (complementary) or instead of (alternative) traditional medicine as usually provided, in the case of ALS, by a neurologist with neuromuscular subspecialty training. CAMs can include diets, meditation, herbs, exercises, and prayer, as well as drugs (2). Some treatments, such as Reiki (3), have been used for many years, whereas others are novel. Novel treatments include off-label prescriptions for existing drugs or therapies, which may have shown promise in preclinical *in vivo* and *in vitro* studies (4).

In this chapter, we will attempt to place the use of CAMs for the treatment of ALS in the context of current scientific knowledge. We will also consider the psychological implications that the search for an alternative treatment can provide, in a complex context, such as ALS. As 'CAMs' is a large umbrella that includes many possible treatments, we will focus in particular detail on the effects of hypnosis and meditation, which have been intensively studied by our teams and have provided encouraging results in clinical trials.

Complementary and alternative medicines for people living with ALS

CAMs are widely used by patients across the globe. In the United States, an estimated 38% of adults use CAMs and usage is higher for women, as well as for people with higher levels of education (5). The overall use of CAMs and the popularity of specific therapies differ between countries (6). The motivations for seeking and using CAMs are complex and multifactorial (7):

- Increasing availability of information on the Internet.
- Increased awareness of other cultures that traditionally use CAMs.
- The perception that CAMs are is easier to understand, safer, and less expensive than conventional medicine.
- CAMs appears to reflect popular ideologies, such as environmentalism.

- A growing recognition that many factors contribute to well-being.
- Distrust of traditional medicine.
- Frustration with the limited effectiveness of conventional medicine for some disease, such as ALS.

Persons with ALS (PALS) will commonly consider and explore CAMs to use as an adjunct to their clinical treatment (8,9), and it is likely that the popularity of CAMs in ALS is related to the lack of satisfactory conventional treatments. In PALS, CAMs often are used as an adjunct to standard treatment delivered by a neurologist.

Information on CAMs is readily available on the Internet, where the quality of evidence is highly variable, ranging from well-organized online repositories of relevant information (e.g. PatientsLikeMe; see Chapter 11), to descriptions of unregulated treatments described anecdotally (10). Patients may spend considerable amounts of time and money on CAMs. A survey of 171 PALS from Germany found that 50% had used CAMs, spending, on average, €4000 on alternative therapies.

It is easy to imagine why PALS take an interest in CAMs. ALS is rapidly progressive, disabling, and ultimately fatal. While symptom management is improving, there are no clinically meaningful disease-modifying therapies (11). Surveys suggest that the specific motivation for CAMs use in ALS include hope for a cure (10% of surveyed patients), improvement in their condition (30%), and slowing of disease progression (50%) (9). As the 'alternative medicine' designation suggests, CAMs generally are not supported by evidence from randomized clinical investigations and claims of efficacy are often spurious or exaggerated, making them controversial and potentially dangerous. Patients with ALS have experienced physical, psychological, and financial harm when seeking CAMs (12,13).

To assist patients and their clinicians with decisions related to CAMs, the ALSUntangled group was formed as part of the North American ALS Research Group (ALSRG). The group's mission is to 'helps patients with amyotrophic lateral sclerosis (ALS) to review alternative and off-label ALS treatments'. The ALSUntangled updates, published in the journal *Amyotrophic Lateral Sclerosis and Frontotemporal Degeneration*, occupy nine of the top ten positions on the 'Most Read' section of the journal's website (accessed 13 January 2017). The popularity of these articles demonstrates significant interest, presumably from patients, as well as clinicians and researchers, in CAMs for treatment of ALS.

To summarize the evidence and highlight potential risks of using CAMs in ALS, the ALSUntangled group has conducted several reviews of CAMs for ALS.[1] A summary is given in 'Complementary and alternative therapies with published preclinical evidence supporting their use for ALS' of those CAMs that (a) are supported by published preclinical and clinical evidence, (b) have been tested in a rigorous randomized controlled trial, and (c) present risks to patients with ALS. A detailed discussion of specific evidence and efficacy is beyond the scope of this chapter, and interested readers are directed to a published summary (14).

---

[1] http://www.alsuntangled.com/completed.html

Complementary and alternative therapies with published preclinical evidence supporting their use for ALS

iPlex (mecasermin rinfabate)

iPlex is a drug which contains recombinant insulin-like growth factor 1 and insulin-like growth factor binding protein-3 (15). There is no evidence that it slows disease progression in patients with ALS.

Aimspro (hyperimmune goat serum)

Aimspro is a drug that was created to assist with the production of antibodies for HIV infection. ALSUntangled does not recommend its use for PALS (16). A well-designed randomized controlled trial of aimspro in diffuse systemic sclerosis suggests that it may be a safe and tolerable treatment for use in humans.

Spirulina (blue-green algae)

Spirulina consists of a specific type of algae that grows in alkaline lakes. Its commercial distributors claim that it contains proteins, pro-vitamin A, mixed carotenoids, phycocyanin, chlorophyll, and gamma linoleic acid 17). There is no evidence that spirulina is effective for ALS and there appears to be a risk of toxicity from its use.

Bee venom (apitoxin)

Bee venom from honeybees contains bioactive compounds, which may modulate neuroinflammation and glutamate toxicity (18). The ALSUntangled group feels that bee venom demonstrates biological effects that may be useful to patients with ALS, but does not recommend its use for patients outside of a research study.

Cannabis

Cannabis plants are used for fibre, oil, and for medicinal and recreational use (19). Cannabis' positive effect on immunomodulation and excitotoxicity suggests that it may be useful for patients with ALS. There is evidence from animal studies that it may slow disease progression, and anecdotal reports suggest that it *could* reduce mood disturbances and improve appetite.

Deanna protocol

The Deanna protocol refers to a combination of nutritional supplements, massage, stretching, aerobic exercises, and range of motion exercises (20). Although it includes a range of therapies designed to target specific phenomena linked to ALS pathogenesis, including glutamate excitotoxicity and oxidative stress, there remains no evidence of its benefit.

Vitamin D

Vitamin D is an essential nutrient that can be synthesized by the human body following exposure to direct sunlight or absorbed in small quantities from food or supplements. Patients with ALS may be at risk of vitamin D deficiency, which if confirmed by testing, would warrant supplementation with vitamin D. There is no evidence that vitamin D supplementation slows disease progression or improves symptoms (21).

Complementary and alternative therapies with supporting evidence from randomized controlled trials

Sodium chlorite NP001

Sodium chlorite NP001 is a salt solution that may lower levels of cytotoxic macrophages in people with ALS, potentially reducing inflammation and damage to motor neurons (22). A phase II, placebo-controlled, ascending dose study found a dose-dependent reduction in the expression of monocyte CD16, which is a marker of monocyte activation/inflammation.

Complementary and alternative therapies that pose a risk to patients

Iplex

Iplex, described above, was offered to patients in Italy in 2007 as part of an expanded access programme and data relating to Iplex users were released in 2009. Of the 110 patients who were exposed to Iplex treatment, 57 discontinued treatment, and 34 of those died (23). The discontinuation and death rates for Iplex treatment appear to be higher than other treatments for ALS. Although it is not clear if this can be attributed to the intervention or other factors (such as more advanced disease progression at initiation of treatments) ALSUntangled places Iplex in the highest risk category offered in their table of evidence, as more than 5% of exposed patients have experienced death or hospitalization.

Stem cell transplants (San Jose Tec)

The San Jose Tec treatment involved the transplant of CD133+ stem cells obtained from peripheral blood, which may be capable of differentiating into neurons (24). There are insufficient safety or efficacy data to support the use of San Jose Tec, and a high mortality rate of 10% (one of ten patients known to have taken the drug) for patients enrolled in the only published trial of this intervention (24).

Stem cell transplants (XCell Centre)

The XCell Centre protocol uses treated material from a bone marrow biopsy, which is taken from the patients and injected into venous blood or cerebrospinal fluid (25). There is no evidence supporting the efficacy of the XCell treatment and it appears to have been implicated in the death or hospitalization of up to 5% of patients (14).

Aimspro

Aimspro, described above, was noted to be associated with a decline in respiratory function in a patient claiming to have ALS who started using Aimspro after non-invasive ventilation (16).

Sodium chlorite WF10 and oral preparation

WF10 is a solution of OXO-K993 containing stabilized chlorite ions. The solution is intended to support the immune system by targeting the macrophage, a type of white blood cell involved in regulating immune function (26). There is some evidence that the oral preparation of sodium chlorite is associated with hospitalization or death of PALS (26).

Propofol

Propofol is an intravenous, short-acting amnestic/hypnotic agent that is primarily used for procedural sedation, or to induce or maintain general anaesthesia. Propofol's mechanisms of action suggest that it may be relevant for treating ALS. There is anecdotal evidence of benefits coincident with propofol use, but these have not been demonstrated using validated instruments or well-designed studies (27). Propofol has many serious risks, including respiratory depression hypotension, and cardiac arrhythmias, and should only be administered by those trained in anaesthesia with appropriate cardiopulmonary monitoring.

Improving the evidence base for complementary and alternative medicine

There is a natural imbalance between the rate at which CAMs are proposed and catch the public eye and the rate at which a robust evidence-base can be developed. The former might happen in a few days; the latter often takes many years. There is a need to address this gap, especially for diseases with fast progression and poor prognosis. Wick and colleagues set out to assess the efficacy of lithium using an innovative methodology which relied on patient self-report for dosage and outcomes using an online patient community (28). Despite some clear methodological disadvantages compared to the gold standard of randomized controlled trials (RCTs), most notably the lack of a control group and randomization, the study did not find a beneficial effect of lithium on disease progression compared to disease progression-matched controls, a find that was supported by RCTs (29,30).

How should clinicians deal with complementary and alternative medicines?

There are many ways in which health professionals can address patient questions about CAMs in their clinical practice. Bedlack and colleagues (31) suggest three models.

Paternalism

In the paternalistic model of doctor–patient relationship, the physician defines the patient's goals and strategies for achieving them. This model of care is problematic with regard to CAMs because doctors do not necessarily have the same goals, values, and notions of acceptable risk/benefit ratios as their patients. Physician-based paternalistic decisions about CAMs are likely to be unacceptable to patients.

Autonomy

Autonomy is a newer model of medical decision making in which the patient plays a central role. Under this model, the patient's goals and methods for achieving them are central, correct, and absolute. This approach may also be problematic because it fails to capitalize on the experience and expertise of the clinician, and because the patient may be misled by unregulated claims made about the safety and potential effectiveness of CAMs, particularly via online sources (32).

Shared decision-making

Paternalism and autonomy represent two poles of a continuum of doctor–patient involvement. In contrast, shared decision making (SDM) represents a combination of patient and clinician input into disease management. In SDM, the patient's values and goals are central, but there is an acknowledgment that the clinician can potentially modify goals and values by providing new information. Shared decision-making is highly valued across specialties and increasingly considered to be the 'ideal' form of medical interaction, but it can be hard to achieve in practice (33). When navigating decisions about CAMs, there is a clear benefit from a shared approach in which the patient's preferences and priorities are taken into account, and the clinician can share his/her knowledge on the quality of evidence underlying different CAMs, and on the likely physiological and psychological effects of specific treatments.

Framework for discussing CAMs with patients

Schofield and colleges have provided recommendations for effectively discussing CAMs in oncology consultations, which may provide a useful framework for neurologists working with PALS (34). They suggest the following steps.

Understand and respect patient perspectives

The first step is to elicit an understanding of a patient's situation and to clarify their preference for information. Open-ended questions with a focus on a patient's psychological or existential preferences may be a good way to begin discussions about CAMs. It is important to be aware of and to respect different information needs of patients and their individual belief systems

Example questions:

'What is your understanding of things at this point?'

'What are your hopes for the future?'

Ask about CAMs

This can be part of the routine history, but may be even more important at key points in the illness trajectory, such as when making treatment decisions and where there is a significant change in condition.

Example questions:

'Are you current doing or consider doing anything else for your condition?'

'Are you taking other medications or treatments?'

'Have you read about any other treatments on the internet, and would you like to discuss what you have read?'

Explore details about CAM use and actively listen

When asking about CAMs, it is important to explore a patient's understanding, to listen carefully to the patient perspective and to guide decisions by asking about their expectations for the CAM they are interested in

Example questions:

'Can you tell me more about the CAM you are interested in please? What does it involve and how often would you use it?'

'What do you hope to gain from trying <this CAM>?'

'How will you know if <this CAM> has been helpful for you?'

Respond to the patient

Patients should be encouraged to express their feelings and clinicians should express empathy and support the desire for hope and control.

Example questions:

'How are you coping with all of this?'

'It is natural for patients to explore all possible options for your treatment, and I fully support you in this process.'

Why support the use of CAMs?

Much is made of the debate between evidence-based medicine and alternative medicine which, from the perspective of modern clinical may seem one-sided (35). It is true that no evidence is available that supports the use of alternative medicine (of course, the presence of such evidence would eventually ensure that the treatment would be no longer referred to as 'alternative'), but there are potentially important reasons not to ignore these treatment options, at least for the psychological implications that these could have.

The large number of PALS who seek and spend large sums of money on CAMs is an indication of their important role in the experience of disease and suggests that they should not be completely disregarded due to their lack of clinical evidence. There is a complex balance to consider when advising PALS on CAM treatments. Clearly, no CAMs should be recommended that have been shown to pose a risk to patients. We recommend that this process should be patient-centred, supportive and iterative.

What is potentially important and useful is the psychological impact of alternative medicine and how seeking alternative treatments may conceivably bolster quality of life not by any measurable improvement in symptoms but by giving patients a feeling of control, empowerment, or hope (36). This must, of course, may be counterbalanced by the potentially devastating consequences of false hope.

Patients living with ALS will often consider supplementary therapies, which are not typically used in conventional medicine. These therapies may vary dramatically with regard to their cost, burden, and the potential for harm. Engaging with these therapies may give patients feelings of control and hope that their disease progression may slow, stop, or even improve (37). Clinicians should adopt a shared decision-making approach to assisting patients with making decisions about CAMs to moderate expectations and ensure patient safety. A wide range of resources is available to assist both patients and their clinicians in making decisions about CAMs, most notably information published by the ALS Untangled group.

Hypnosis and ALS

What is hypnosis and how does it work

Hypnosis is a very ancient medical practice. The first historical record of the use of healing suggestions is the Egyptian Ebers Papyrus, written in about 1500 BC. Since then similar practices have been described in classical Greece, Rome, and throughout history, up to modern psychotherapy and medicine.

Although there are many definitions of hypnosis, it can be defined as a state of highly focused awareness on one or more stimuli, characterized by a reduction of normal critical thinking in regard to acceptable instructions and suggestions (38). Hypnosis is a natural psychophysiological phenomenon that can occur spontaneously in a large number of situations. For instance, natural hypnosis can rise by watching television, reading an absorbing book, performing monotonous or repetitive activities, or playing a musical instrument. In medical literature, in contrast, hypnosis is traditionally described as an administered clinical procedure, consisting of different steps:

- In a first preliminary phase, the hypnotic process is described to the patient and explicit consent to proceed is obtained. This is a very important phase, as while it rightfully informs the patient, it also fulfils the goal of increasing the compliance. Contrary to common myths, no suggestions or instructions will be accepted or performed if they are not acceptable to the patient and if the hypnotist is not trusted.

- The next step, typically referred as 'hypnotic induction', consists of inducing a trance-like state in the patient. This can be accomplished through a great number of techniques, the most common of which are gaze manipulation (e.g. fixation or repetitive movement), administration of monotonous and repetitive stimuli (e.g. constant speech, metronomes, flashing lights), confusion (using sentences that confound the mental processes, such as 'now the part of you that is apart from the part listening to my voice … can just begin to relax …', and other dissociation-based mind–body techniques (e.g. arm drop, levitation, or catalepsy).

- Once the hypnotic trance is obtained (it can be assessed by different manifestations, such as eyes fluttering, altered respiration, and facial muscle relaxation), the hypnotist can deliver specific suggestions, such as analgesia, relaxation, wellness, calm, serenity. The extreme focus on a single idea, or a few ideas, a condition labelled *monodeism*, can generate actual physiological alterations. For instance, by suggesting to a hypnotized patient that his hand is resting in a bucket of ice, significant analgesia and peripheral vasoconstriction can be measured in the patient's hand; in other words, the body reacts just as if the situation were real.

- The last step consists in leading the patient back to a fully awake, normal state of consciousness. This is traditionally obtained by slowly counting from 10 to 1 (or the reverse), and the suggestion that at the end of the count the patient will be fully awake. While this phase is not strictly necessary, as any patient would spontaneously return to his usual state of consciousness given enough time, this procedure has the goal of informing the patient that the treatment has concluded, and offers a good setting for post-hypnotic induction.

While this sequence may provide a logical understanding of the hypnotic process, in actual clinical use, the borders between various steps are blurred, and most often inductions and suggestions are provided simultaneously. Furthermore, when working with trained patients, or with specific techniques, such as many Ericksonian ones, a formal induction might even not be used at all. Despite contradictory information in the classic literature, the clinical experience of one of the authors' clinical (Palmieri) suggests that the hypnotic process is almost always successful. While there are individual predispositions to trance, every session conducted by a sufficiently skilled hypnotist can lead to a positive experience for the patient, and at least minor beneficial effects.

From the hypnotist's point of view, inducing a hypnotic trance is a very peculiar experience, which entails a unique intimacy with the patient. Specifically, the therapeutic alliance (*rapport*) reached through trance induction is characterized by great velocity and intensity, in comparison to the one experienced in traditional psychotherapy, with the obvious distinctions between the two phenomena.

Hypnosis-based treatment in ALS: Theoretical premises and clinical application

As previously mentioned, hypnosis is a non-pharmacological methodology that can be employed with almost any patient by someone with appropriate training. It has low costs and virtually no side effects. Interestingly for ALS, hypnosis has shown valuable efficacy in the treatment of secondary symptoms that accompany many neurological diseases, as well as in the treatment of a number of psychopathological conditions.

Studies have shown the efficacy of hypnosis in the treatment of anxiety and depression, especially when concurrent with a physical illness (39–41). Hypnosis also has been shown to be efficacious for acute or chronic pain (42), phobia (43), and psychosomatic symptoms (44). Furthermore, hypnosis was found to be a valuable tool to reduce the impact of symptoms in many neurological conditions, such as multiple sclerosis (45), Parkinson's disease (46), stroke (47), peripheral nerve lesions (48), quadriplegia (49), dystonia (50), and headache (51). Finally, a few promising studies have also reported that hypnosis was successfully employed to modulate the immune system in healthy people (52) and cancer patients (53).

In patients with ALS, the treatment of psychological symptoms has proven particularly difficult, given the disease's unique features. In those patients with bulbar involvement, traditional speech-based psychological techniques cannot be optimally employed. In the search for potential solutions to these shortcomings, mind–body based techniques, including hypnosis, could represent an interesting option. In fact, while most hypnotic induction methods require some degree of movement, it is possible to induce hypnosis without any muscular activity from the patient. Furthermore, once a hypnotic trance is achieved, it is very easy to teach the subject how to spontaneously return to such state of consciousness, a process called 'self-hypnosis' (54), and reactivate the positive suggestions learned from the hypnotist. This latter point can be particularly relevant when the patient's verbal communication abilities are minimal. During this stage, self-hypnosis skills may provide patients with a way to autonomously cope with pain and fear.

Empirical result of a longitudinal study on patients

Based on these theoretical considerations and the promising data of a pilot study (55), the long-term effects of a hypnosis-based intervention were investigated in a recent study by Kleinbub and colleagues (56). In this study, 15 people with ALS attended four weekly hypnotic sessions in their homes. Each session was conducted by a trained hypnotist accompanied by a psychologist who administered all the questionnaires, but who did not remain in the same room during the treatment. Each hypnosis session consisted of three phases:

- ◆ The first one was a standardized hypnotic induction based on well-established ideodynamic (ideomotor) techniques (57) and focused on mind–body relaxation, lasting about 20 min.
- ◆ The second, core phase, lasting 30–45 minutes, consisted of the administration of therapeutic metaphors, guided visual imagery, and direct and indirect suggestions individually tailored on the basis of the needs of each patient.
- ◆ The final phase of each session, lasting about 10 minutes, consisted of anchoring suggestions aimed to teach self-hypnosis, followed by a slow, guided return to a state of full consciousness.

While the individual suggestions and metaphors were specifically chosen on a per-patient basis, according to their evolving clinical condition, personality, and history, the four sessions were based on fixed themes, common to every patient. In the first hypnotic session, the suggestions were orientated to a safe and quiet place where the patient could symbolically rest and recover in deep relaxation. In the second session, the suggestions were focused on the awareness of individual thoughts, emotions, and body perceptions (e.g. breathing rate). In the third session, the suggestions were directed to a change of time focus, imagining the members of various generations of a family and then projecting them and their heirs into the future, in a sort of 'life chain'. The fourth, concluding session, focused on metaphors associated with positive emotions and resilience.

The results, analysed through Bayesian mixed models regressions, showed a strong effect of the treatment on anxiety, while depression levels of the sample were already low. Longitudinal depression, and anxiety scores and their cut-offs are shown in Fig. 5.1.

Similar results were found in regard to QoL scores (Fig. 5.2), where the treatment was associated with an increase in self-reported well-being, the only exception being the bulbar subscore. Of note is that, on the last follow-up, the scores had begun to drop back toward the baseline. This contrasts with anxiety scores, for which improvement was maintained 3 months after the end of the treatment. This may indicate a limit in the duration of the beneficial effect of the intervention on QoL and could signal the need for an ongoing care programme.

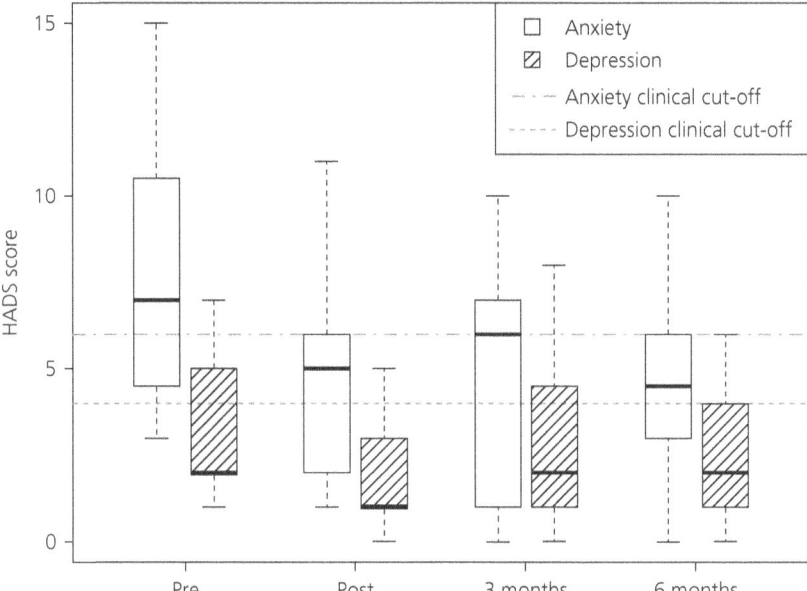

Fig. 5.1 Anxiety and depression scores of ALS patients at baseline, and immediately, 3 months, and 6 months after the 1-month treatment. Bottom and top sections of the box represent, respectively, the first and third quartiles; the band inside the box represents the median; and the whiskers represent the lowest or highest observation within 1.5 times the interquartile ranges from the bottom and top of the box, respectively.

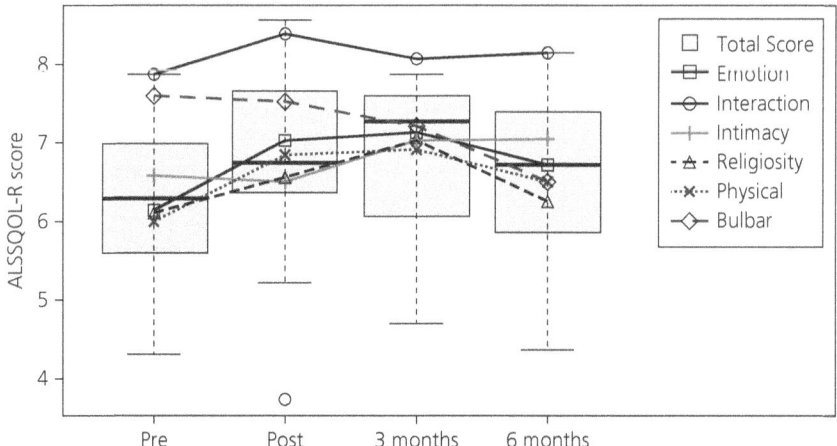

Fig. 5.2 Quality of Life scores of ALS patients at the various time points. The box plots refer to the ALSSQOL-R total scores, while the lines describe the individual subscale mean scores. Gains were generally lost by 6 months post-intervention. See text for details.

Aside from its own inherent importance, the achievement of higher quality of life appears to be associated with a decrease in negative symptoms, such as suffering, sense of burden, and hopelessness (58). Recent evidence suggests that these psychological components could also impact the disease progression. The first support for a relationship between psychological status and physical outcomes in ALS was provided by a seminal study by McDonald and colleagues (59), who found that patients with psychological distress showed a significantly greater risk of mortality than those with higher psychological well-being. Similarly, other studies (60, 61) found that mood and personality traits had a strong influence on the survival rate of ALS patients. Recently, another study (62) of a large sample of people with ALS demonstrated that a mindful attitude could attenuate the progression of the disease, further reinforcing the importance of efficacious psychological support for these patients. The hypothesis that hypnosis may have an effect on the progress of functional impairment was therefore also tested using the ALS-Functional Rating Scale—Revised (ALS-FRS-R) (63). The ALS-FRS-R was assessed before the intervention (T0) and at the last follow-up, six months after the end of the treatment (T3). These scores were compared with control data obtained by selecting a sample of 15 patients with motor neuron disease who were matched for baseline ALS-FRS-R score, age, gender, onset site, and time since symptoms onset. A difference score was computed by subtracting the ALSFRS-R score at 6 months from that at baseline (lower values indicating poorer function), and data from the treatment and control groups (Fig. 5.3) were statistically compared (by means of Bayesian estimation). Results showed substantial evidence in favour the treated group. While the magnitude of the difference was small (4.63 points), this

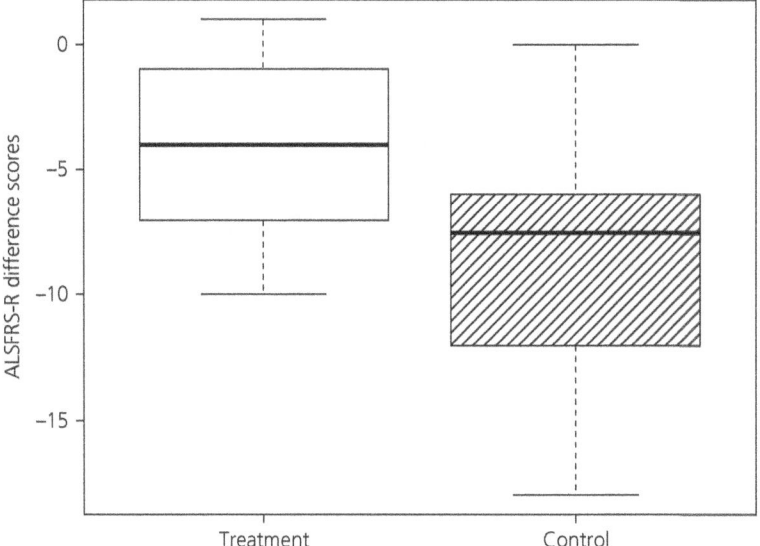

Fig. 5.3 Change in ALSFRS-R scores from baseline of ALS patients 6 months after hypnosis and of controls.

effect was significant. Hypnosis slowed disease progression in the treated ALS patients, compared with non-treated ones.

This association can be interpreted from at least two different perspectives. First of all, changes in the central nervous system during hypnosis have been documented by neuroimaging and psychophysiological studies, and there are many sites in the nervous system in which the overall neural output to skeletal muscle can be modified (64, 65). Specifically, hypnosis can have effects on biological measures such as pain threshold or inflammatory states (for an exhaustive review see 45), that have been connected to ALS progression (66). Secondly, specific suggestions for muscular relaxation could have played a role, independently from the hypnotic phenomenon per se, in training patients not to overload, and thus to partially preserve, the still innerved muscular fibres. The two hypotheses are not mutually exclusive, and the precise mechanisms underlying these changes have yet to be discovered.

From a psychodynamic perspective, each of the themes of the hypnotic suggestions that were employed in these studies was designed to have an influence at both the conscious and unconscious levels in patients, to promote long-term benefits. For instance, the vivid hypnotic recall of positive imagery of the past and the projection of these symbolic representations into the future (suggestion promoted in the third hypnotic session), can be seen as a process that allows the patient to restructure the experience of the self in a coherent and significant temporal dimension. These images, while evoking a feeling of hope, trigger support functions, ideas of protection and help, and therefore may reactivate internal representations of secure attachment. Indeed, the persistent decrease in anxiety levels could have been partially related to the hypnotic suggestion of sources of protection (first session), conceived in the attachment theory framework (67, 68).

Secondary psychological effects on ALS caregivers

The psychological effects of ALS are not confined to the patients. The symptoms of the disease result in a high burden on family and other caregivers. While not always considered in research, this dimension is crucial in the perspective of psychological intervention in ALS. Scientific and clinical literature has previously shown the strong reciprocal association between patients' and caregivers' well-being (69–72). While the intervention was offered only to the patients, a possible indirect psychological effect on the caregivers was explored. Specifically, anxiety and depression of the primary caregivers (usually the spouse, a son or a daughter), were assessed at the same time-points as for the patients (see Fig. 5.4).

As in the patient sample, anxiety was the most prominent symptom at baseline. Data analysis confirmed the hypothesis of an indirect effect of the patient treatment on the caregivers, in particular for anxiety. Most notably, whereas the greatest improvement in patients was observed right after the treatment (T1), the highest decrease in the caregivers' anxiety was observed in the subsequent follow-up, 3 months later, strengthening the interpretation of a positive systemic consequence of an efficacious treatment on patients, with an effect lasting at least up to 6 months. Depression, on the other hand, was below the clinical threshold for almost all caregivers throughout the study. One of the only two participants in this sample showing depressive symptoms, showed

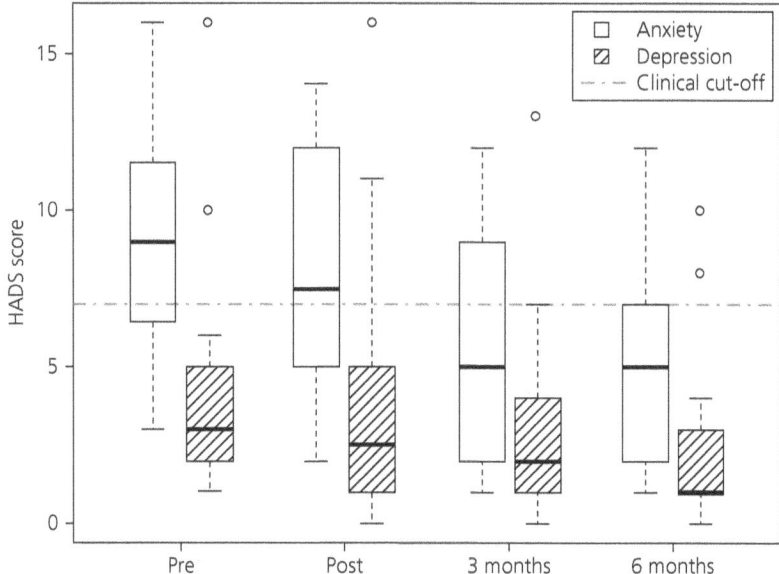

Fig. 5.4 Caregiver's anxiety and depression scores at baseline (T0), immediately after the 1-month treatment (T1), and at 3 (T2) and 6 (T3) months after the end of the intervention.

a constant improvement in the later follow-ups, whereas the other one's score dropped below the clinical threshold after the treatment. However, the symptoms resurfaced after 6 months. These observations suggest that hypnosis treatment on patients affected by ALS may have a positive effect on caregivers' depressive symptoms as well, but further study is needed. Of course, the lack of a control group prevents causal inferences.

The study showed satisfying results and represented an interesting adventure, on a human level, for both the researchers and the patients that participated. Some touching episodes made a strong impression in the memory of the researchers. People reflected on their lives, and learned, through a collaborative effort, the way to find new perspectives through which their experiences were made meaningful despite their disease. For example, a woman in an advanced stage waited for the visit of the researchers as 'if it were a party, a birthday', and always instructed her daughters to prepare cakes and sweets. Her hospitality was exceptional. 'I know that I won't live long', she said. 'It's not important how long one lives, but how! Thank you for having brought back the memories of my most beautiful days, and of who I was … Of who I still am! I am not ALS, I am everything that I experienced until now. I feel peaceful'.

Meditation and ALS

What is meditation?

The term 'meditation' refers to a broad set of practices that focus the attention inwards. The object of the focusing process could be the breath, a mantra, thoughts, feelings, and sensations, emotions, an area of the body, or other stimuli. Regardless of the type of technique, the primary aim is generally to find a calm centre in ourselves, to quiet the mind, and to be aware in the present (73). Self-awareness is generally proposed as a critical component for deep healing to take place (74). Meditative techniques have been reported to improve mindfulness, concentration, and self-transcendence (75), together with several benefits in terms of psychological and physical well-being (76,77). Meditation techniques have been an important part of many spiritual traditions for thousands of years, and have been incorporated in the Western medical and healing practice since the second half of the twentieth century.

Approaches to meditation are varied, and not easily classified, but a first distinction could be between concentrative and mindfulness techniques. The former uses an object of focus of attention, such as a mantra (e.g. the word 'ohm'), breathing, or an external stimulus. The training consists in keeping the focus on the object, disengaging from distractions and from the usual mental processes. Mindfulness meditation promotes being in the present moment, with a non-judgmental attitude (78). Meditators learn to prevent the mind from wandering into chains of association, with different techniques that help them stay in a mindful state of attention. Eventually, meditators tend to develop an awareness of their thoughts and feelings, without being controlled by emotional reactions that could arise as a response to these beliefs. The results of long and successful mindfulness meditation training could be a mind that just observes thoughts, feelings, and sensations, without letting them create emotions and other thoughts. Another kind of meditation is 'guided meditation', in which contents are approached from a mindful perspective, rather than an analytic one. The guide could be a chant, a mandala (a graphical geometric pattern, generally made of circles or squares), or images related to complex universal experiences (e.g. death, suffering, compassion). Generally, meditation training includes a combination of all these three elements (concentration, mindfulness, or guidance), with different emphases on each.

There are many types of meditation programmes, which vary with respect to the type of mental activity suggested (e.g. attention, feeling, reasoning, memory), the use of mental faculties (e.g. active or passive), the objects to which meditation is directed (e.g. cognition, emotions, body, God), the amount of requested/recommended training, and the emphasis, or not, on religion and/or spirituality (79). In Western countries, sometimes meditation practices are integrated with larger complementary and alternative programmes, which may include other treatments (e.g. dietary, exercise).

There are two main reasons for practicing meditation (77). One is to overcome psychological or emotional issues, using the practice as a form of therapy, aimed to improve self-regulation. The other is the wish to achieve a better understanding of life, to gain wisdom and to enlarge consciousness. Of course, these two aims often overlap, and most practitioners pursue both goals to different extents (80). Both these reasons are highly relevant to the ALS field.

Benefits of meditation

Meditation-based interventions are increasingly being used for the promotion of quality of life and the reduction of distress (77), demonstrating positive effects in both clinical and non-clinical samples (81). Benefits include improvements in terms of psychological well-being, reducing negative emotions, stress, anxiety, and depression, and increasing reported levels of happiness, self-confidence, and general effectiveness (73). This training also seems to lead to changes on the physical level (e.g. improved immune system, slowed heart rate), sometimes with a reduction of symptoms in chronic patients. For example, meditation appeared to be effective in pain management (78).

Meditation and ALS

There are several clinical and theoretical reasons to support the idea that meditation could be a helpful instrument for people with ALS and their caregivers (82, 83).

Awareness

The focus on the present moment and acceptance, which is generally emphasized in meditation practice, could help people with ALS to cope with their emotions and reactions to the illness. Long-term meditation practice facilitates the awareness of the present moment, resulting in an attitude to pay attention to what 'I am now' or 'how I feel now', suppressing beliefs about what 'I am *not* doing'. In people with ALS, these beliefs can easily become 'what I cannot do anymore', promoting negative thoughts and emotions.

Prevention of mental rumination

As reported by previous studies (e.g. 84), sadness and depression may occur more easily in people with ALS than in the general population. Meditation has a general positive effect on the mood. Furthermore, it helps to prevent mental rumination, which is the process of repetitively, passively thinking about aspects of a 'negative' experience. Rumination is one of the main psychological components that sustain depressive thoughts (85). Meditation training allows one to de-centre the mind from the rumination process, moving the focus from the depressive loop to other aspects, or simply observing and accepting this mental process, without being trapped in it.

Death and spirituality

A mindful approach to life, promoted by long-term meditation practice, seems to change the perception of death and mortality (86). Expert meditators generally have a more receptive consideration of death, in comparison with non-meditators (87). That leads to a reduction in personal strife and avoidance. In terminal illnesses such as ALS, the perception of one's own mortality often represents a major issue (88), because of the fear of an approaching death. Meditation can provide a valuable tool to better deals with these fears. It can also represent the beginning of a 'spiritual journey', motivated by the need to find answers to existential questions.

Self-dialogue in the locked-in stage

Advanced stages of ALS often include a 'locked-in' condition, where no residual movement is possible, but the brain remains active. Meditation is sometimes referred to as 'self-dialogue' (89), as the process of being in contact with thoughts and feelings, with awareness and acceptance, is a central component of most meditations practices. As a result, the quality of the inner dialogue improves, with a positive impact on self-acceptance and, in general, on the person's well-being. Moreover, meditation training also increases the acceptance of being physically immobile for long periods. Those who experienced meditation for the first time, often report uncomfortable feelings related to the need to maintain the same position for a long period. The training often addresses these feelings, incorporating them and resulting in psychological comfort. Since many people with ALS lack movement, it is possible that this kind of acceptance training can improve their experience. Unfortunately, both these ideas (inner dialogue and stillness acceptance) are very hard to prove experimentally, as it is not easy to understand the subjective experience of a person who cannot move at all.

Caregivers

Meditation practice could be particularly helpful for the caregivers. The burden experienced by them is well-studied, but limited interventions have been explored to address it. One the issues that often caregivers experience is the shift of identity, focused on being a caregiver. Meditation training can help put them in contact with their own needs and emotions, even if some have been 'neglected' because of their role as a caregiver (90). Furthermore, as there is a connection between the existential well-being of the patient and that of the caregiver (91), the effects of meditation on this aspect could also benefit the other component of the dyad.

A structured meditation programme for people with ALS and their caregivers

The potential of meditation in ALS care has recently received attention, as one of our research groups developed an ALS-specific protocol (83), adapting the classic Mindfulness-Based Stress Reduction (MBSR) programme. The MBSR is a structured clinical protocol, developed by Jon Kabat-Zinn in the 1980s (78), which is rooted in the Theravada Buddhism meditation tradition. It includes meditation and yoga exercises, and consists of eight-weekly group meetings (2-hour classes), a 1-day retreat, and homework. The MBSR is probably the most common structured meditation protocol used in Western clinical settings. The interest in the protocol has significantly grown over the last three decades, as it seems efficacious in reducing stress and mood disturbances in people with different clinical conditions, including cancer, pain, cardiac diseases, and multiple sclerosis (92).

The adaptation of the classic MBSR to the clinical peculiarities of ALS required substantial changes to the original protocol. For example, physical impairment may hinder the execution of yoga exercises. While the emphasis is on the process of the movement, rather than its outcome, the perception of physical limitations can produce negative emotions (e.g. sense of inadequacy). Another challenge deals with emotional reactions. Sometimes people with ALS, as well as their caregivers, face severe anger or sadness (82). These feelings may 'detonate' during the meetings, as the person is put in contact with his/her own emotions. Furthermore, meditation may result in contact with avoided part of the psychological/emotional experience, such as fear or rage. A conscious elaboration of underlying emotions is considered a healthy process (93), but it requires advanced clinical skills from the professionals who lead the course.

The meditation protocol is open to both ALS patients and caregivers, who join the sessions together, in the same group. It has a slightly shorter duration than the original MBSR, with sessions that last about 90 minutes and it does not incorporate the 1-day retreat. To better deal with the intense emotive tension that can arise in the course, there are two trainers (the original MBSR has only one). The presence of a co-trainer aims to reduce the risk of burnout and it allows better management of a crisis situation, with the possibility of dividing the group or focusing the attention on somebody with particular needs.

The language of the protocol has been adapted, with topics, metaphors, and sharing moments that deal with meaningful content for patients and caregivers. The emphasis is put on the acceptance of the discomfort related to physical limitations, and on the appreciation of what can be experienced, despite the illness progression. Participants are encouraged to explore the impact that physical limitations may have on their emotions, with particular attention on the expression of anger (e.g. aggression feelings against the caregiver).

Meditation and awareness exercises are provided in a form that is suitable for people with ALS. For example, the original MBSR includes a mindful eating exercise, which consists of guided attention to the consumption of a raisin. To avoid swallowing difficulty, the ALS meditation protocol uses a lump of sugar.

The role of awareness of breathing is central in many meditation practices, as is represents an easy anchoring to the sensations experienced in the present moment. As ALS can progressively impair respiratory function, focusing on breathing could be emotionally triggering, impairing the exercise. The protocol includes breathing awareness exercises only for those who have successfully started to accept their own emotions. Instead of breathing exercises, the protocol initially focuses on the body scan practice. This is an exercise that requires the individual to pay attention to the feelings that arise from the body, with a non-judgmental attitude.

Instead of Yoga exercises, the meditation protocol includes awareness of minimal movements, derived from the Feldenkrais method (94). These exercises consist of the awareness of subtle movements of finger or eye muscles. Also, musical stimuli are included in the protocol, as a way to promote feelings and sensations. Different meditation sessions are based on visualization exercises, which also include motor imagery tasks (imagining making a movement, with no actual muscle activation).

Effects of the ALS meditation protocol

The efficacy of the protocol has been tested in a randomized clinical trial, with both qualitative and quantitative assessments. Marconi and colleagues (36) interviewed 26 people with ALS and 18 caregivers who joined the ALS meditation protocol. Both patients and caregivers reported a subjective improvement of their own wellbeing, with a general reduction of anxiety and a general improvement in their mood. Acceptance of the illness seemed to be one of the main effects, with a positive impact

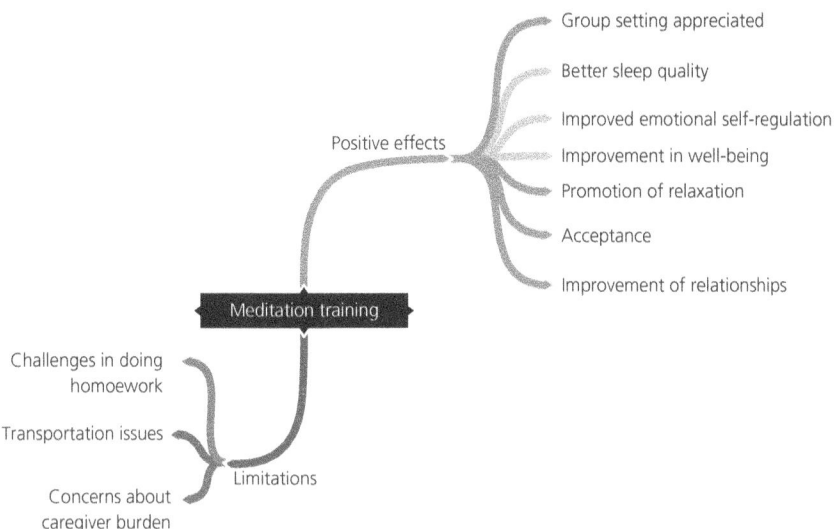

Fig. 5.5 Positive effects and limitations of the meditation training according to the participants' experiences.

on quality of life. Participants reported that accepting the illness lead to a reframing of their illness perception, which was no longer perceived as something that 'absorbed' the whole person. Caregivers seemed particularly satisfied by the chance to be in contact with their emotions and the 'permission' that they gave to themselves to explore and experience them, without judgment. Participants also indicated that the protocol helped them to better manage their own emotions, providing helpful coping strategies. In general, participants were very satisfied with the protocol, although many of them reported problems in doing the homework. This was particularly true for the caregivers, who were generally occupied in care activities for many hours during the day, sometimes in combination with work or other family duties. Positive effects and limitations that were reported by the participants are summarized in Fig. 5.5.

Results from a randomized clinical trial, conducted over 4 years, with 100 ALS patients, confirmed the positive impact of the meditation programme (95). When compared with usual multidisciplinary care, meditation training leads to a significantly higher quality of life over a 12-month follow-up (Fig. 5.6). Furthermore, patients who joined the meditation training experienced lower levels of anxiety and depression (Fig. 5.7–5.8). The effects of the training, therefore, appeared to be beneficial to people with ALS, who learned a different way to cope with stress and beliefs related to the illness. One possible mediator for the effect of meditation training is the cultivation of mindfulness, which has been largely reported to promote psychological well-being, tolerance of distress, and resilience (see Chapter 4). Acceptance and non-judgmental attitudes were also promoted during the training, leading the patient to achieve a less anxious attitude toward their clinical condition. The trial did not address the question about the effects of the training on the patients' functioning. Therefore, the potential

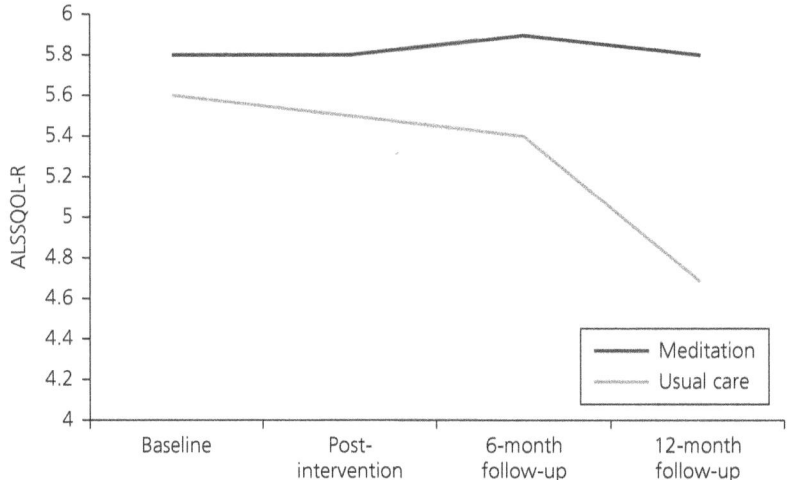

Fig. 5.6 Quality of life course in the meditation group or in the usual care group.

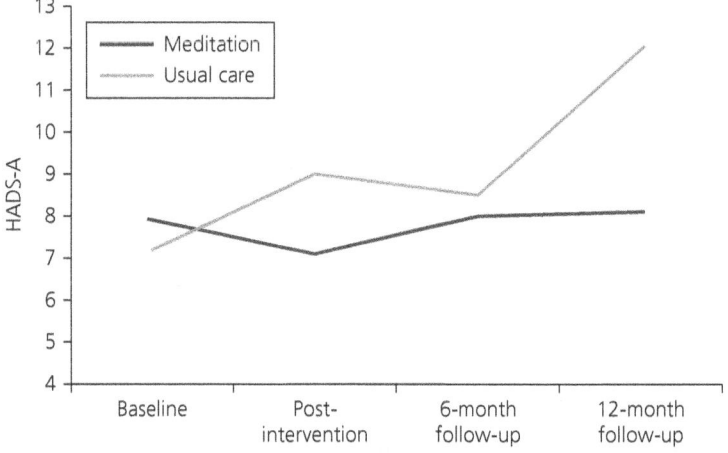

Fig. 5.7 Anxiety course in the meditation group or in the usual care group.

effect of meditation on the course of the disease remains unresolved. Future studies will have to address this intriguing question.

Conclusions

The field of CAMs can provide multiple options for people with ALS. Many of these options have not been supported by scientific studies, and some of them may be danger-ous. Physicians should be aware of current scientific knowledge, incorporating this con-stantly changing flow of information in their clinical practice. For example, preliminary data about hypnosis and meditation suggest that these two treatment options could, at

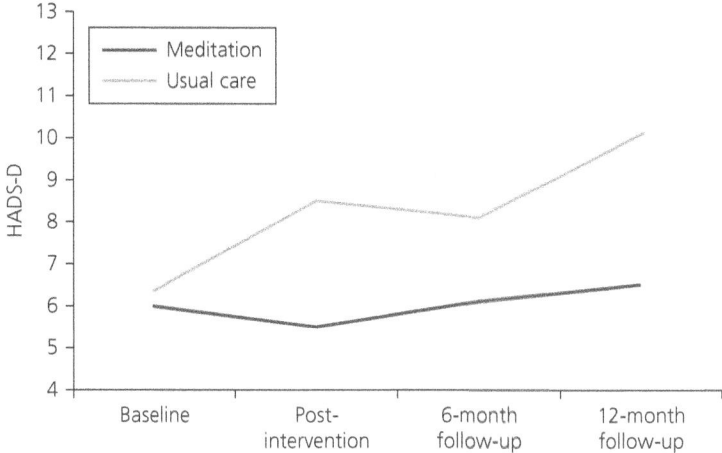

Fig. 5.8 Depression course in the meditation group or in the usual care group.

the very least, improve the quality of life of the patients (and of their caregivers). No harms or side effects have been reported by the studies that have used these interventions. It is in the interests of patients, caregivers, and also health professionals that these types of interventions be discussed. Those that are not harmful, and may be beneficial, should be promoted within the ALS community. These interventions could be provided in clinical, as well as community settings. For example, patient associations could facilitate the provision of these treatments by providing a setting for group meetings.

Together with the direct effects of 'alternative' treatments on patient and caregiver well-being, self-efficacy is another property that makes CAMs so relevant in the ALS field. People with ALS do not have many 'weapons' to fight the illness. The 'ammunition' provided by CAMSs can improve patients' perceived control, which is an essential component of psychological well-being (37). Therefore, our recommendation for physicians and health care professionals is to be mindful about the psychological importance of these treatment options, incorporating what we know from the literature into true patient-centred care.

References

1. Eisenberg, D.M., Kessler, R.C., Foster, C., Norlock, F.E., Calkins, D.R., and Delbanco, T.L. (1993) Unconventional medicine in the United States—prevalence, costs, and patterns of use. *New England Journal of Medicine*, **328**(4), 246–52.

2. Angell, M. and Kassirer, J.P. (1998) Alternative medicine-the risks of untested and unregulated remedies. *New England Journal of Medicine*, **339**, 839–40.

3. García, D.Á., Nicolás, I.M., and Hernández, P.J.S. (2016) Clinical approach to fibromyalgia: synthesis of evidence-based recommendations, a systematic review. *Reumatología Clínica* (English Edition), **12**(2), 65–71.

4. Feng, H-L., Leng, Y., Ma, C-H., Zhang, J., Ren, M., and Chuang, D-M. (2008) Combined lithium and valproate treatment delays disease onset, reduces neurological deficits and

prolongs survival in an amyotrophic lateral sclerosis mouse model. *Neuroscience*, **155**(3), 567–72.

5. **Clarke, T.C., Black, L.I., Stussman, B.J., Barnes, P.M., and Nahin, R.L.** (2015) Trends in the use of complementary health approaches among adults: United States, 2002–2012. *National Health Statistics Reports*, **2015**(79), 1.

6. **Ernst, E.** (2000) Prevalence of use of complementary/alternative medicine: a systematic review. *Bulletin of the World Health Organization*, **78**(2), 258–66.

7. **Ventola, C.L.** (2010) Current issues regarding complementary and alternative medicine (CAM) in the United States: Part 1: the widespread use of CAM and the need for better-informed health care professionals to provide patient counseling. *Pharmacy and Therapeutics*, **35**(8), 461.

8. **Bedlack, R.S., Pastula, D., Welsh, E., Pulley, D., and Cudkowicz, M.E.** (2008) Scrutinizing enrollment in ALS clinical trials: room for improvement? *Amyotrophic Lateral Sclerosis*, **9**(5), 257–65.

9. **Wasner, M., Klier, H., and Borasio, G.D.** (2001) The use of alternative medicine by patients with amyotrophic lateral sclerosis. *Journal of the Neurological Sciences*, **191**(1), 151–4.

10. **Bedlack, R.S., Silani, V., and Cudkowicz, M.E.** (2009) IPLEX and the telephone game: the difficulty in separating myth from reality on the internet. *Amyotrophic Lateral Sclerosis*, **10**(3), 182–4.

11. **Miller, R.G., Jackson, C.E., Kasarskis, E.J.**, et al. (2009) Practice parameter update: the care of the patient with amyotrophic lateral sclerosis: drug, nutritional, and respiratory therapies (an evidence-based review). Report of the Quality Standards Subcommittee of the American Academy of Neurology. *Neurology*, **73**(15), 1218–26.

12. **Chew, S., Khandji, A.G., Montes, J., Mitsumoto, H., and Gordon, P.H.** (2007) Olfactory ensheathing glia injections in Beijing: misleading patients with ALS. *Amyotrophic Lateral Sclerosis*, **8**(5), 314–16.

13. **Piepers, S. and van den Berg, L.H.** (2010) No benefits from experimental treatment with olfactory ensheathing cells in patients with ALS. *Amyotrophic Lateral Sclerosis*, **11**(3), 328–30.

14. **ALSUntangled Group** (2015) ALSUntangled: introducing the Table of Evidence. *Amyotrophic Lateral Sclerosis and Frontotemporal Degeneration*, **16**(1–2), 142.

15. **ALSUntangled Group** (2009) ALSUntangled update 1: Investigating a bug (Lyme Disease) and a drug (Iplex) on behalf of people with ALS. *Amyotrophic Lateral Sclerosis*, **10**(4), 248.

16. **ALSUntangled Group** (2010) ALSUntangled No. 7: Investigating hyperimmune goat serum (Aimspro) for ALS. *Amyotrophic Lateral Sclerosis*, **11**(6), 571.

17. **ALSUntangled Group** (2011) ALSUntangled No. 9: Blue-green algae (Spirulina) as a treatment for ALS. *Amyotrophic Lateral Sclerosis*, **12**(2), 153–5.

18. **ALSUntangled Group** (2011) ALSUntangled 13: Bee venom. *Amyotrophic Lateral Sclerosis*, **12**(6), 471–2.

19. **ALSUntangled Group** (2012) ALSUntangled No. 16: Cannabis. Amyotrophic Lateral Sclerosis. 2012;**13**(4), 400–4.

20. **ALSUntangled Group, Fournier, C., Bedlack, B.**, et al. (2013) ALS Untangled No. 20: the Deanna protocol. *Amyotrophic Lateral Sclerosis and Frontotemporal Degeneration*, **14**(4), 319.

21. **ALSUntangled Group** (2014) ALSUntangled No. 24: Vitamin D. *Amyotrophic Lateral Sclerosis and Frontotemporal Degeneration*, **15**(3–4), 318.

22. **Miller, R.G., Zhang, R., Block, G.,** et al. (2014) NP001 regulation of macrophage activation markers in ALS: A phase I clinical and biomarker study. *Amyotrophic Lateral Sclerosis and Frontotemporal Degeneration*, **15**(7–8), 601–9.

23. **ALSUntangled Group**. (2009) ALSUntangled Update 1: Investigating a bug (Lyme Disease) and a drug (Iplex) on behalf of people with ALS. *Amyotrophic Lateral Sclerosis*, **10**(4), 248–50.

24. **Martinez, H.R., Gonzalez-Garza, M.T., Moreno-Cuevas, J.E.,** et al. (2009) Stem-cell transplantation into the frontal motor cortex in amyotrophic lateral sclerosis patients. *Cytotherapy*, **11**(1), 26–34.

25. **ALSUntangled Group**. (2010) ALSUntangled update 4: investigating the XCell-Center. *Amyotrophic Lateral Sclerosis*, **11**(3), 337.

26. **ALSUntangled Group** (2013) ALSUntangled No. 19: Sodium chlorite. *Amyotrophic Lateral Sclerosis and Frontotemporal Degeneration*, **14**(3), 236.

27. **ALSUntangled Group** (2013) ALSUntangled No. 22: Propofol. *Amyotrophic Lateral Sclerosis and Frontotemporal Degeneration*, **14**(7–8), 640.

28. **Wicks, P., Vaughan, T.E., Massagli, M.P.,** and **Heywood, J.** (2011) Accelerated clinical discovery using self-reported patient data collected online and a patient-matching algorithm. *Nature Biotechnology*, **29**(5), 411–14.

29. **Aggarwal, S.P., Zinman, L., Simpson, E.,** et al. (2010) Safety and efficacy of lithium in combination with riluzole for treatment of amyotrophic lateral sclerosis: a randomised, double-blind, placebo-controlled trial. *Lancet Neurology*, **9**(5), 481–8.

30. **Chio, A., Borghero, G., Calvo, A.,** et al. (2010) Lithium carbonate in amyotrophic lateral sclerosis lack of efficacy in a dose-finding trial. *Neurology*, **75**(7), 619–25.

31. **Bedlack, R.S., Joyce, N., Carter, G.T., Paganoni, S.,** and **Karam, C.** (2015) Complementary and alternative therapies in amyotrophic lateral sclerosis. *Neurologic Clinics*, **33**(4), 909–36.

32. **Bedlack, R.** and **Hardiman, O.** (2009) ALSUntangled (ALSU): a scientific approach to off-label treatment options for people with ALS using tweets and twitters. *Amyotrophic Lateral Sclerosis*, **10**(3), 129–30.

33. **Charles, C., Gafni, A.,** and **Whelan, T.** (1997) Shared decision-making in the medical encounter: what does it mean?(or it takes at least two to tango). *Social Science & Medicine*, **44**(5), 681–92.

34. **Schofield, P., Diggens, J., Charleson, C., Marigliani, R.,** and **Jefford, M.** (2010) Effectively discussing complementary and alternative medicine in a conventional oncology setting: communication recommendations for clinicians. *Patient Education and Counseling*, **79**(2), 143–51.

35. **Singh, S.** and **Ernst, E.** (2008) *Trick or Treatment: The Undeniable Facts about Alternative Medicine*. London: WW Norton & Company.

36. **Marconi, A., Gragnano, G., Lunetta, C.,** et al. (2016) The experience of meditation for people with amyotrophic lateral sclerosis and their caregivers—a qualitative analysis. *Psychology, Health & Medicine*, **21**(6), 762–8.

37. **Pagnini, F., Bercovitz, K.,** and **Langer, E.** (2016) Perceived control and mindfulness: Implications for clinical practice. *Journal of Psychotherapy Integration*, **26**(2), 91.

38. Green, J.P., Barabasz, A.F., Barrett, D., and Montgomery, G.H. (2005) Forging ahead: the 2003 APA Division 30 definition of hypnosis. *International Journal of Clinical and Experimental Hypnosis*, **53**(3), 259–64.

39. Shih, M., Yang, Y-H., and Koo, M. (2012) A meta-analysis of hypnosis in the treatment of depressive symptoms: a brief communication. *International Journal of Clinical and Experimental Hypnosis*, **57**(4), 431–42.

40. Willemsen, R., Haentjens, P., Roseeuw, D., and Vanderlinden, J. (2010) Hypnosis in refractory alopecia areata significantly improves depression, anxiety, and life quality but not hair regrowth. *Journal of the American Academy of Dermatology*, **62**(3), 517–18.

41. Plaskota, M., Lucas, C., Pizzoferro, K., Saini, T., Evans, R., and Cook, K. (2012) A hypnotherapy intervention for the treatment of anxiety in patients with cancer receiving palliative care. *International Journal of Palliative Nursing*, **18**(2), 69–75.

42. Dillworth, T. and Jensen, M.P. (2010) The role of suggestions in hypnosis for chronic pain: A review of the literature. The Open Pain Journal, **3**(1), 39.

43. Crawford, H.J. and Barabasz, A.F. (1993) Phobias and intense fears: Facilitating their treatment with hypnosis. In: Rhue, J.W. & Lynn, S.J. (eds), *Handbook of Clinical Hypnosis*, pp. 311–37. Washington, DC: American Psychological Association.

44. Barber, T.X. (1978) Hypnosis, suggestions, and psychosomatic phenomena: A new look from the standpoint of recent experimental studies. *American Journal of Clinical Hypnosis*, **21**(1), 13–27.

45. Jensen, M.P., Adachi, T., Tomé-Pires, C., Lee, J., Osman, Z.J., and Miró, J. (2015) Mechanisms of hypnosis: toward the development of a biopsychosocial model. *International Journal of Clinical and Experimental Hypnosis*, **63**(1), 34–75.

46. Wain, H.J., Amen, D., and Jabbari, B. (1990) The effects of hypnosis on a parkinsonian tremor: case report with polygraph/EEG recordings. *American Journal of Clinical Hypnosis*, **33**(2), 94–8.

47. Holroyd, J. and Hill, A. (1989) Pushing the limits of recovery: hypnotherapy with a stroke patient. *International Journal of Clinical and Experimental Hypnosis*, **37**(2), 120–8.

48. Pajntar, M., Jeglič, A., Štefančič, M., and Vodovnik, L. (1980) Improvements of motor response by means of hypnosis in patients with peripheral nerve lesions. *International Journal of Clinical and Experimental Hypnosis*, **28**(1), 16–26.

49. Lucas, D., Stratis, D., and Deniz, S. (1981) From the clinic: Hypnosis in conjunction with corrective therapy in a quadriplegic patient: a case report. *American Corrective Therapy Journal*, **35**(5), 116.

50. Benedittis, G.D. (1996) Hypnosis and spasmodic torticollis-report of four cases: A brief communication. *International Journal of Clinical and Experimental Hypnosis*, **44**(4), 292–306.

51. Ezra, Y., Gotkine, M., Goldman, S., Adahan, H.M., and Ben-Hur, T. (2012) Hypnotic relaxation vs amitriptyline for tension-type headache: Let the patient choose. *Headache: The Journal of Head and Face Pain*, **52**(5), 785–91.

52. Whitehouse, W.G., Dinges, D.F., Orne, E.C., et al. (1996) Psychosocial and immune effects of self-hypnosis training for stress management throughout the first semester of medical school. *Psychosomatic Medicine*, **58**(3), 249–63.

53. Hidderley, M. and Holt, M. (2004) A pilot randomized trial assessing the effects of autogenic training in early stage cancer patients in relation to psychological status and immune system responses. *European Journal of Oncology Nursing*, **8**(1), 61–5.

54. **Brann, L., Owens, J.,** and **Williamson, A.** (2015) *The Handbook of Contemporary Clinical Hypnosis: Theory and Practice.* Oxford: John Wiley & Sons; 2015.

55. **Palmieri, A., Kleinbub, J.R., Calvo, V.,** et al. (2012) Efficacy of hypnosis-based treatment in amyotrophic lateral sclerosis: A pilot study. *Frontiers in Psychology,* **3,** 465.

56. **Kleinbub, J.R., Palmieri, A., Broggio, A.,** et al. (2015) Hypnosis-based psychodynamic treatment in ALS: a longitudinal study on patients and their caregivers. *Frontiers in Psychology,* **6,** 624.

57. **Bernheim, H.** (1900) *Suggestive Therapeutics: A Treatise on the Nature and Uses of Hypnotism.* New York, NY: GP Putnam's sons.

58. **MacLeod, C.** and **Clarke, P.J.** (2015) The attentional bias modification approach to anxiety intervention. *Clinical Psychological Science,* **3**(1), 58–78.

59. **McDonald, E.R., Wiedenfeld, S.A., Hillel, A., Carpenter, C.L.,** and **Walter, R.A.** (1994) Survival in amyotrophic lateral sclerosis: The role of psychological factors. *Archives of Neurology,* **51**(1), 17–23.

60. **Johnston, M., Earll, L., Giles, M., McClenahan, R., Stevens, D.,** and **Morrison, V.** (1999) Mood as a predictor of disability and survival in patients newly diagnosed with ALS/MND. *British Journal of Health Psychology,* **4**(2), 127–36.

61. **Krampe, H., Bartels, C., Victorson, D.,** et al. (2008) The influence of personality factors on disease progression and health-related quality of life in people with ALS. *Amyotrophic Lateral Sclerosis,* **9**(2), 99–107.

62. **Pagnini, F., Phillips, D., Bosma, C., Reece, A.,** and **Langer, E.** (2015) Mindfulness, physical impairment and psychological well-being in people with amyotrophic lateral sclerosis. *Psychology & Health,* **30**(5), 503–17.

63. **Cedarbaum, J.M., Stambler, N., Malta, E.,** et al. (1999) The ALSFRS-R: A revised ALS functional rating scale that incorporates assessments of respiratory function. *Journal of the Neurological Sciences,* **169**(1), 13–21.

64. **Faymonville, M-E., Boly, M.,** and **Laureys, S.** (2006) Functional neuroanatomy of the hypnotic state. *Journal of Physiology, Paris,* **99**(4), 463–9.

65. **Raz, A., Fan, J.,** and **Posner, M.I.** (2006) Neuroimaging and genetic associations of attentional and hypnotic processes. *Journal of Physiology, Paris,* **99**(4), 483–91.

66. **Lam, L., Halder, R.C., Montoya, D.J.,** et al. (2015) Anti-inflammatory therapies of amyotrophic lateral sclerosis guided by immune pathways. *American Journal of Neurodegenerative Disease,* **4**(2), 28.

67. **Bowlby, J.** (1977) Attachment theory and its therapeutic implications. *Adolescent Psychiatry,* **6,** 5–33.

68. **Mikulincer, M., Shaver, P.R., Bar-On, N.,** and **Ein-Dor, T.** (2010) The pushes and pulls of close relationships: attachment insecurities and relational ambivalence. *Journal of Personality and Social Psychology,* **98**(3), 450.

69. **Pagnini, F., Rossi, G., Lunetta, C.,** et al. (2010) Burden, depression, and anxiety in caregivers of people with amyotrophic lateral sclerosis. *Psychology, Health & Medicine,* **15**(6), 685–93.

70. **Pagnini, F., Banfi, P., Lunetta, C.,** et al. (2012) Respiratory function of people with amyotrophic lateral sclerosis and caregiver distress level: a correlational study. *BioPsychoSocial Medicine,* **6**(1), 1.

71. **Palmieri, A., Abrahams, S., Sorarù, G.,** et al. (2009) Emotional lability in MND: Relationship to cognition and psychopathology and impact on caregivers. *Journal of the Neurological Sciences,* **278**(1), 16–20.

72. **Palmieri, A., Soraru, G., Albertini, E.,** et al. (2010) Psychopathological features and suicidal ideation in amyotrophic lateral sclerosis patients. *Neurological Sciences,* **31**(6), 735–40.

73. **Monk-Turner, E.** (2003) The benefits of meditation: Experimental findings. *Social Science Journal,* **40**(3), 465–70.

74. **Neff, K.** (2003) Self-compassion: An alternative conceptualization of a healthy attitude toward oneself. *Self and Identity,* **2**(2), 85–101.

75. **Goyal, M., Singh, S., Sibinga, E.M.,** et al. (2014) Meditation programs for psychological stress and well-being: a systematic review and meta-analysis. *Journal of the American Medical Association: Internal Medicine,* **174**(3), 357–68.

76. **Brow, K.W.** and **Ryan, R.M.** (2003) The benefits of being present: mindfulness and its role in psychological well-being. *Journal of Personality and Social Psychology,* **84**(4), 822.

77. **Sedlmeier, P., Eberth, J., Schwarz, M.,** et al. (2012) The psychological effects of meditation: A meta-analysis. *Psychological Bulletin,* **138**(6), 1139.

78. **Kabat-Zinn, J.** (1990) *Full Catastrophe Living: Using the Wisdom of your Body and Mind to Face Stress, Pain, and Illness.* New York, NY: Delacorte.

79. **Shear, J.** (2006) *The Experience of Meditation: Experts Introduce the Major Traditions.* St Paul, MN: Paragon House.

80. **Coleman, J.W.** (2002) *The New Buddhism: The Western Transformation of an Ancient Tradition.* Oxford: Oxford University Press.

81. **Davis, D.M.** and **Hayes, J.A.** (2011) What are the benefits of mindfulness? A practice review of psychotherapy-related research. *Psychotherapy (Chicago),* **48**(2), 198–208.

82. **Pagnini, F.** (2013) Psychological wellbeing and quality of life in amyotrophic lateral sclerosis: A review. *International Journal of Psychology,* **48**(3), 194–205.

83. **Pagnini, F., Di Credico, C., Gatto, R.,** et al. (2014) Meditation training for people with amyotrophic lateral sclerosis and their caregivers. *Journal of Alternative and Complementary Medicine,* **20**(4), 272–5.

84. **Pagnini, F., Manzoni, G.M., Tagliaferri, A.,** and **Gibbons, C.J.** (2015) Depression and disease progression in amyotrophic lateral sclerosis: A comprehensive meta-regression analysis. *Journal of Health Psychology,* **20**(8), 1107–28.

85. **Papageorgiou, C.** and **Wells, A.** (2003) An empirical test of a clinical metacognitive model of rumination and depression. *Cognitive Therapy and Research,* **27**(3), 261–73.

86. **Niemiec, C.P., Brown, K.W., Kashdan, T.B.,** et al. (2010) Being present in the face of existential threat: The role of trait mindfulness in reducing defensive responses to mortality salience. *Journal of Personality and Social Psychology,* **99**(2), 344.

87. **Ball, M.S.** and **Vernon, B.** (2015) A review on how meditation could be used to comfort the terminally ill. *Palliative and Supportive Care,* **13**(05), 1469–72.

88. **Bolmsjö, I.** (2001) Existential issues in palliative care: interviews of patients with amyotrophic lateral sclerosis. *Journal of Palliative Medicine,* **4**(4), 499–505.

89. **Germer, C.K., Siegel, R.D.,** and **Fulton, P.R.** (2013) *Mindfulness and Psychotherapy.* New York, NY: Guilford Press.

90. **Oster, C.** and **Pagnini, F.** (2012) Resentment, hate, and hope in amyotrophic lateral sclerosis. *Frontiers in Psychology,* **3**, 530.

91. **Pagnini, F., Lunetta, C., Rossi, G.,** et al. (2011) Existential well-being and spirituality of individuals with amyotrophic lateral sclerosis is related to psychological well-being of their caregivers. *Amyotrophic Lateral Sclerosis,* **12**(2), 105–8.

92. **Bohlmeijer, E., Prenger, R., Taal, E.,** and **Cuijpers, P.** (2010) The effects of mindfulness-based stress reduction therapy on mental health of adults with a chronic medical disease: a meta-analysis. *Journal of Psychosomatic Research*, **68**(6), 539–44.

93. **Ginot, E.** (2015) *The Neuropsychology of the Unconscious: Integrating Brain and Mind in Psychotherapy*. Norton Series on Interpersonal Neurobiology. London: WW Norton & Company.

94. **Hillier, S.** and **Worley, A.** (2015) The effectiveness of the feldenkrais method: A systematic review of the evidence. *Evidence-Based Complementary and Alternative Medicine*, Article ID 752160.

95. **Pagnini F, Marconi A, Tagliaferri A, Manzoni GM, Gatto R, Fabiani V,** et al. (2017) Meditation Training for People with Amyotrophic Lateral Sclerosis: A Randomised Clinical Trial. European Journal of Neurology. 24(4):578–86.

Chapter 6

Genetic counselling: Psychological impact and concerns

Bryan J. Traynor and Adriano Chiò

Background

There is a growing awareness among both clinicians and patients concerning the predictive power of modern genomics. Nevertheless, interpretation of genetic results is often nuanced and it can be challenging to put this information into the correct context for patients. For this reason, genetic counselling has emerged as a means of quantifying genetic risk and for helping patients understand the implications of their genetic test results. In this chapter, we will discuss, in general terms, the importance of genetic counselling, describe what is involved in the process of genetic counselling and how it is delivered to patients, and outline how advances in sequencing technology are changing the scope of genetic counselling. We will also describe the relevance of genetic counselling as it pertains to amyotrophic lateral sclerosis (ALS) and we will end with a vision of the future of genetic counselling.

Why is genetic counselling necessary?

Genetic counselling is the process involving the communication of information about genetic testing and risks to the individual and/or the family (1). As in all things in modern medicine, genetic counselling is an expensive endeavour and this cost must be justified. A useful starting point is to ask why genetic counselling is necessary. A related question centres on why the medical profession considers genetic testing to be fundamentally different in nature compared with routine blood tests, such as blood cholesterol or glucose measurements.

First, there has been an explosion in our knowledge of the human genome and the role that genetics plays in both common and rare diseases over the last decade (2). Interpretation of this huge volume of genetic data is becoming more and more challenging. Genetic counsellors are rigorously trained in the interpretation of such genetic tests. A key aspect of their training is the ability to find and evaluate information on variants and genes in published literature and online databases, a skill that is neither trivial nor straightforward.

Secondly, improved awareness among the public has fuelled a demand for genetic testing and genetic knowledge. Commercial entities, like 23&Me, provide consumers with the opportunity to have their genomes rapidly assessed for known pathogenic variants and risk factors at low cost (3). While genomic technologies have clearly improved our capacity to generate large datasets, our ability to interpret the biological consequences of detected variants lags behind (4). Today, it is not unusual for an individual to purchase genetic testing from a commercial vendor and then to bring the results of these studies to their medical care providers for interpretation. Neurology has been at the forefront of this genetic revolution, primarily due to the large number of genetic disorders that exist within this specialty.

What special considerations are associated with genetic testing?

There are key aspects of genetic information that require special attention in comparison to other types of medical data. The most obvious is that the genetic knowledge is irrevocable. Once the patient learns of their genetic status, they cannot unlearn it. Furthermore, genetic information has wider implications for other members of the family and, at least for now, most genetic mutations are not treatable. By extension, psychological distress arising from this knowledge is open-ended. Studies have shown that expert genetic counselling decreases the chance of psychological distress, presumably as it educates patients and their families, and effectively manages expectations (5). This fact alone has being a driving force in the emergence of genetic counselling as an entity, and has been discussed extensively in the published literature (6–8).

Genetic mutations are not typically amenable to medical intervention. As a consequence, most genetic testing fails the World Health Organization requirement of screening tools for 'sufficient yield', as patients are not brought to any form of treatment as a result of the test (9). Indeed, the lack of change in treatment or outcome is a frequently cited reason among patients, asymptomatic relatives, and medical care professionals for not proceeding with genetic testing (10). The development of effective and safe gene therapy may dramatically shift the risk/benefit balance in the future (see section on 'The future of genetic counselling').

Genetic test results can have profound emotional, psychological, ethical, and legal ramifications on the family unit, since related individuals may be at risk of inheriting the pathogenic mutation (11, 12). There is ongoing ethical debate as to whether non-tested family members should or should not automatically be informed of genetic test results. Presently, the 'right not to know' is considered to be a basic principle of human clinical genetics recognized by most international regulatory statements and legislation (12–16). In our opinion, this approach is likely to be challenged in the future.

How do patients access genetic counselling?

Genetic counselling is usually provided by genetic counsellors and there are currently 4000 genetic counsellors working in the USA. These numbers are likely to continue to grow commensurate with rising demand (17). Most have a Masters of Science degree in genetic counselling and are certified by the American Board of Genetic Counseling (18). In addition to theoretical and practical genetics, the education of genetic counsellors emphasizes the management of a patient's psychological well-being, and may even be considered as psychologists specializing in genetics. In genetic clinics, genetic counsellors play a central role in patient assessment with the overall aim of providing information and support to families. They also receive referrals from other physicians who may not routinely employ genetic testing and, in those instances, serve as a resource to advise physicians on which genetic tests are most appropriate. In other models, commercial gene testing companies employ genetic counsellors who liaise with consumers and physicians to educate patients, to provide test results to the patient, and to help interpret the data.

Genetic counselling is usually performed in two steps. In the initial visit, the patient meets with the genetic counsellor prior to the genetic testing. The genetic counsellor will describe the role of genetic testing in quantifying disease risk. This is an opportunity for the patient to learn about the genetics of their particular disorder, what genetic tests might be available and the recommendations of published guidelines for genetic testing if available. A central aspect of this visit is to educate the patient as to what positive and negative results might mean for them. Such a discussion will include how this information may affect their family.

Patients are encouraged to ask questions and to consider the financial, psychological and medical implications of their testing. For example, patients need to be made aware that genetic testing can be expensive and insurance companies do not always reimburse the full cost. The Genetic Information Nondiscrimination Act of 2008 (GINA) prohibits the use of genetic information in health insurance and employment (19, 20). Nevertheless, patients may discuss issues such as the inclusion of their genetic results in their medical record or whether to inform their primary care physician of the results. Indeed, the protections afforded by GINA do not extend to long-term care insurance or to life insurance. The overarching aim of this first meeting is to provide the patient with the information necessary for them to make an informed decision as to whether they want to move forward with the genetic testing.

Assuming that the patient opts to undergo genetic testing, a second face-to-face consultation is usually held after the results are available. This provides an opportunity for the results of the genetic testing to be returned to the patient in a safe, controlled environment, to help the patient understand the implication of their results and to interpret them in an appropriate context. Clearly, a positive test may have enormous implications for an individual and their family. Perhaps contrary to expectation, patients may view a negative test unfavourably, as it may mean that their own diagnosis remains uncertain. It is the role of the genetic counsellor to anticipate these scenarios and to mitigate the associated psychological distress.

Special care is required in the case of presymptomatic individuals seeking genetic testing. The typical scenario is that a young member of a family known to carry a particular genetic mutation wishes to undergo genetic testing for that variant. Often this request occurs in the context of a significant life event, such as reaching the age of majority, impending marriage, or potential reproduction. Again, a positive result may have significant implications for that person, even though they do not have symptoms. Nevertheless, many genetic mutations do not have complete penetrance and so not every individual carrying that mutation may go on to develop the disease. Such uncertainty can be challenging for individuals to deal with and it is the task of the genetic counsellor to educate and guide the patient through these choppy waters.

Paradoxically, a negative test may also be associated with a feeling of guilt, especially if siblings or other family members have tested positive. Such 'survivor' guilt may be equally challenging to deal with (21).

The influence of technology on genetic counselling

The advent of next-generation sequencing has revolutionized how genetic research is performed. This technology is increasingly entering into clinical practice (22), and this has increased the importance of genetic counselling. This methodology provides information across the entire patient's exome or genome, and typically generates a large number of variants (in the range of 100,000) for each individual. Although the pathogenic mutation can often be identified within this long list, the functional consequence of some variants may be difficult to interpret. The term 'variant of unknown significance' has arisen in the field (23), but a concrete example might be more illustrative. Imagine that next generation sequencing identifies a variant in a gene known to cause familial ALS in a patient with ALS. This variant is not found in online databases of human polymorphisms totalling about 70,000 individuals, suggesting that it is very rare. However, no one else in the patient's family has been diagnosed with ALS, or they have been diagnosed with ALS, but DNA is not available. It is not possible to show the variant segregates with disease within the family in that scenario. *In silico* predictions of pathogenicity give some clue as to whether the variant is pathogenic or benign based on the biochemical properties of amino acid change, conservation across species, comparison with other mutations in the human genome, etc. However, these tools are estimates at best and can be unreliable (24). In the end, the physician and genetic counsellor can tell the patient that they carry a rare variant in a known ALS gene, but that it is not possible to say whether that particular variant is the cause of their disease. Understandably, this uncertainty about whether or not a variant is the cause of their disease or not can be a source of significant psychological distress for the patient and their family. Future studies may elucidate the effect of the variant, but that is an open-ended setting that can be frustrating for both patient and the physician. It is the role of the genetic counsellors to explain the findings to the patient, and to help the patient and their family respond appropriately to the uncertainty surrounding their genetic diagnosis.

Societal attitudes are also changing how genetic information is perceived. Individuals can cheaply access their personal genome information through direct-to-consumer companies. Increasing amounts of biological information about genes and even about individual variants is available on the Internet. While self-empowerment of individuals concerning their health is to be welcomed, care must be taken to avoid causing them unnecessary psychological distress. Ready access to genetic counselling can help alleviate these issues.

ALS genetics

Genetic factors play a significant role in ALS aetiology and pathogenesis, and to date, more than 25 genes linked to ALS have been identified. These genes are discussed in greater detail in Marangi and Traynor, Brain Research 2015 (25). The following section represents a brief summary of that article focused on the key ALS genes.

Overall, the genetic cause of approximately two-thirds of familial ALS and of about 10% of sporadic disease has been identified (26). Genetic mutations are clearly responsible for the remaining one-third of familial disease, whereas genome-wide data suggest that genetic factors contribute to at least 23% of sporadic ALS (27). Locus, allelic, and clinical heterogeneity of ALS are the main factors complicating the discovery and validation of new genes, since a single gene may be involved in a very limited number of cases (25). Furthermore, the relative impact of various genes may be quite disparate among different populations. For example, the hexanucleotide repeat expansion of *C9orf72* is a common cause of ALS and frontotemporal dementia in the Caucasian population, but is relatively rare in African and Asian populations (28).

The following is a list of the main *ALS* genes that have been discovered to date presented in order of their discovery.

SOD1

Autosomal dominant mutations in *SOD1* were the first identified genetic cause of ALS (29). Since then, over 150 different mutations have been reported in this gene, and they account for 12–20% of FALS cases and are found in about 1% of apparently sporadic cases (25,30,31). It is not clear whether all of the reported variants in *SOD1* are pathogenic or instead represent incidental findings in affected subjects (32).

TARDBP (TDP-43)

TAR DNA-binding protein 43 (TDP-43) was identified as a major component of ubiquitin-positive cytoplasmic inclusions that are the neuropathological hallmark of the disease (33). Not surprisingly, mutations in the *TARDBP* gene (encoding the TDP-43 protein) were soon after identified in both sporadic and familial ALS cases (25,34,35). *TARDBP* mutations are found in about 4% of FALS cases and in a far smaller percentage of sporadic cases (30, 31).

FUS

Mutations were identified in *FUS*, a protein that shares functional homology with TDP-43, shortly after the discovery of TARDBP as a cause of familial ALS (25,36,37). Mutations in this gene account for ~5% of FALS and for about 1% of SALS (30, 31, 38, 39). Mutations in this gene are mostly associated with limb-onset ALS in young men, although FTD has also been reported in patients carrying *FUS* mutations.

OPTN

Optineurin (*OPTN*) mutations have long been described as a cause of primary open angle glaucoma (40). Autosomal dominant and recessive mutations in *OPTN* have been reported in FALS cases (41). Mutations in this gene appear to be a more common cause of ALS in Asian populations (42), and are a less common cause of ALS among Caucasian populations (25).

VCP

This was the first *ALS* gene found by exome sequencing and accounts for 1–2% of familial ALS cases (43). Mutations in *VCP* were already known to underlie a clinical syndrome characterized by FTD, inclusion body myopathy, and Paget's disease of the bone (IBMPFD) (25).

UBQLN2

UBQLN2 maps to chromosome X (44). Even though *UBQLN2* mutations are a rare cause of ALS, its role in the pathogenesis of ALS is supported by the presence of ubiquilin-2 within the neuronal inclusions that are the pathological hallmark of ALS pathology (25, 26).

C9orf72 repeat expansion

The pathogenic hexanucleotide repeat expansion in the *C9orf72* gene was identified as the cause of 9p21-linked ALS and FTD in 2011 (45,46). The *C9orf72* repeat expansion is the most frequent genetic cause of both FALS (about 40%) and familial FTD (about 25%) (28). The discovery also demonstrated that ALS and FTD form a neurodegenerative disease spectrum. The co-existence of cognitive dysfunction in ALS patients complicates genetic counselling as it limits the ability of patients to understand the consequences of what they are been told. In this scenario, genetic counsellors typically request that the patient's caregiver or next of kin be present during the session. The identification of the same repeat expansion in a sizeable portion of sporadic ALS cases provided the first proof that genetics could underlie this more common form of disease (25).

Other familial ALS genes

Mutations in other genes that have been identified as a cause of familial ALS including *PFN1* (involved in maintenance of cytoskeletal structure)(47); *MATR3* (another RNA/DNA binding protein)(48); *CHCHD10* (important in mitochondrial stability and observed in ALS alone and in frontotemporal dementia, cerebellar ataxia, and myopathy(49–51); and *TBK1* (52).

Genetic counselling recommendations for ALS

Several sets of guidelines have been published for ALS. Key questions addressed by these criteria centre on who should be tested and what genes should be screened. For example, in 2012, the European Federation of Neurological Societies (EFNS) issued guidelines indicating that DNA analysis should be limited to 'cases with a known family history of ALS, and in sporadic ALS cases with the characteristic phenotype of the recessive D90A mutation' and not performed in 'cases with sporadic ALS with a typical classical ALS phenotype' (12,53). However, our understanding of ALS genetics has evolved considerably since then, making these criteria essentially outmoded. More recently, the ITALSGEN consortium published consensus guidelines for genetic testing in ALS patients arising from a recent workshop that sought input from neurologists, geneticists, psychologists and ethicists (12).

Genetic screening guidelines matter, not just for providing guidance to physicians, patients, and families, but also because reimbursement policies for genetic testing and counselling are often based on these criteria (12). For example, genetic testing in apparently sporadic cases is not reimbursed in many countries including the USA. Nevertheless, scientific research shows that the distinction between familial ALS and sporadic ALS is not as clear-cut as previously thought (54).

Which patients should undergo genetic testing?

There is near complete agreement that ALS patients reporting a family history of ALS or FTD should be offered genetic testing. In contrast, most criteria do not recommend genetic testing of sporadic ALS patients in clinical practice (12). A possible exception to this criterion is testing for the *C9orf72* repeat expansion. In fact, there are more sporadic ALS patients due to the *C9orf72* repeat expansion than there are familial ALS patients due to the same expansion:

- 40% of familial ALS patients carry the repeat expansion;
- 10% of ALS cases are familial in nature;
- thus, familial ALS patients carrying the repeat expansion account for 4% of all ALS cases.

In contrast, 7–8% of sporadic ALS patients carry the same expansion, accounting for ~6% of all ALS cases (28).

Should genetic testing be offered to asymptomatic at-risk subjects?

The usefulness of genetic testing for asymptomatic at-risk subjects in the clinical setting is presently unknown and is typically not offered to subjects (12). At-risk relatives of an ALS patient with a known genetic mutation who seek genetic testing should be referred for formal genetic counselling (12,55–57).

What genes should be tested?

Two-thirds of the known mutations in ALS patients are found in four genes, namely *C9ORF72, SOD1, TARDBP*, and *FUS* (12). Therefore, these genes should be considered for initial screening in cases of familial ALS. *C9ORF72* testing is the only genetic test that is routinely pursued in sporadic ALS cases, as mutations in other genes are rarely identified in cases without a family history (12). Phenotypic clues may suggest mutations in specific genes. For example, a family history of Paget's disease of the bone or inclusion myopathy would prioritize sequencing of the *VCP* gene for mutations (43); a personal or family history of frontotemporal dementia would point towards *C9orf72* repeat expansion as a culprit; and a personal history of early onset sensorineural deafness in an ALS patient may be consistent with Brown–Vialetto–Van Laere syndrome leading to *SLC52A2* and *SLC52A3* being screened for mutations (58–60).

If these four genes are negative, additional genetic analysis can be performed. Alternatively, exome sequencing in a CLIA-certified laboratory can be considered (12).

The future of genetic counselling

The role of genomics in clinical medicine will continue to grow over the next decade, and may eventually dominate the practice of health care. Gene therapy tailored to the specific underlying defect of the individual patient has the potential to become a powerful force. Indeed, early stage clinical trials involving antisense oligonucleotides against mutated *SOD1* have already been completed (61), and similar gene therapy approaches may be feasible for the *C9orf72* repeat expansion (62). Cataloguing human genetic variations and understanding their functional consequences will be an additional necessary step to a realization of this scenario. The 100,000 Genomes Project in the United Kingdom (63) and President Obama's Precision Medicine Initiative (64) will probably have a significant impact in this regard. In the middle of this, the role of genetic counselling will come to the fore in explaining genetic results, and their implications to patients and their families.

References

1. Javaher P, Kaariainen H, Kristoffersson U, et al. (2008) EuroGentest: DNA-based testing for heritable disorders in Europe. *Community Genetics*, **11**(2), 75–120.

2. Lander, E.S. (2011) Initial impact of the sequencing of the human genome. *Nature*, **470**(7333), 187–97.

3. 23andMe (2017) Get to know you. Health and ancestry start here. [Available at: https://www.23andme.com/ (accessed 21 July 2017).

4. Edwards, S.L., Beesley, J., French, J.D., and Dunning, A.M. (2017) Beyond GWASs: illuminating the dark road from association to function. *American Journal of Human Genetics*, **93**(5), 779–97.

5. Eijzenga, W., Hahn, D.E., Aaronson, N.K., Kluijt, I., and Bleiker, E.M. (2014) Specific psychosocial issues of individuals undergoing genetic counseling for cancer—a literature review. *Journal of Genetic Counseling*, **23**(2), 133–46.

6. Burke, W., Pinsky, L.E., and Press, N.A. (2001) Categorizing genetic tests to identify their ethical, legal, and social implications. *American Journal of Medical Genetics*, **106**(3), 233–40.

7. Duncan, R.E., Gillam, L., Savulescu, J., Williamson, R., Rogers, J.G., and Delatycki, M.B. (2008) 'You're one of us now': young people describe their experiences of predictive genetic testing for Huntington disease (HD) and familial adenomatous polyposis (FAP). *American Journal of Medical Genetics Part C: Seminars in Medical Genetics*, **148C**(1), 47–55.

8. Klitzman, R., Thorne, D., Williamson, J., Chung, W., and Marder, K. (2007) Disclosures of Huntington disease risk within families: Patterns of decision-making and implications. *American Journal of Medical Genetics Part A*, **143A**(16), 1835–49.

9. Wilson, J.M.G. and Jungner, G. (1968) *Principles and Practice of Screening for Disease.* Geneva: World Health Organization.

10. Riesgraf, R.J., Veach, P.M., MacFarlane, I.M., and LeRoy, B.S. (2015) Perceptions and attitudes about genetic counseling among residents of a midwestern rural area. *Journal of Genetic Counseling*, **24**(4), 565–79.

11. Fong, J.C., Karydas, A.M., and Goldman, J.S. (2012) Genetic counseling for FTD/ALS caused by the C9ORF72 hexanucleotide expansion. *Alzheimers Research Therapy*, **4**(4), 27.

12. **Chio, A., Battistini, S., Calvo, A.,** et al. (2014) Genetic counselling in ALS: Facts, uncertainties and clinical suggestions. *Journal of Neurology, Neurosurgery & Psychiatry*, **85**(5), 478–85.

13. **Rahman, B., Meiser, B., Sachdev, P.,** et al. (2012) To know or not to know: An update of the literature on the psychological and behavioral impact of genetic testing for Alzheimer disease risk. *Genetic Testing and Molecular Biomarkers*, **16**(8), 935–42.

14. **Nicolas, P.** (2009) Ethical and juridical issues of genetic testing: A review of the international regulation. *Critical Reviews in Oncology and Hematology*, **69**(2), 98–107.

15. **Andorno, R.** (2004) The right not to know: an autonomy based approach. *Journal of Medical Ethics*, **30**(5), 435–9; discussion 9–40.

16. **Zinberg, R.E.** (2006) Genetic testing: Is there a right not to know? *MCN American Journal of Maternal and Child Nursing*, **31**(3), 144.

17. **Pain, E.** (2016) Genetic counseling: A growing area of opportunity http://www.sciencemag.org/careers/2016/06/genetic-counseling-growing-area-opportunity2016 (accessed 21 July 2017).

18. **American Board of Genetic Counselling** (2016) Available at: http://www.abgc.net/ABGC/AmericanBoardofGeneticCounselors.asp (accessed 21 July 2017).

19. **The Genetic Information Nondiscrimination Act of 2008** (2008) [Available at: https://www.eeoc.gov/laws/statutes/gina.cfm (accessed 23 October 2017).

20. **U.S. Equal Opportunity Employment Commission** (2016) EEOC issues final rules on employer wellness programs. Available at: https://www.eeoc.gov/eeoc/newsroom/release/5-16-16.cfm (accessed 23 October 2017).

21. **Graceffa, A., Russo, M., Vita, G.L.,** et al. (2009) Psychosocial impact of presymptomatic genetic testing for transthyretin amyloidotic polyneuropathy. *Neuromuscular Disorders*, **19**(1), 44–8.

22. **Bowdin, S., Ray, P.N., Cohn, R.D.,** and **Meyn, M.S.** (2014) The genome clinic: a multidisciplinary approach to assessing the opportunities and challenges of integrating genomic analysis into clinical care. *Human Mutation*, **35**(5), 513–19.

23. **Green, R.C., Berg, J.S., Grody, W.W.,** et al. (2013) ACMG recommendations for reporting of incidental findings in clinical exome and genome sequencing. *Genetic Medicine*, **15**(7), 565–74.

24. **Grimm, D.G., Azencott, C.A., Aicheler, F.,** et al. (2015) The evaluation of tools used to predict the impact of missense variants is hindered by two types of circularity. *Human Mutation*, **36**(5), 513–23.

25. **Marangi, G.** and **Traynor, B.J.** (2015) Genetic causes of amyotrophic lateral sclerosis: new genetic analysis methodologies entailing new opportunities and challenges. *Brain Research*, **1607**, 75–93.

26. **Renton, A.E., Chio, A.,** and **Traynor, B.J.** (2014) State of play in amyotrophic lateral sclerosis genetics. *Nature, Neuroscience*, **17**(1), 17–23.

27. **Keller, M.F., Ferrucci, L., Singleton, A.B.,** et al. (2014) Genome-wide analysis of the heritability of amyotrophic lateral sclerosis. *Journal of the American Medical Association Neurology*, **71**(9), 1123–34.

28. **Majounie, E., Renton, A.E., Mok, K.,** et al. (2012) Frequency of the C9orf72 hexanucleotide repeat expansion in patients with amyotrophic lateral sclerosis and frontotemporal dementia: a cross-sectional study. *Lancet Neurology*, **11**(4), 323–30.

29. **Rosen, D.R., Siddique, T., Patterson, D.,** et al. (1993) Mutations in Cu/Zn superoxide dismutase gene are associated with familial amyotrophic lateral sclerosis. *Nature*, **362**(6415), 59–62.

30. Chio, A., Traynor, B.J., Lombardo, F., et al. (2008) Prevalence of SOD1 mutations in the Italian ALS population. *Neurology*, **70**(7), 533–7.

31. Millecamps, S., Salachas, F., Cazeneuve, C., et al. (2010) SOD1, ANG, VAPB, TARDBP, and FUS mutations in familial amyotrophic lateral sclerosis: Genotype-phenotype correlations. *Journal of Medical Genetics*, **47**(8), 554–60.

32. Andersen, P.M. (2006) Amyotrophic lateral sclerosis associated with mutations in the CuZn superoxide dismutase gene. *Current Neurology and Neuroscience Reports*, **6**(1), 37–46.

33. Neumann, M., Sampathu, D.M., Kwong, L.K., et al. (2006) Ubiquitinated TDP-43 in frontotemporal lobar degeneration and amyotrophic lateral sclerosis. *Science*, **314**(5796), 130–3.

34. Sreedharan, J., Blair, I.P., Tripathi, V.B., et al. (2008) TDP-43 mutations in familial and sporadic amyotrophic lateral sclerosis. *Science*, **319**(5870), 1668–72.

35. Kabashi, E., Valdmanis, P.N., Dion, P., et al. (2008) TARDBP mutations in individuals with sporadic and familial amyotrophic lateral sclerosis. *Nature Genetics*, **40**(5), 572–4.

36. Vance, C., Rogelj, B., Hortobagyi, T., et al. (2009) Mutations in FUS, an RNA processing protein, cause familial amyotrophic lateral sclerosis type 6. *Science*, **323**(5918), 1208–11.

37. Kwiatkowski, T.J., Jr, Bosco, D.A., Leclerc, A.L., et al. (2009) Mutations in the FUS/TLS gene on chromosome 16 cause familial amyotrophic lateral sclerosis. *Science*, **323**(5918), 1205–8.

38. Brown, J.A., Min, J., Staropoli, J.F., et al. (2012) SOD1, ANG, TARDBP and FUS mutations in amyotrophic lateral sclerosis: A United States clinical testing lab experience. *Amyotrophic Lateral Sclerosis*, **13**(2), 217–22.

39. Lattante, S., Conte, A., Zollino, M., et al. (2012) Contribution of major amyotrophic lateral sclerosis genes to the etiology of sporadic disease. *Neurology*, **79**(1), 66–72.

40. Rezaie, T., Child, A., Hitchings, R., et al. (2002) Adult-onset primary open-angle glaucoma caused by mutations in optineurin. *Science*, **295**(5557), 1077–9.

41. Maruyama, H., Morino, H., Ito, H., et al. (2010) Mutations of optineurin in amyotrophic lateral sclerosis. *Nature*, **465**(7295), 223–6.

42. Sugihara, K., Maruyama, H., Kamada, M., Morino, H., and Kawakami, H. (2011) Screening for OPTN mutations in amyotrophic lateral sclerosis in a mainly Caucasian population. *Neurobiology of Aging*, **32**(10), 1923 e9–10.

43. Johnson, J.O., Mandrioli, J., Benatar, M., et al. (2010) Exome sequencing reveals VCP mutations as a cause of familial ALS. *Neuron*, **68**(5), 857–64.

44. Deng, H.X., Chen, W., Hong, S.T., et al. (2011) Mutations in UBQLN2 cause dominant X-linked juvenile and adult-onset ALS and ALS/dementia. *Nature*, **477**(7363), 211–15.

45. Renton, A.E., Majounie, E., Waite, A., et al. (2011) A hexanucleotide repeat expansion in C9ORF72 is the cause of chromosome 9p21-linked ALS-FTD. *Neuron*, **72**(2), 257–68.

46. DeJesus-Hernandez, M., Mackenzie, I.R., Boeve, B.F., et al. (2011) Expanded GGGGCC hexanucleotide repeat in noncoding region of C9ORF72 causes chromosome 9p-linked FTD and ALS. *Neuron*, **72**(2), 245–56.

47. Wu, C.H., Fallini, C., Ticozzi, N., et al. (2012) Mutations in the profilin 1 gene cause familial amyotrophic lateral sclerosis. *Nature*, **488**(7412), 499–503.

48. Johnson, J.O., Pioro, E.P., Boehringer, A., et al. (2014) Mutations in the Matrin 3 gene cause familial amyotrophic lateral sclerosis. *Nature Neuroscience*, **17**(5), 664–6.

49. **Muller, K., Andersen, P.M., Hubers, A.,** et al. (2014) Two novel mutations in conserved codons indicate that CHCHD10 is a gene associated with motor neuron disease. *Brain*, **137**(Pt 12), e309.

50. **Bannwarth, S., Ait-El-Mkadem, S., Chaussenot, A.,** et al. (2014) A mitochondrial origin for frontotemporal dementia and amyotrophic lateral sclerosis through CHCHD10 involvement. *Brain*, **137**(Pt 8), 2329–45.

51. **Johnson, J.O., Glynn, S.M., Gibbs, J.R.,** et al. (2014) Mutations in the CHCHD10 gene are a common cause of familial amyotrophic lateral sclerosis. *Brain*, **137**(Pt 12), e311.

52. **Cirulli, E.T., Lasseigne, B.N., Petrovski, S.,** et al. (2015) Exome sequencing in amyotrophic lateral sclerosis identifies risk genes and pathways. *Science*, **347**(6229), 1436–41.

53. **EFNS Task Force on Diagnosis and Management of Amyotrophic Lateral Sclerosis, Andersen, P.M., Abrahams, S.,** et al. (2012) EFNS guidelines on the clinical management of amyotrophic lateral sclerosis (MALS)—revised report of an EFNS task force. *European Journal of Neurology*, **19**(3), 360–75.

54. **Conte, A., Lattante, S., Luigetti, M.,** et al. (2012) Classification of familial amyotrophic lateral sclerosis by family history: Effects on frequency of genes mutation. *Journal of Neurology, Neurosurgery & Psychiatry*, **83**(12), 1201–3.

55. **Fanos, J.H., Gronka, S., Wuu, J., Stanislaw, C., Andersen, P.M.,** and **Benatar, M.** (2011) Impact of presymptomatic genetic testing for familial amyotrophic lateral sclerosis. *Genetic Medicine*, **13**(4), 342–8.

56. **Paulsen, J.S., Nance, M., Kim, J.I.,** et al. (2013) A review of quality of life after predictive testing for and earlier identification of neurodegenerative diseases. *Progress in Neurobiology*, **110**, 2–28.

57. **McCluskey, L.** (2006) Presymptomatic genetic testing for ALS. *Virtual Mentor*, **8**(1), 16–19.

58. **Green, P., Wiseman, M., Crow, Y.J.,** et al. (2015) Brown–Vialetto–Van Laere syndrome, a ponto-bulbar palsy with deafness, is caused by mutations in c20orf54. *American Journal of Human Genetics*, **86**(3), 485–9.

59. **Johnson, J.O., Gibbs, J.R., Van Maldergem, L., Houlden, H.,** and **Singleton, A.B.** (2010) Exome sequencing in Brown–Vialetto–van Laere syndrome. *American Journal of Human Genetics*, **87**(4), 567–9; author reply 9–70.

60. **Yamamoto, S., Inoue, K., Ohta, K.Y.,** et al. (2009) Identification and functional characterization of rat riboflavin transporter 2. *Journal of Biochemistry*, **145**(4), 437–43.

61. **Miller, T.M., Pestronk, A., David, W.,** et al. (2013) An antisense oligonucleotide against SOD1 delivered intrathecally for patients with SOD1 familial amyotrophic lateral sclerosis: A phase 1, randomised, first-in-man study. *Lancet Neurology*, **12**(5), 435–42.

62. **Fernandes, S.A., Douglas, A.G., Varela, M.A., Wood, M.J.,** and **Aoki, Y.** (2013) Oligonucleotide-based therapy for FTD/ALS caused by the C9orf72 repeat expansion: A perspective. *Journal of Nucleic Acids*, **2013**, 208245.

63. **Siva, N.** (2015) UK gears up to decode 100,000 genomes from NHS patients. *Lancet*, **385**(9963), 103–4.

64. **Collins, F.S.** and **Varmus, H.** (2015) A new initiative on precision medicine. *New England Journal of Medicine*, **372**(9), 793–5.

Chapter 7

Resilience and coping strategies in ALS patients and caregivers

Stephanie H. Felgoise and Michelle L. Dube

Introduction

Amyotrophic lateral sclerosis (ALS) has a profound impact on the lives of persons with ALS (PALS) and their caregivers. As ALS progresses, PALS and their caregivers must continually adjust to changing roles in their personal lives (1). These experiences are often compounded by a loss of employment and subsequent financial strains (2), emotional challenges including depression, anxiety, and guilt (3–5), and a disruption in social relationships related to increased social withdrawal and isolation (6,7). The effects of ALS seep into all aspects of PALS' lives and the lives of their caregivers and families (3,8).

The ALS caregiving role can progress at different rates and become overwhelming, with a majority of caregivers dedicating an average of 12 hours per day to their caregiving responsibilities (9). Caregiving demands can include physical tasks such as transferring and dressing, offering emotional support, and managing finances, appointments, and medical equipment (9). ALS caregivers must learn to balance these newfound responsibilities with non-caregiving duties and family role responsibilities (10,11). Some ALS caregivers report feeling physically unwell, exhausted, and fatigued (11–13). Depression, burden, anxiety, and distress have been reported (8,12,14). Caregivers often have decreased social engagement and loss of productivity at work (7–8,14). Over time, these biopsychosocial challenges can affect the quality of life of both PALS and caregivers (3,9,15).

Quality of Life

Quality of life (QoL) has been discussed in detail in Chapter 2. Within the context of ALS, it is understandable that the disease can shape PALS' and caregivers' perception of their physical, psychosocial, religious/spiritual, and environmental functioning (15). Indeed, reductions in QoL are well documented in the ALS literature (8,16–17). Evidence is mixed regarding the impact PALS and their caregivers have on each other's QoL. Some studies have reported a high concordance between the QoL of PALS and their caregivers indicating that the well-being of caregiver has the potential to influence PALS' QoL and vice versa (18,19), whereas Weller (20) did not demonstrate a reciprocal relationship between PALS-caregiver dyads. In the presence of an incurable illness such as ALS, there is an assumption that all patients and caregivers will exhibit clinically significant rates of depression that will increase with disease progression; however, while PALS demonstrate similar clinical evolution, there is individual variability in the way individuals experience and live with ALS (15). For some, an ALS diagnosis signifies the beginning of chronic distress that may last for the duration of the illness (21), some identify healthy ways to cope, while others use maladaptive strategies (22,23). For others, depression may ensue following the initial diagnosis, but soon thereafter, they maintain high QoL and continue living rewarding, meaningful, and purposeful lives (17, 24,25). This heterogeneity in adjustment has led researchers to believe that individual factors, such as virtues and coping style, may contribute to positive adjustment, or resilience, in PALS (19,26). Selected instruments for assessing QoL, and the constructs assessed, can be found in Table 7.1.

Resilience

The exploration of resilience within the context of chronic illness has flourished since the recent growth of the positive psychology movement (27,28). There are a multitude of definitions for the construct 'resilience'(29); for the purposes of this chapter, resilience is defined as the capacity to maintain physical, psychological, social, spiritual, and environmental well-being in the face of adverse life events (28,30). Resilience does not imply an absence of difficulty or emotional upset nor does it represent an inherent personality trait (30,31). Rather, it is a lifelong process in which an individual develops core strengths and virtues that amass into a repertoire of behaviours and cognitions that help to sustain an individual in the face of adversity (29,31). As such, research in resilience involves the identification of vulnerability and protective factors that increase or decrease the likelihood of negative life outcomes (32). Vulnerability factors increase the probability of negative effects, whereas protective factors decrease the likelihood of negative outcomes. Such protective factors may include adequate coping skills and social support, optimism, and high self-efficacy (32).

Coping

Embedded within this definition of resilience is the capacity to cope with difficult life events. Coping, more broadly, is defined as a purposeful attempt to reduce, prevent, or control stress, and/or manage difficult situations (28,31). Within the coping literature, a distinction is made between coping resources and coping strategies (28). Coping strategies include the adaptive or maladaptive techniques or skills attempted or used to overcome obstacles in everyday life. Increasing adaptive coping strategies is often the focus of intervention for chronically- or terminally-ill patients and families (28,31). Coping resources are the individual characteristics that influence how an individual copes. They are the resources a person draws upon to manage obstacles, and can include personality characteristics, self-efficacy, health, and social support (28). Coping resources include changeable and unchangeable, adaptive and maladaptive variables and can promote or inhibit the availability of coping strategies (28). As such, an individual who has greater coping resources will have a larger repertoire of coping strategies from which to choose. The literature indicates that coping strategies differ in individuals with various

Table 7.1 Review of select measures of QoL, coping, and resilience factors

Measure	Construct(s) Assessed
Quality of life	
ALS Specific Quality of Life—Revised (ALSSQOL-R; Felgoise et al., 2011)(49)	Overall and domain-specific QoL for individuals with ALS
McGill Quality of Life Questionnaire (MQOL; Cohen et al., 2017)(112)	Multiple dimensions and overall QoL of people with a life-threatening illness
Quality of Life Inventory (QOLI; Frisch, 1994)(32)	Well-being and satisfaction with life across 16 domains ('Sweet Sixteen')
World Health Organization Quality of Life-BREF (WHOQOL-BREF; The WHOQOL Group, 1998)(113)	Physical, psychological, social, and environmental QoL
Coping	
Ways of Coping Questionnaire (WCQ; Folkman & Lazarus, 1988) (99)	Coping processes; thoughts and actions used to cope with stressful situations
Ways of Coping Checklist (WCC; Folkman & Lazarus, 1980)(100)	Coping based on the authors' stress and coping theory
Brief COPE (Carver, 1997)(101)	Dispositional and situational coping styles
Motor Neuron Disease Coping Scale (MNDCS; Lee et al., 2001) (102)	Coping strategies in PALS across six domains
Hope	
State Hope Scale (Snyder et al., 1996)(103)	State hope
Hope Scale (Snyder et al., 1991)(103)	Dispositional hope
Optimism	
Life Orientation Test-Revised (LOT-R; Scheier, Carver, & Bridges, 1994)(105)	Generalized optimism versus pessimism
Problem solving	
Social Problem Solving Inventory-Revised (SPSI-R) (D'Zurilla et al., 2002)(42)	Problem solving abilities (positive and negative)
Religiosity/spirituality	
Idler Index of Religiosity (IIR; Idler, 1987) (106)	Private and public religiousness
Brief Multidimensional Measure of Religiosity/Spirituality (BMMRS; Fetzer Institute, 1999)(107)	Health-relevant domains of religiousness and spirituality
Social Support and Relationships	
Social Support Questionnaire (SSQ; Sarason et al., 1983)(108)	Quantity and quality of self-perceived social support
Dyadic Adjustment Scale (DAS; Spanier, 1976)(109)	Couples' relationship satisfaction

(Continued)

Table 7.1 Continued

Measure	Construct(s) Assessed
Revised Dyadic Adjustment Scale (RDAS; Busby et al., 1995)(110)	Quality of marital relationships
Marital Adjustment Test (MAT; Locke & Wallace, 1959)(111)	Marital satisfaction and wellbeing

Source: Felgoise, S.H., Walsh, S.M., Stephens, H.E., Brothers, A., and Simmons, Z. The ALS Specific Quality of Life-Revised (ALSSQOL-R) User's Guide. 2011. Available at: http://www.pennstatehershey.org/c/document_library/get_file?uuid=b9de0a6a-9c1d-4f77-bdf0-5c6c846e018e&groupId=22147.

levels of resilience (33), within and across disease states (6,34), including ALS (35). Therefore, coping is viewed as one of many factors that contribute to resilience (28,31). Dyadic coping is a process by which individuals' coping styles interact and affect each others' in a partnered relationship. It has been described as the interplay between verbal and non-verbal stress signals exchanged between two individuals (36). Partners can be equally supportive to each other; have agreed on unequal coping responsibility; or engage in maladaptive dyadic coping in which the inequality raises hostility, ambivalence, or negativity in one or both partners. Handling of stressful situations and marital well-being are maximized with effective dyadic coping (37), which often requires effective use of individual coping strategies. Dyadic coping strategies are important to examine in the relationships of PALS, given their increased level of dependence for care.

Coping strategies have been classified, defined, and measured in numerous ways in the literature (38).Most commonly, cognitive, behavioural, and religious techniques are referenced. Examples of cognitive techniques include positively appraising situations; actively directing thoughts toward the past; rationalizing; trivializing; maintaining optimism and a fighting spirit (6). Behavioural strategies include active problem-solving efforts; seeking social support; seeking information; using humour; and activity engagement. Religious coping is sometimes considered a cognitive (religious thoughts, faith) strategy, behavioural (actively praying) strategy, or as an altogether separate category of these cognitive and behavioural coping strategies. Research suggests that a strong and secure attachment to God may be a resilience factor and positively impact psychological adjustment to a chronic or acute disease. In contrast, a poor attachment may have a negative impact in a number of ways, including obtaining social support and having a positive outlook on the disease (39). In a study of 147 patients with motor neuron disease, coping accounted for the most variance in QoL, mediated by anxiety and depression, in which 59% of QoL was predicted by a structural equation model of anxiety, coping, depression, fatigue, social withdrawal, and QoL (40). All of these strategies can be conceptualized through the Social Problem-Solving Model (41). Selected instruments for assessing coping, and the constructs assessed, can be found in Table 7.1.

Social Problem Solving Model and ALS

The Social Problem-Solving Model of Coping (42) is well known in the clinical health psychology literature (see (43) for a review). Social problem solving, and the component processes have been identified as key variables in understanding coping and resilience in PALS and their lay-caregivers. Understanding this model and clinical applications has potential benefits for those affected by ALS.

Problems are essentially a 'perceived or real imbalance' between the demands of the environment and one's personal resources (42). Coping attempts are any efforts made to reduce, prevent, control, or minimize stress (43), and effective problem-solving coping is defined as using a rational and systematic set of coping skills to change the problematic situation, one's reaction to it, or both. Effective coping results in finding solutions that maximize positive outcomes and minimize negative consequences of the problem-solving effort, while solving the problem. The theory of social problem solving (43) suggests problems consist of major life events (which are often unchangeable, such as a diagnosis of ALS), and daily problems, some of which result from the major life event (i.e. difficulty with ambulation, impaired communication, or eating); how one copes with these problems has been shown to affect distress and emotional well-being, and may lead to more or less additional problems, and ultimately affect overall QoL.

Social problem solving as an empirically-tested model of coping includes problem orientation variables, behavioural response styles, and social problem-solving skills (44). Problem orientation is the way people view their world. Persons holding a positive problem orientation most often view problems as solvable, and as challenges, while maintaining a hopeful, optimistic disposition about the problem(s) and their ability to solve it/them. Maintaining a negative problem orientation inhibits and interferes with effective problem solving, as persons with this orientation often view their ability to solve problems as limited, and hopeless. Problem orientation variables originate and are affected from cognitive variables that are modifiable through cognitive and behavioural interventions designed to help persons address and minimize cognitive distortions or unrealistic, inaccurate, or maladaptive ways of thinking about problematic situations, and oneself. Specifically, persons' appraisal; attributions and attributional style; perceptions of problems, solutions, and their solvability; and self-efficacy for coping greatly affect their motivation to solve problems in daily living, and to do so effectively. Research has shown control of negative affectivity and maintenance of a positive disposition, such as a positive problem orientation, is critical for setting and reaching goals, and solving problems effectively, achieving happiness, and ultimately having a positive QoL((32, p. 33).

Behavioural response styles are patterns of behaviour that are often developed over time based on social learning, reinforcement from the environment (people and circumstances), and probably temperament to some degree. These include an impulsive/careless approach to problem solving, in which any or all aspects of the problem-solving process may be circumvented and a solution may be implemented with little consideration of the potential consequences. This style of coping is generally ineffective, and leads to maladaptive outcomes. Similarly, an avoidant style of coping generally does not result in solving problems effectively, as any or all aspects of the problem-solving process may be minimized or unattended to entirely, and may also have significant negative consequences for individuals. A rational problem-solving style is optimal, and reflects a systematic way of thinking about problems in daily living. Persons with rational problem solving styles of coping systematically consider all aspects of the problem, the problem-solving goal, and obstacles to achieving the desired outcome. While adaptive or maladaptive behavioural response styles may develop naturally overtime, rational problem-solving skills can be taught and learned, and impulsive/careless or avoidant coping styles can be modified, countered, or extinguished with social problem-solving therapy and/or skills training (43). Having a positive problem orientation, and strong or adaptive social problem-solving skills are considered protective or resilience factors (45), and are associated with other resilience factors, such as hope, positive affect and optimism (i.e. (46)), happiness, and satisfaction with life or positive well-being (47). Such resilience factors are critical to best helping PALS and their caregivers cope with the many challenges of the disease and its daily impact.

Resilience Factors

Resilience factors have been examined in the ALS patient and caregiving literature (48–50). There are multiple pathways to resilience and a variety of internal and external factors have been identified as potential protective factors (51) that promote positive adjustment to ALS and the caregiving experience. Such resilience factors include hope, optimism, social problem solving, spirituality and religiosity, and social support and relationship satisfaction, as discussed below. Selected instruments for assessing these factors, and the constructs assessed, can be found in Table 7.1.

Hope

Hope is a feeling of expectation and desire for a certain outcome. Embedded within the construct of hope is goal-attainment, which is comprised of two inter-related cognitive sets: agency and pathways (52). Agency refers to the perceived ability to initiate and maintain a course of action to reach a stated goal, whereas pathways refer to the perceived ability to generate and revise a plan of action to attain a goal (52). Agency and pathways are different ways of thinking about goals, whereby agency can be viewed as the motivational component of hope and pathways reflects the planning or problem-solving component. Higher agency (e.g. 'I *can* reach my goal') and higher pathways (e.g. 'I know *how* to reach my goal') are associated with higher hope. Consistent with this theory, PALS with high hope should have the ability to effectively utilize their resources to confront the ALS diagnosis and manage living with it.

Hope has been described as a 'driving force' that facilitates positive adjustment to ALS in both PALS and their caregivers and is crucial to maintaining QoL (53). For PALS in particular, hope is a source of strength that sustains them through life with ALS, whereby the process of seeking hope allowed PALS to persevere in spite of their diagnosis (54). A study conducted by Rabkin and colleagues (25) identified an inverse relationship between depressive symptoms and hopefulness. This study also examined wish to die and findings demonstrated that PALS who had no wish to die had higher scores on measures of their capacity for pleasure, hope, and overall QoL than patients who endorsed a wish to die (25). In other studies, hope was associated with less hate and resentment toward ALS and increased motivation to follow medical advice (55). The literature demonstrates that hope is generally not related to physical functioning or demographic variables (48) and the meaning of hope can vary across individuals. For example, PALS identified several themes relevant to hope such as: hope for a cure, social support, search for information, spiritual beliefs, limiting the impact on others, adapting to changing capacities, living in the moment, and self-transcendence (48).

As is true for PALS, ALS caregivers also demonstrate hopeful thinking. Hope has shown its potential to buffer against the negative impact of ALS on caregivers' QoL. Felgoise and colleagues (49) examined resilience factors in a sample of ALS caregivers and identified hope as the best overall predictor of physical, psychological, social, and environmental QoL. Findings indicated that hope was a better predictor of positive adjustment than optimism, social problem solving, and spirituality/religiosity. Hope can take many forms within the ALS caregiving population and is not restricted to having hope for the patient, a cure, or related ideas. Rabkin et al. (26) reported that caregivers expressed hope in terms of believing in their ability to make it through the caregiving experience, looking forward to regaining one's life and identity, and recognizing that their role as caregiver was time-limited and not permanent (26). As such, hope can serve as a strong motivator for ALS caregivers.

Optimism

Optimism refers to a generalized expectancy that good things will happen (56). In the context of ALS, optimism has been associated with positive adjustment and is considered an important factor in coping (22) Nelson et al. (57) conducted a study with 100 PALS to identify factors related to QoL. A majority of PALS reported that positive personality factors such as optimism, humour, and flexibility helped to facilitate coping. Optimism has also been associated with self-esteem and self-worth (58), increased willingness to participate in alternative or contemporary therapies and fewer symptoms of depression (23). Another study identified an association between levels of optimism and the wish to die among PALS; those who expressed a wish to die reported less optimism, less comfort in religion, and greater hopelessness (19). Notable in this study is the cluster of resilience factors mentioned, which may indicate that certain resilience factors promote other resilience variables. Although less studied in the caregiving population, optimism can influence the experiences of ALS caregivers. For example, optimism promoted caregivers' acceptance of the ALS diagnosis and its associated losses (13). In this regard, caregivers with greater optimism had a tendency to positively reframe losses by shifting their focus on abilities rather than disabilities (13). Moreover, findings from a study conducted by Felgoise and colleagues (49) revealed that optimism contributed to ALS caregiver's QoL in the psychological, social, and environmental domains.

Problem solving

As previously discussed, the ability to effectively problem solve has also been identified as a predictor of QoL (35,59). Horowitz (60) revealed that poor social problem-solving skills were positively correlated with depression in PALS, and negative problem orientation predicted nearly 30% of the total variance for depression. The author concluded that negative problem orientation rather than physical functioning (i.e. physical and bulbar) predicted higher levels of depression in PALS. Collaborative problem solving between caregivers and healthcare providers promoted PALS' sense of autonomy and also contributed to predicting QoL in PALS in another study (61)). The literature also indicates that PALS who used less active or positive methods of coping reported more symptoms of depression and anxiety than those who endorsed an active/positive coping style (22).

In a sample of 75 ALS caregivers, social problem solving was identified as the best predictor of QoL and psychological morbidity (62). Caregivers using a positive problem orientation and rational response style demonstrated the best overall QoL and the lowest overall psychological morbidity in this study. Similarly, Rabkin et al. (26) reported that depressed caregivers had a tendency to rely on avoidance strategies rather than devising a plan of action. Effective problem solving can also have a significant positive impact on caregivers' physical and psychological QoL (49). The ALS caregiving population has reported that problem solving provides a sense of control and helps them to cope with the emotional impact of watching their loved ones live with ALS (13).

Spirituality and religiosity

ALS provides a unique opportunity to examine the role of spirituality and religiosity in patient and caregiver adjustment to adversity. Religiosity refers to the affiliation with an organized system of beliefs, practices, and rituals that facilitates connection to the sacred or divine (63,64). Spirituality is existential in nature and involves a search for meaning and purpose in life through any type of life experience (63). This may include a search for a higher power, but is generally independent of a particular doctrine or institutional context. A number of studies have shown that religiosity and spirituality contribute to positive outcomes in PALS and their caregivers (50,62,65).

Studies on ALS have reported correlations between organized religion and/or spiritual activities and higher QoL, psychological well-being, social satisfaction, and hopefulness, and a more optimistic outlook on the disease process (66–68). Weller (20) reported a significant inverse relationship between PALS' negative emotions and level of forgiveness, daily spiritual practices, subjective ratings of overall religiosity, and public and private religious activities. Religiosity and spirituality can have differential impacts on PALS. For example, one study suggested that religious faith sustained PALS and helped them to avoid despair, whereas personal spirituality helped them to make sense of their experience with ALS (50). The ALS literature focusing on religiosity indicates that religious beliefs and practice can assist PALS with the coping process. In particular, PALS have indicated that their religious beliefs enabled them to see value in their remaining time and accept their illness and losses (61). Similarly, religious beliefs also guided PALS in interpreting the meaning of the illness experience while also providing them with a source of comfort and serenity (57,69). Stutzki et al. (70) reported that religiosity predicted PALS who were likely to consider assisted suicide or euthanasia. In regard to spirituality, stronger spiritual beliefs were also associated with less interest in hastening death in a sample of PALS (71) and also correlated with decision-making about medical technology, greater hope, and fewer concerns about death (62,67).

The positive effects of PALS' religiosity and/or spirituality can extend to the caregiver. A study demonstrated that higher levels of existential well-being in PALS was associated with higher QoL in their caregivers, and lower levels of depression, anxiety, and burden (72). Stewart Allen (73) also reported PALS' self-ratings of existential well-being were positively correlated with caregiver existential well-being and support. Furthermore, caregivers' level of spirituality and religiousness have also been identified as predictors of their QoL and life satisfaction (62,65). In particular, private religiousness and greater spirituality are positively related to QoL (62,65).

Social support and relationship satisfaction

Social relationships and support networks appear to play an important role in the adjustment to living with ALS. Social support can emanate from multiple sources including spouses, family, friends, and healthcare providers (25,74,75). The positive effects of social support on the experiences of PALS has been explored in the literature. For example, Matuz and colleagues (74) indicated that high levels of perceived social support significantly predicted higher QoL and fewer depressive symptoms in PALS. These authors concluded that a supportive and uncritical social environment promoted effective coping, encouraged positive health behaviours, and diminished physiological response to stress in a sample of PALS. A qualitative study revealed that family relationships strongly influenced PALS' attitudes towards life and their decisions regarding symptoms management (76). Persons with ALS have also reported that support provided by healthcare professionals helped facilitate coping (61,76). These positive experiences were cultivated by providers who listened and provided information to PALS while also respecting PALS' wishes and choices through the use of collaborative problem solving (62).

Social support also promotes resilience among ALS caregivers(77,78). For example, a study that examined life factors contributing to depression and burden identified social support as the only protective factor in caregivers' lives as it was associated with lower levels of burden (11). Additionally, caregivers who connected with other ALS caregivers reported that these experiences provided a sense of fellowship, emotional support, and increased understanding of the caregiving experience (5). Positive outcomes have also been associated with caregivers' connection with family, friends, and professional caregivers (12,77,79).

Satisfaction with social support can also influence the marital relationships of PALS and their caregivers (79,80). Marital relationship satisfaction has not received as much empirical attention as social support; however, the available literature suggests that this construct is equally important insofar as PALS and their caregivers can influence each other's QoL and oftentimes patient-caregiver dyads are spouses or partners. Living with ALS involves intense emotional experiences that can influence the relationship between patient and caregiver (81). There is evidence to suggest that these intensive experiences can strengthen relationships among patient-caregivers and their families, with some caregivers describing deeper connections and mutual support as rewarding aspects of caregiving (77). One study reported that the personal relationship between patient and caregiver gave meaning to the illness experience in which the act of giving and receiving care represented an intimate and relational experience associated with spousal role fulfilment (10). Further, Rodriguez (82) revealed high levels of physical, emotional, and social intimacy in PALS-caregiver couples and indicated that factors such as gender, age, duration of symptoms, and physical and bulbar functioning were not predictors of level of, desire for, or satisfaction with intimate relationships. Similarly, the literature indicates that marital satisfaction is not associated with caregivers' perception of their competency in fulfilling their caregiving role and responsibilities (73). Adequate social support can mitigate negative effects of ALS on the marital relationship satisfaction (79,80). As such, support from friends and family can have a positive impact on the QoL of patient and caregiver individually, as well as on their marital relationship (80).

Therapeutic interventions: Current practices and future directions

Resilience can be built, encouraged, and reinforced by support persons and professionals across disciplines. Research is limited in this area; however, a few studies have noted PALS and their caregivers appear to benefit from dignity therapy (83), Buddhist psychology and mindfulness-based interventions (84,85), and the development of strong, supportive communication styles with healthcare providers (1,8). Key therapeutic interventions that are empirically-supported for other medical populations (i.e. cancer, spinal-cord injuries, renal disease), such as social problem-solving therapy (41,43). Quality of Life Therapy (QOLT) (32), and grief therapy using a constructivist approach (86) seem indicated for effective use with PALS and caregivers, though not yet specifically tested in these populations. Overall, the therapies and interventions described below are consistent in their goal to improve resilience and coping.

Communication

The communication of the diagnosis can be among the most impactful experiences for PALS and their caregivers (87,88). If the news is delivered in a clear, supportive manner, with sufficient opportunities to ask questions, and to discuss fears and concerns, the receipt of the diagnosis can be somewhat relieving for some patients (89). For others, receiving the diagnosis can be traumatic (1,8), especially if the diagnosis was delayed, delivered in an unsupportive manner or without attention to psychological needs. Patients have reported not understanding the disease or how to manage it accurately, and did not receive necessary information from their healthcare providers (1). Information was often obtained from others on the internet. Thus, physicians may provide a primary intervention by learning to deliver 'bad' news optimally. The SPIKES technique, originally designed for delivery of bad news relating to a cancer diagnosis, has a useful formula that is generalizable for communicating effectively with PALS (90). Recognizing the impact the initial conversations with PALS and their caregivers may have on their coping and other resilience factors, hopelessness, and overall psychological disposition, it is highly recommended that a counsellor or psychologist be present during the delivery of the diagnosis or shortly thereafter, to provide psychosocial support and resources.

Dignity therapy

Dignity therapy is a brief approach (averaging 12 hours) to psychosocial patient care based on an empirically-validated model of dignity in terminally-ill people in which persons discuss 'issues that matter most or that they would most want remembered about their life' (83, p. 32). Therapy sessions follow a semi-structured interview that focuses on this content. The goal of therapy is to generate a transcript that is synthesized, edited, and returned to the patient to share with or leave for family members or friends after death. Caregivers can be guided through a similar process. Creating this legacy document was viewed as a positive experience for persons with motor neuron diseases and caregivers, independently in a study of Italian participants. Dignity therapy reportedly helped patients and caregivers attend to 'unfinished business,' 'feel like themselves,' and recognize their capability of 'filling an important role.' However, while viewed as acceptable and feasible, the study of persons with motor neuron disease and caregivers did not show effectiveness for either sample in improving QoL, spiritual wellbeing, caregiver burden, or decreasing distress or hopelessness. Perhaps these findings are due to low distress in the samples overall. Or, it is possible that Dignity Therapy does not directly reduce distress, but rather builds resilience and is a form of positive coping and meaning making, and is therefore well received. Further studies specifically with PALS and caregivers seem warranted to determine the reasons participants reviewed this intervention as important and helpful, and the ways in which they felt helped.

Buddhist psychology and mindfulness-based interventions

Buddhist philosophy purports that the life cycle consists of life, death, and rebirth in a cyclical and continuous process, and not in a dualistic fashion of life-death, as held in Western traditions (84). Buddhist followers also believe that 'life is suffering' and includes sickness, aging, and death ((84), p. 663). Acceptance of all aspects of life and experiences are to be mindfully observed and used to grow as a human being (84).

According to Buddhist tradition, persons' six senses (sixth is thinking) and reactions to the experiences of these senses create cognitions and affect that lead to cravings or aversions. Behaviours respond to these cravings and aversions and create 'relationships among cognition, affect, actions, and their effects' (84, p. 661). Persons are encouraged to be mindful of their experiences through their senses and their reactions to them. Compassion and self-compassion are critical components to allowing this process to unfold.

The emphasis of this philosophy as applied to grief work is that the process should not be pathologized, and grieving and bereaved individuals should be empowered to observe and be mindful of their own growth process and ever-changing relationships held previously and currently with the deceased (in the case of caregivers, and in the dying process for PALS) (84). Mindfulness-based approaches based on Buddhist philosophy are in contrast to Western philosophy is viewed as task-orientated. For instance, some suggest Western philosophies require bereaved individuals to 'work through' grief and 'get over the loss' or 'move on.'

Thus, new age therapies such as Acceptance and Commitment Therapy (85), and other mindfulness-based approaches would aim to help PALS and caregivers to experience their emotions and losses in a non-judgmental way and accept their life and impending death with compassion and comfort. This approach is consistent with building and increasing resilience. Mindfulness has just recently gained attention in the ALS literature (90) and has been found to be predictive of better psychological well-being and QoL in a longitudinal observational study (see also Chapter 4). Furthermore, PALS who reported more mindfulness had a slower disease progression over four months.

The Dual Process Model (91) borrows from Buddhist and Western philosophies. This model suggests effective intervention for persons in grief is to facilitate both loss-oriented coping (through emotional expression and experiencing or 'being') and restoration-oriented coping (i.e. learning new roles and skills to adjust to the resultant changes of loss, or 'doing') (91). 'Being' allows for meaning making of the loss and related experiences by 'bridging' the experiencing and the explaining of these events and losses (84). 'Doing' reflects efforts toward tasks that are goal-oriented and is consistent with a Western approach to grief work.

Several therapies that may be effective for PALS and caregivers may be consistent with the Dual Process Model: Social Problem-solving Therapy (PST) and Contemporary PST, Constructivist Approach to Grief Therapy (86), and QOLT (32). Each of these models of therapy contain aspects of problem solving and a focus on strengths, meaning, and an individualized approach to improving well-being and resilience. For PALS and their caregivers, these therapies offer models to address current salient problems, construction of short-term and long-term goals, consider future concerns, develop an understanding of the current circumstances in the context of one's own life, and process emotional reactions to the diagnosis and experience of living with ALS.

Social problem-solving therapy

SPS Therapy aims to help individuals and couples decrease their emotional distress, improve their problem-solving skills, increase their sense of control, and improve their overall QoL (41). This social competence model has been empirically-validated as an effective treatment for persons with cancer and their significant others. It has also been modified and applied to numerous other medical populations (42). SPS is designed to increase coping, which could be accomplished by changing problematic situations, one's reaction to the situations, or both. As such, the model allows for specific ALS-related problems to be considered, one's emotional reaction to the diagnosis, experiences, and losses associated with ALS. This therapeutic intervention was originally designed as a ten session protocol, but has also been used partially on the phone, in groups, and as an adjunctive therapy to others. As such, it is flexible to meet individual needs. Variations of SPS therapy and skills training have also been used in primary care medical settings successfully with older adults (92,93), veterans (94), and depressed adults (95), therefore, it is likely to be adapted to an ALS patient-care environment.

The core sessions of SPS include key elements of cognitive-behavioural therapy: development of a therapeutic relationship and safe environment, and agenda setting, and use of cognitive behavioural principles and techniques. Sessions include focusing on introduction and assessment, problem orientation (emphasis on worldview and emotions), behavioural response style, and rational problem solving skills (problem definition and formulation, generation of alternatives, decision making, and solution implementation and verification) (41). Because SPS is a reciprocal process and not always linear, problem orientation variables are discussed and revisited throughout therapy. The structure of this therapy allows integration of other techniques and interventions, couples work, and development of short-term and long-term goals and plans for living with ALS, and end-of-life care and topics, if so desired. In keeping with The Dual Process Model, tasks of problem solving, and emotional acceptance and coping can be well-addressed, while examining meaning in one's life in the past, present, and future. Contemporary SPS (43) incorporates all aspects of SPS in the context of four tool kits:

- multitasking and cognitive overload;
- emotional dysregulation and maladaptive problem solving;
- healthy thinking and positive imagery;
- planful problem solving.

The core principles are the same, with additional attention to cognitive skills, motivation, and increased emphasis on mindfulness-based approaches to coping. While this model has been less the focus of research, it is also likely adaptable for PALS and caregivers.

Constructivist Grief Therapy

Constructivist Grief therapy is based on principles consistent with cognitive behaviour therapy and is steeped in personal construct theory (96). The primary goal of constructivist grief therapy is to help individuals cope by finding and creating new meaning and a new conceptualization for their change in life circumstances, anticipated, tangible or intangible loss. This therapeutic approach recognizes the significant and permanent changes brought about by loss, and highlights an acceptance of one's reality changing forever. In this process, sense making, benefit finding, and identity change are examined and encouraged. Persons are guided through the process of constructing new purpose in their lives, and establishing new relationships with their lost loved ones, or lost functions, for example. The bereaved or persons anticipating loss begin to think of their life in a new way, in light of the loss.

Constructivist Grief Therapy suggests the hardest losses to accept and cope with are those that don't 'make sense,' arguably, such as a diagnosis of ALS. People try to find reasons, ask 'why'—'why this, why this person/me?'... to try to create understanding, predictability, and meaning. Each PALS and their family members may construct different personal answers to these ultimately unanswerable questions. Research suggests participants in constructivist grief therapy experience personal growth, increased resilience, independence, confidence, improved social relationships and appreciation for life. Thus, the individual and purposeful structure of this therapy may be well suited for PALS and their caregivers.

Quality of life therapy

QOLT (32) is an empirically-supported theoretically derived therapy based on the principles of positive psychology, cognitive and behavioural therapies, and consistent with behavioural medicine. The strength of this therapy as it applies to PALS and caregivers is its emphasis on evaluating and addressing aspects of one's life across 16 key domains. These 16 domains include: health, self-esteem, goals and values/spiritual life, money, work, play, learning, creativity, helping, love, friends, children, relatives, home, neighbourhood, and community (32, p. 23).

QOLT is purported to be useful as a life coaching approach, or therapeutic adjuvant or primary protocol. Rather than approaching therapy from a problem reduction viewpoint, QOLT focuses on building and strengthening resilience. As PALS and caregivers are constantly experiencing changes in ambulation, ability to travel, communicate, or enjoy activities of daily living, QOLT encourages problem solving to increase and enhance areas of life that may be important and modifiable, given physical, cognitive, and emotional changes. Likewise, caregivers may evaluate and modify the 'Sweet 16' as life circumstances change over the course of the PALS illness and decline, and after their loved ones' death. QOLT provides specific interventions for each area affecting QoL that can facilitate dyadic coping, individual coping, development of new resilience, and improvement in QoL overall. The overarching goals of QOLT that undoubtedly apply to PALS and caregivers are as follows: '(1) increasing and improving "inner abundance" and experience, 2) increasing the amount of "quality time" the client experiences, and (3) increasing the client's meaning and purpose in life' (32, p. vii).

Summary

Considerable advances have been made in our understanding of the biopsychosocial-spiritual challenges confronted by PALS and their caregivers (8,97). Despite these challenges, some PALS and caregivers report positive adjustment and appear to demonstrate resilience in the face of adversity. The resilience literature reveals that factors such as hope, optimism, and social support can promote well-being and facilitate coping (49,57). Exploration of these protective factors is critical to understanding how to best help PALS and their caregivers cope with the many challenges of the disease and its daily impact((8)). In the absence of a cure, psychosocial-spiritual interventions aimed at understanding or bolstering resilience and coping are important foci of investigation. For instance, identifying ways to increase resilience, specifically through the development of social problem-solving skills, may lead to improved QoL for this population. As such, this review highlighted interventions aimed at enhancing resilience factors and coping, such as social problem solving therapy, QOLT, and mindfulness-based techniques. These interventions have been studied in other medical populations (32,43); however, limited attention has been given to the study of psychosocial-spiritual interventions within the ALS population (8,98). Future research is needed to address this significant gap in the literature.

References

1. **Cipolletta, S.** and **Amicucci, L.** (2014) The family experience of living with a person with amyotrophic lateral sclerosis: A qualitative study. *International Journal of Psychology*, **50**(4), 288–94.

2. **Obermann, M.** and **Lyon, M.** (2015) Financial cost of amyotrophic lateral sclerosis: A case study. *Amyotrophic Lateral Sclerosis and Frontotemporal Degeneration*, **16**, 54–7.

3. **Averill, A.J., Kasarskis, E.J.**, and **Segerstrom, S.C.** (2007) Psychological health in patients with amyotrophic lateral sclerosis. *Amyotrophic Lateral Sclerosis*, **8**(4), 243–54.

4. **Chen, Z., Guo, X., Zheng, Z.**, et al. (2015) Depression and anxiety in amyotrophic lateral sclerosis: Correlations between the distress of patients and caregivers. *Muscle & Nerve*, **51**(3), 353–7.

5. **Ozanne, A.O., Graneheim, U.H., Persson, L.**, and **Strang, S.** (2011) Factors that facilitate and hinder the manageability of living with amyotrophic lateral sclerosis in both patients and next of kin. *Journal of Clinical Nursing*, **21**(9–10),1364–73.

6. **Hecht, M.J., Hillemacher, T., Grasel E.**, et al. (2002) Subjective experience and coping in ALS. *Amyotrophic Lateral Sclerosis and Other Motor Neuron Disorders*, **3**(4), 225–32.

7. **Tramonti, F., Barsanti, I., Bongioanni, P., Bogliolo, C.**, and **Rossi, B.** (2014) A permanent emergency: A longitudinal study on families coping with amyotrophic lateral sclerosis. *Families, Systems & Health*, **32**(3), 271–9.

8. **Pagnini, F., Rossi, G., Lunetta, C.**, et al. (2010) Burden, depression, and anxiety in caregivers of people with amyotrophic lateral sclerosis. *Psychological Health Medicine*, **15**(6), 685–93.

9. **Aoun, S.M., Connors, S.L., Priddis, L., Breen, L.**, and **Colyer, S.** (2012) Motor neurone disease family carers' experiences of caring, palliative care and bereavement: An exploratory qualitative study. *Palliative Medicine*, **26**(6), 842–50.

10. **Lerum, S.V., Solbraekke, K.N.**, and **Frich, J.C.** (2016) Family caregivers' accounts of caring for a family member with motor neurone disease in Norway: A qualitative study. *BMC Palliative Care*, **15**(1), 22.

11. **Qutub, K., Lacomis, D., Albert, S.M.**, and **Feingold, E.** (2014) Life factors affecting depression and burden in amyotrophic lateral sclerosis caregivers. *Amyotrophic Lateral Sclerosis and Frontotemporal Degeneration*, **15**(3–4), 292–7.

12. **Aoun, S.M., Bentley, B., Funk, L., Toye, C., Grande, G.**, and **Stajduhar, K.J.** (2013) A 10-year literature review of family caregiving for motor neurone disease: Moving from caregiver burden studies to palliative care interventions. *Palliative Medicine*, **27**(5), 437–46.

13. **Oyebode, J.R., Smith, H.**, and **Morrison, K.** (2013) The personal experience of partners of individuals with motor neuron disease. *Amyotrophic Lateral Sclerosis and Frontotemporal Degeneration*, **14**, 39–43.

14. **Burke, T., Elamin, M., Galvin, M., Hardiman, O.**, and **Pender, N.** (2015) Caregiver burden in amyotrophic lateral sclerosis: A cross-sectional investigation of predictors. *Journal of Neurology*, **262**,1526–32.

15. **Simmons, Z.** (2015) Patient-perceived outcomes and quality of life in ALS. *Neurotherapeutics*, **12**, 394–402.

16. **Kubler, A., Winter, S., Ludolph, A.C., Hautzinger, M.**, and **Birbaumer, N.** (2005) Severity of depressive symptoms and quality of life in patients with amyotrophic lateral sclerosis. *Neurorehabilitation and Neural Repair*, **19**(3), 182–93.

17. **Roach, A.R., Averill, A.J., Segerstrom, S.C.**, and **Kasarakis, E.J.** (2009) The dynamics of quality of life in ALS patients and caregivers. *Annals of Behavioural Medicine*, **37**, 197–206.

18. **Chio, A., Gauthier, A., Montuschi, A.**, et al. (2004) A cross-sectional study on determinants of quality of life in ALS. *Journal of Neurology, Neurosurgery & Psychiatry*, **75**(11), 1597–601.

19. **Rabkin, J.G., Wagner, G.J.**, and **Del Bene, M.** (2000) Resilience and distress among amyotrophic lateral sclerosis patients and caregivers. *Psychosomatic Medicine*, **62**(2), 271–9.

20. **Weller, A.B.** (2009) Caregiver religiosity, spirituality, and positive emotion as predictors of psychological well-being in amyotrophic lateral sclerosis patients. *PCOM Psychology Dissertations*, **145**, 1–149. Available at: http://digitalcommons.pcom.edu/psychology_dissertations/145 (accessed 25 July 2017).

21. **Ganzini, L., Johnston, W.S., and Hoffman, W.F.** (1999) Correlates of suffering in amyotrophic lateral sclerosis. *Neurology*, **52**(7), 1434–40.

22. **Larsson, B.J., Nordin, K., Askmark, H., and Nygren, I.** (2014) Coping strategies among patients with newly diagnosed amyotrophic lateral sclerosis. *Journal of Clinical Nursing*, **23**(21–22), 3148–55.

23. **Larsson, B.J., Nordin, K., and Nygren, I.** (2016) Coping with amyotrophic lateral sclerosis; from diagnosis and during disease progression. *Journal of Neurological Sciences*, **361**, 235–42.

24. **Mock, S. and Boerner, K.** (2010) Sense making and benefit finding among patients with amyotrophic lateral sclerosis and their primary caregivers. *Journal of Health Psychology*, **15**(1), 115–21.

25. **Rabkin, J.G., Goetz, R., Factor-Litvak, P.,** et al. (2015) Depression and wish to die in a multi-center cohort of ALS patients. *Amyotrophic Lateral Sclerosis and Frontotemporal Degeneration*, **16**(3–4), 265–73.

26. **Rabkin, J.G., Albert, S.M., Rowland, L.P., and Mitsumoto, H.** (2009) How common is depression among ALS caregivers? A longitudinal study. *Amyotrophic Lateral Sclerosis*, **10**, 448–55.

27. **Aspinwall, L.G. and Tedeschi, R,G.** (2010) The value of positive psychology for health psychology: Progress and pitfalls in examining the relation of positive phenomena to health. *Annals of Behavioural Medicine*, **39**, 4–15.

28. **Muller, R., Ward, P.R., Winefield, T., Tsourtos, G., and Lawn, S.** (2009) The importance of resilience to primary care practitioners: An interactive psycho-social model. *Australasian Medicine*, **1**(1), 1–15.

29. **Limardi, S., Stievano, A., Rocco, G., Vellone, E., and Alvaro, R.** (2015) Caregiver resilience in palliative care: A research protocol. *Journal of Advanced Nursing*, **72**(2), 421–33.

30. **Luthar, S.S. and Cicchetti, D.** (2000) The construct of resilience: Implications for interventions and social policies. *Developmental Psychopathology*, **12**(4), 857–85.

31. **Leipold, B. and Greve, W.** (2009) Resilience: A conceptual bridge between coping and development. *European Psychology*, **14**(1), 40–50.

32. **Frisch, M.B.** (2013) *Quality of Life Therapy: Applying a Life Satisfaction Approach to Positive Psychology and Cognitive Therapy*, 2nd edn. Hoboken, NJ: John Wiley & Sons, Inc;.

33. **Joyce, P.Y., Smith, R.E., and Vitaliano, P.P.** (2005) Stress-resilience, illness, and coping: A person-focused investigation of young women athletes. *Journal of Behavioural Medicine*, **28**(3), 257–65.

34. **Ahlstrom, G. and Wenneberg, S.** (2002) Coping with illness-related problems in persons with progressive muscular diseases: The Swedish version of the Ways of Coping Questionnaire. *Scandinavian Journal of Caring Sciences*, **16**(4), 368–75.

35. **Montel, S., Albertini, L., Desnuelle, C., and Spitz, E.** (2012) The impact of active coping strategies on survival in ALS: The first pilot study. *Amyotrophic Lateral Sclerosis*, **13**(6), 599–601.

36. **Bodenmann, G.** (2005) Dyadic coping and its significance for marital functioning. In: Revenson, T., Kayser, K., and Bodenmann, G. (eds) Couples Coping with

Stress: Emerging Perspectives on Dyadic Coping, pp. 33–50. Washington, DC: American Psychological Association.

37. **Wunderer, E.** and **Schneewind, K.A.** (2008). The relationship between marital standards, dyadic coping, and marital satisfaction. *European Journal of Social Psychology*, **38**, 462–76.

38. **Skinner, E.A., Edge, K., Altman, J.,** and **Sherwood, H.** (2003) Searching for the structure of coping: A review and critique of category systems for classifying ways of coping. *Psychology Bulletin*, **129**(2), 216–69.

39. **Cassibba, R., Papagna, S., Calabrese, M.T., Costantino, E., Paterno, A.,** and **Granqvist, P.** (2014) The role of attachment to God in secular and religious/spiritual ways of coping with a serious disease. *Mental Health and Religious Culture*, **17**(3), 252–61.

40. **Gibbons, C., Thornton, E., Ealing, J.,** et al. (2013) The impact of fatigue and psychosocial variables on quality of life for patients with motor neuron disease. *Amyotrophic Lateral Sclerosis and Frontotemporal Degeneration*, **14**(7–8), 537–45.

41. **Nezu, A.M., Nezu, C.M., Friedman, S.H., Faddis, S.,** and **Houts, P.S.** (1999) *Helping Cancer Patients Cope: A Problem-solving Approach.* Washington, DC: APA Press.

42. **D'Zurilla, T.J., Nezu, A.M.,** and **Maydeu-Olivares, A.** (2002) *Social Problem-solving Inventory-revised (SPSI-R).* North Tonawanda, NY: Multihealth Systems, Inc.

43. **Nezu, A.M., Nezu, C.M.,** and **D'Zurilla, T.J.** (2013) *Problem-solving Therapy: A Treatment Manual.* New York, NY: Springer Publishing Company, LLC.

44. **Nezu, A.M., Nezu, C.M.,** and **D'Zurilla, T.J.** (2007) *Solving Life's Problems: A 5-step Guide to Enhanced Well-being.* New York, NY: Springer.

45. **Bell, A.C.** and **D'Zurilla, T.J.** (2009). The influence of social problem-solving ability on the relationship between daily stress and adjustment. *Cognitive Therapeutic Research*, **33**, 439–48.

46. **Webster Nelson, D.** and **Sim, E.K.** (2014) Positive affect facilitates social problem solving. *Journal of Applied Social Psychology*, **44**(10), 635–42.

47. **Chang, E.C., D'Zurilla, T.J.,** and **Sanna, L.J.** (2009) Social problem solving as a mediator of the link between stress and psychological well-being in middle-adulthood. *Cognitive Therapeutic Research*, **33**(1), 33–49.

48. **Fanos, J.H., Gelinas, D.F., Foster, R.S., Postone, N.,** and **Miller, R.G.** (2008) Hope in palliative care: From narcissism to self-transcendence in amyotrophic lateral sclerosis. *Journal of Palliative Medicine*, **11**(3), 470–5.

49. **Felgoise, S.H., Dube, M.L., Chakraborty, B.,** and **Simmons, Z.** (2016) Resilience factors: Predictors of quality of life in family caregivers of patients with amyotrophic lateral sclerosis. Manuscript submitted for publication.

50. **O'Brien, M.R.** and **Clark, D.** (2015) Spirituality and/or religious faith: A means for coping with the effects of amyotrophic lateral sclerosis/motor neuron disease? *Palliative Support Care*, **13**(6), 1603–14.

51. **Seligman, M.E.** and **Csikszentmihalyi, M.** (2000) Positive psychology: An introduction. *American Psychologist*, **55**(1), 5–14.

52. **Snyder, C.R.** (2002) Hope theory: Rainbows in the mind. *Psychology Inquiry*, **13**(4), 249–75.

53. **Mitsumoto, H.** and **Del Bene, M.** (2000) Improving the quality of life for people with ALS: The challenge ahead. *Amyotrophic Lateral Sclerosis and Other Motor Neuron Disorders*, **1**(5), 329–36.

54. **Brown, J.** and **Addington-Hall, J.** (2008) How people with motor neurone disease talk about living with their illness: A narrative study. *Journal of Advanced Nursing*, **62**(2), 200–8.

55. **Oster, C.** and **Pagnini, F.** (2012) Resentment, hate, and hope in amyotrophic lateral sclerosis. *Frontiers in Psychology*, **3**, 530.

56. **Carver, C.S.**, **Scheier, M.F.**, and **Segerstrom, S.C.** (2010) Optimism. *Clinical Psychological Review*, **30**, 879–89.

57. **Nelson, N.D.**, **Trail, M.**, **Van, J.N.**, **Appel, S.H.**, and **Lai, E.C.** (2003) Quality of life in patients with amyotrophic lateral sclerosis: Perceptions, coping resources, and illness characteristics. *Journal of Palliative Medicine*, **6**(3), 417–24.

58. **King, S.J.**, **Duke, M.M.**, and **O'Connor, B.A.** (2009) Living with amyotrophic lateral sclerosis/motor neurone disease (ALS/MND): Decision-making about 'ongoing change and adaptation.' *Journal of Clinical Nursing*, **18**(5), 745–54.

59. **Ng, L.** and **Khan, F.** (2011). Identification of personal factors in motor neurone disease: A pilot study. *Rehabilitation Research and Practice*, Article ID 871237. doi:10.1186/s12955-015-0214-8

60. **Horowitz, M.D.** (2008) Does social problem-solving moderate the relationship between physical functioning and depression in ALS patients? *PCOM Psychology Dissertations*, **64**, 1–83.

61. **Foley, G.**, **O'Mahony, P.**, and **Hardiman, O.** (2007) Perceptions of quality of life in people with ALS: Effects of coping and health care. *Amyotrophic Lateral Sclerosis*, **8**(3), 164–9.

62. **Murphy, V.**, **Felgoise, S.H.**, **Walsh, S.M.**, and **Simmons, Z.** (2009) Problem solving skills predict quality of life and psychological morbidity in ALS caregivers. *Amyotrophic Lateral Sclerosis*, **10**(3), 147–53.

63. **Hill, P.**, **Pargament, K.**, **Hood, R.**, et al. (2000) Conceptualizing religion and spirituality: Points of commonality, points of departure. *Journal of the Theory of Social Behaviour*, **30**(1), 51–77.

64. **Tsang, J.** and **McCullough, M.** (2004) Measuring religious constructs: A hierarchical approach to construct organization and scale selection. In: Lopez, S. and Snyder, C. (eds) *Positive Psychological Assessment: A Handbook of Models and Measures*, pp. 345–60. Washington, DC: American Psychological Association.

65. **Calvo, A.**, **Moglia, C.**, **Ilardi, A.**, et al. (2011) Religiousness is positively associated with quality of life of ALS caregivers. *Amyotrophic Lateral Sclerosis*, **12**, 168–71.

66. **Dal Bello-Haas, V.**, **Andrews-Hinders, D.**, **Bocian, J.**, **Mascha, E.**, **Wheeler, T.**, and **Mitsumoto, H.** (2000) Spiritual well-being of the individual with amyotrophic lateral sclerosis. *Amyotrophic Lateral Sclerosis*, **1**(5), 337–41.

67. **Murphy, P.L.**, **Albert, S.M.**, **Weber, C.M.**, **Del Bene, M.L.**, and **Rowland, L.P.** (2000) Impact of spirituality and religiousness on outcomes in patients with ALS. *Neurology*, **55**(10), 1581–4.

68. **Walsh, S.M.**, **Bremer, B.A.**, **Felgoise, S.H.**, and **Simmons, Z.** (2005) Religiousness is related to quality of life in patients with ALS. *Neurology*, **60**(9), 1527–9.

69. **McLeod, J.E.** and **Clarke, D.M.** (2007) A review of psychosocial aspects of motor neurone disease. *Journal of Neurological Sciences*, **258**, 4–10.

70. **Stutzki, R.**, **Weber, M.**, **Reiter-Theil, S.**, **Summen, U.**, **Borasio, G.D.**, and **Jox, R.J.** (2014) Attitudes towards hastened death in ALS: A prospective study of patients and family caregivers. *Amyotrophic Lateral Sclerosis and Frontotemporal Degeneration*, **15**(1–2), 68–76.

71. **Rabkin, J.G.**, **Albert, S.M.**, **Del Bene, M.L.**, et al. (2005) Prevalence of depressive disorders and change over time in late-stage ALS. *Neurology*, **65**(1), 62–7.

72. **Pagnini, F., Lunetta, C., Rossi, G.,** et al. (2011) Existential well-being and spirituality of individuals with amyotrophic lateral sclerosis is related to psychological well-being of their caregivers. *Amyotrophic Lateral Sclerosis*, **12**(2), 105–8.

73. **Stewart Allen, J.** (2004) Caregivers' relationship satisfaction and perception of competency as predictors of quality of life for ALS patients. *PCOM Psychology Dissertations*, **133**, 1–139. Available at: http://digitalcommons.pcom.edu/psychology_dissertations/133 (accessed 25 July 2017).

74. **Matuz, T., Birbaumer, N., Hautzinger, M.,** and **Kubler, A.** (2015) Psychosocial adjustment to ALS: A longitudinal study. *Frontiers in Psychology*, **6**, 1197.

75. **Neudert, C., Wasner, M.,** and **Borasio, G.D.** (2004) Individual quality of life is not correlated with health-related quality of life or physical function in patients with amyotrophic lateral sclerosis. *Journal of Palliative Medicine*, **7**(4), 551–7.

76. **Hogden, A., Greenfield, D., Nugus, P.,** and **Kiernan, M.C.** (2010). What influences patient decision-making in amyotrophic lateral sclerosis multidisciplinary care? A study of patient perspectives. *Patient Preference and Adherence*, **6**, 829–38.

77. **Weisser, F.B., Bristowe, K.,** and **Jackson, D.** (2015) Experiences of burden, needs, rewards and resilience in family caregivers of people living with motor neurone disease/amyotrophic lateral sclerosis: A secondary thematic analysis of qualitative interviews. *Palliative Medicine*, **29**(8), 737–45.

78. **Goldstein, L.H., Atkins, L., Landau, S., Brown, R.G.,** and **Leigh, P.N.** (2006) Longitudinal predictors of psychological distress and self-esteem in people with ALS. *Neurology*, **67**(9), 1652–8.

79. **O'Connor, E.J., McCabe, M.P.,** and **Firth, L.** (2008) The impact of neurological illness on marital relationships. *Journal of Sex and Marital Therapy*, **34**(2), 115–32.

80. **Atkins, L., Brown, R.G., Leigh, P.N.,** and **Goldstein, L.H.** (2010) Marital relationships in amyotrophic lateral sclerosis. *Amyotrophic Lateral Sclerosis*, **11**(4), 344–50.

81. **Boerner, K.** and **Mock, S.E.** (2011) Impact of patient suffering on caregiver well-being: The case of amyotrophic lateral sclerosis patients and their caregivers. *Psychology & Health Medicine*, **17**(4), 457–66.

82. **Rodriguez, J.L.** (2010) Understanding the impact of physical functioning on the experience, desire, and satisfaction of physical, emotional and social intimacies in persons with amyotrophic lateral sclerosis (ALS). *PCOM Psychology Dissertations*, **118**, 1–155.

83. **Aoun, S.M., Chochinov, H.M.,** and **Kristjanson, L.J.** (2015) Dignity therapy for people with motor neuron disease and their family caregivers: A feasibility study. *Journal of Palliative Medicine*, **18**, 31–7.

84. **Wada, K.** and **Park, J.** (2009) Integrating Buddhist psychology into grief counseling. *Death Studies*, **33**(7), 657–83.

85. **Hayes, S.C., Strosahl, K.D.,** and **Wilson, K.G.** (1999) *Acceptance and Commitment Therapy*. New York, NY: Guilford Press.

86. **Gillies, J.** and **Neimer, R.A.** (2006) Loss, grief, and the search for significance: Reconstruction in bereavement toward a model of meaning. *Journal of Constructivist Psychology*, **19**(1), 31–65.

87. **O'Brien, M.R., Whitehead, B., Jack, B.A.,** and **Mitchell, J.D.** (2011) From symptom onset to a diagnosis of amyotrophic lateral sclerosis/motor neuron disease (ALS/MND): Experiences of people with ALS/MND and family carers-A qualitative study. *Amyotrophic Lateral Sclerosis*, **12**(2), 97–104.

88. McCluskey, L., Casarett, D., and Siderowf, A. (2004) Breaking the news: A survey of ALS patients and their caregivers. *Amyotrophic Lateral Sclerosis and Other Motor Neuron Disorders*, **5**(3), 131–5.

89. Hennessey, A. (2016) Neurologists' emotional experiences in caring for individuals with amyotrophic lateral sclerosis: An exploratory study. *PCOM Psychology Dissertations/ 400*. Available at: http://digitalcommons.pcom.edu.ezproxy.pcom.edu:2048/psychology_dissertations/400/ (accessed 04 October 2017).

90. Pagnini, F., Phillips, D., Bosma, C.M., Reece, A., and Langer, E. (2015) Mindfulness, physical impairment and psychological well-being in people with amyotrophic lateral sclerosis. *Psychology & Health*, **30**(5), 503–17.

91. Strobe, M. and Schut, H. (1999) The dual process model of coping with bereavement: Rationale and description. *Death Studies*, **23**(3), 197–224.

92. Enguidanos, S., Kogan, A.C., Keefe, B., Geron, S.M., and Katz, L. (2011) Patient-centered approach to building problem solving skills among older primary care patients: Problems identified and resolved. *Journal of Gerontology and Social Work*, **54**(3), 276–91.

93. Wernher, I., Bjerregaard, F., Tinsel, I., et al. (2014) Collaborative treatment of late-life depression in primary care (GermanIMPACT): Study protocol of cluster-randomized controlled trial. *Trials*, **15**, 351.

94. Kasckow, J., Klaus, J., Morse, J., et al. (2014) Using problem solving therapy to treat veterans with subsyndromal depression: A pilot study. *International Journal of Geriatric Psychiatry*, **29**(12), 1255–61.

95. Bambling, M. and King, R. (2013). Extended problem solving treatment for depression. *Counselling and Psychotherapy Research*, **13**(4), 317–23.

96. Kelly, G.A. (1970) A summary statement of a cognitively-oriented comprehensive theory of behaviour. In: Mancuso, J.C. (ed.), *Readings for a Cognitive Theory of Personality*, pp. 27–58. New York, NY: Holt, Rinehart, and Winston.

97. Pagnini, F. (2013) Psychological wellbeing and quality of life in amyotrophic lateral sclerosis: A review. *International Journal of Psychology*, **48**(3), 194–205.

98. Gould, R.L., Coulson, M.C., Brown, R.G., Goldstein, L.H., Al-Chalabi, A., and Howard, R.J. (2015) Psychotherapy and pharmacotherapy interventions to reduce distress or improve well-being in people with amyotrophic lateral sclerosis: A systematic review. *Amyotrophic Lateral Sclerosis and Frontotemporal Degeneration*, **16**(5–6), 293–302.

99. Folkman, S. and Lazarus, R.S. (1988) *Ways of coping questionnaire: Research edition*. Palo Alto, CA: Consulting Psychologists Press.

100. Folkman, S. and Lazarus, R.S. (1980) An analysis of coping in a middle-aged community sample. *Journal of Health and Social Behaviour*, **21**(3), 219–39.

101. Carver, C.S. (1997) You want to measure coping but your protocols too long: Consider the brief COPE. *International Journal of Behavioural Medicine*, **4**(92): 92–100.

102. Lee, J.N., Rigby, S.A., Burchardt, F., Thornton, E.W., Dougan, C., and Young C.A. (2001) Quality of life issues in motor neurone disease: the development and validation of a coping strategies questionnaire, the MND Coping Scale. *Journal of Neurological Sciences*, **15**(191), 79–85.

103. Snyder, C.R., Sympson, S.C., Ybasco, F.C., Borders, T.F., Babyak, M.A., and Higgins, R.L. (1996) Development and validation of the State Hope Scale. *Journal of Personal and Social Psychology*, **70**(2), 321–35.

104. **Snyder, C.R., Harris, C., Anderson, J.R.,** et al. (1991) The will and the ways: development and validation of an individual-differences measure of hope. *Journal of Personal and Social Psychology,* **60**(4), 570–85.

105. **Scheier, M.F., Carver, C.S., and Bridges, M.W.** (1994) Distinguishing optimism from neuroticism (and trait anxiety, self-mastery, and self-esteem): a reevaluation of the Life Orientation Test. *Journal of Personal and Social Psychology,* **67**(6), 1063–78.

106. **Idler, E.L.** (1987) Religious involvement and the health of the elderly: some hypotheses and an initial test. *Social Forces,* **66**(1), 226–8.

107. **Fetzer Institute/ National Institute on Aging Working Group.** (1999) *Multidimensional measurement of religiousness/ spirituality for use in health research: a report of the Fetzer Institute/ National Institute on Aging Working Group.* Kalamazoo, MI: Fetzer Institute.

108. **Sarason, I.G., Levine, H.M., Basham, R.B., and Sarason, B.R.** (1983) Assessing social support: the Social Support Questionnaire. *Journal of Personal and Social Psychology,* **44**(1), 127–39.

109. **Spanier, G.B.** (1976) Measuring dyadic adjustment: new scales for assessing the quality of marriage and similar dyads. *Journal of Marriage and Family,* **38**(1), 15–28.

110. **Busby, D.M., Crane, D.R., Larson, J.H., and Christensen, C.** (1995) A revision of the Dyadic Adjustment Scale for use with distressed and nondistressed couples: construct hierarchy and multidimensional scales. *Journal of Marriage and Family,* **21**, 289–308.

111. **Locke, H.J.** and **Wallace, K.M.** (1994) Short marital adjustment and prediction tests: their reliability and validity. *Journal of Marriage and Family,* **21**(3), 251–5.

112. **Cohen, S.R., Sawatzky, R., Russell, L.B., Shahidi, J., Heyland, D.K.,** and **Gadermann, A.M.** (2017) Measuring the quality of life of people at the end of life: The McGill Quality of Life Questionnaire-Revised. *Palliative Medicine,* **31**(2), 120–9.

113. The WHOQOL Group. (1998) Development of the World Health Organization WHOQOL-BREF quality of life assessment. *Psychological Medicine,* **28**(3), 551–8.

Chapter 8

Cognitive and behavioural dysfunction in ALS and its assessment

Sharon Abrahams and Christopher Crockford

Introduction

It is now evident that a significant proportion of people with ALS (PALS) will experience changes in behaviour and cognition in addition to progressive physical symptoms. In its extreme form this presents as a frontotemporal dementia (FTD) with a characteristic behavioural syndrome and personality change. A further significant proportion show specific changes that can be detected through neuropsychological assessment and the remainder show motor system involvement only. These different manifestations of ALS constitute a clinical spectrum from ALS without cognitive and behavioural dysfunction to FTD (see Fig. 8.1). Cognitive and behaviour change are integral facets of the disease, and may impact on daily activities, caregivers, families, and clinical interventions. This chapter describes the presentation of cognitive and behavioural symptoms in PALS, and how clinicians can assess these symptoms.

The presentation of cognitive and behavioural dysfunction in PALS

The ALS-FTD spectrum: Evolving understanding

ALS has been traditionally viewed as a disease that spares non-motor functions. This is somewhat paradoxical given that descriptions of non-motor symptoms in PALS emerged in the 1880s, not long after Charcot's initial report in 1874 (1). Similarly, a link with FTD was described as early as 1924 (2). Yet, research delineating the profile of cognition and behaviour in ALS has only gained momentum over the last 30 years. The neglect of these symptoms may be partly explained by several factors:

- the presentation of ALS is variable, with frank dementia in only a few;
- in PALS there may be fewer demands placed on cognitive performance as increasing physical disability typically prevents working and undertaking other activities;
- the pronounced physical disability of some individuals with ALS masks symptoms and makes measurement difficult;
- the sparing of cognitive functions was seen as a saving grace by patients, caregivers, and clinicians, and so served to perpetuate this misrepresentation.

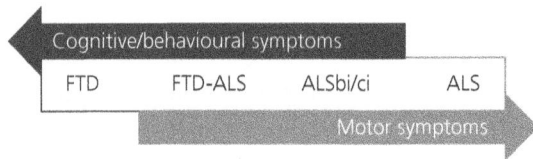

Fig. 8.1 ALS-FTD spectrum.

Recent advances have established that ALS is on a spectrum with FTD with clinical, genetic, and pathological overlap and variable involvement of the frontal and temporal lobes of the brain. FTD, also known as frontotemporal lobar degeneration, is an umbrella term describing three distinct syndromes. Behavioural variant frontotemporal dementia (bvFTD) is the most common form in ALS, and is characterized by signature changes in personality, social conduct, and executive functions (3). Progressive non-fluent aphasia and semantic dementia are two forms of progressive aphasia, which are also described in some PALS, although the latter is rarely seen. Approximately 15% of PALS have concurrent bvFTD, and a similar proportion of patients with bvFTD will also develop ALS during the course of their dementia. The prevalence of specific and more subtle cognitive or behavioural impairments appears to be between 30 and 50% of patients with ALS as determined by a number of large clinic- and population-based studies (4,5). A large multicentre USA study of 274 ALS patients revealed that only 39.2% performed normally on cognitive testing, with 54.2% defined as mild cognitive impairment (6). Similar rates are found from European studies, with 13.8% of a sample of 160 Irish patients fulfilling criteria for FTD, while a further 34.1% showed some cognitive impairment (7); of 207 Italian patients, 12.6% had ALS-FTD, while 37.2% had cognitive impairment (8). An overlap between ALS and FTD has long been suspected, but the findings of a spectrum of cognitive and behavioural impairment ranging from no impairments to dementia, and more recently common pathological changes in the brain and common genetic mutations in a proportion of cases has established that the two are interlinked (9) (see Fig. 8.1).

Cognition in PALS

Neuropsychological or cognitive assessment measures a range of thinking abilities including memory, language, visuoperception, and executive functions. In ALS the most pronounced deficits are found on tests of letter fluency and executive functions, but more recently changes in language and social cognition have been described as highly prevalent (9). This has been confirmed by a recent meta-analysis across studies (10). However, an issue that continues to influence findings is the use of tests that do not accommodate for disability (such as slowed writing) and which may therefore exaggerate the appearance of performance deficits.

Verbal fluency

Verbal fluency is a commonly used clinical assessment and involves the generation of a list of words beginning with a specified letter (letter fluency) or a list of semantically related words (category fluency) in a specified time. Letter fluency is the most widely recognized marker of cognitive impairment in PALS (11–15) and deficits in this measure often occur with other deficits of executive functions (7). To accommodate for physical disability in ALS, verbal fluency can be calculated using a verbal fluency index (VFI) (14); following the word generation condition, where the patient is asked write or say as many words as possible in a given time, he/she is then asked to re-read, or copy out the previously generated words. Using this measure the authors have demonstrated a consistent impairment independent of motor disability. The VFI is calculated using the following equation:

$$\text{Vfi} = \frac{\text{Time for word generation test} - \text{time taken to read or copy words}}{\text{total number of words generated}}$$

Successful performance on tests of verbal fluency requires an interactive involvement of language, short-term memory, and executive abilities. Individuals need to access their lexical store, and continuously monitor their performance to avoid rule breaks and repetition. Performance relies on intrinsically generating words, the formation of strategies, and switching between strategies to continue to produce words. Abrahams et al. (14) conducted an in-depth investigation of the verbal fluency deficits in PALS to determine whether intrinsic response generation, phonological loop functions (short-term verbal memory), or simple word retrieval were responsible for the impairment. In this study, the deficits were found in fluency tests, and not in tests of phonological loop functions or simple word retrieval, indicating that the difficulty in this sample of patients lay in higher order executive processes, rather than in language or memory. This is consistent with the findings that letter fluency deficits are strong markers for frontal lobe dysfunction as revealed through brain imaging studies (12,13,16–18).

Executive functions

Executive functioning describes a broad range of higher order cognitive abilities that allow individuals to determine goals, formulate ways of achieving those goals, and adapt to changing circumstances to achieve those goals. As such, these abilities include decision making, planning, attention (including divided attention used when multi-tasking), and monitoring performance, adjusting behaviour on the basis of feedback and problem solving.

Attention is a fundamental component of executive functions, allowing an individual to focus and sustain that focus on relevant information, while ignoring other irrelevant information. Impairment of selective attention, or an inability to focus on one stimulus in the presence of multiple competing stimuli, has been demonstrated in ALS (19–21). The Stroop Test is a commonly used measure of attention, which requires individuals to read a list of colour words, each presented in a different colour, as quickly as possible. The ability to complete this task requires you to selectively attend to either the word or the colour, and inhibit the conflicting information. While some researchers found PALS made more inhibitory errors (19,22,23), others did not, particularly when controlling for speech disability (11,15). Tests of divided attention necessary for multitasking are also sensitive to ALS (18). Here, patients held a sequence of numbers in mind, while performing a simple visual processing speed task. Patients were able to undertake the visual task as rapidly as healthy controls, but showed a disproportionate decrement in performance when the two tasks were combined. Deficits on this test were also specifically related to white matter dysfunction in regions of the frontal lobes using diffusion tensor magnetic resonance imaging techniques.

Working memory is a core facet of executive functions, and allows people to store, process, and manipulate information on a short-term basis. Working memory is different from short-term memory in that it allows you to 'work' with information, rather than simply store it. A common task used to assess working memory is backward digit span, in which participants must repeat a series of numbers of increasing length in reverse order. While some authors reported deficient performance in PALS (24,25), others did not. Other more demanding tests of working memory have also been shown to be impaired in ALS including the N-Back test. Here, a participant must hold in mind a series of letters, numbers, or shapes sequentially, and identify a match between the current item and an item two or three positions back (26).

Executive functions also allow people to form concepts and to think flexibly. Concept formation is often tested through the ability to categorize or group distinct objects. Impairment in this ability has been demonstrated in ALS using card sorting tests, in which the participant must group distinct cards and determine an overarching rule of membership (e.g. these cards have curved edges and these have straight edges) (27,28). The Wisconsin Card Sorting Test is a traditional measure of this function. Here, the participant not only classifies cards into four groupings, but once these are established, the tester changes the rule and the participant must shift to thinking of a new way to classify the cards (set-shifting). A recent meta-analysis of this test demonstrated that PALS completed fewer categorization trials, made more errors, and took longer to learn new rules compared with controls (29). PALS were also more likely to continue to choose a previously correct rule. This failure to shift mental set is called perseveration and can also be seen in everyday behaviour, where a person will continue to conduct an activity that is no longer appropriate to the situation and will not be able to adapt flexibly to a changing environment.

Social cognition

Social cognition is an umbrella term that describes the cognitive processes necessary for successful negotiation of social situations. Social cognition encompasses fundamental components of emotion processing and recognition, such as responding to a sad event, or recognizing emotions in others such as happiness, sadness, fear, or disgust. It also includes more complex processes involved in the interpretation of the thoughts and actions of others (also known as theory of mind (ToM)) and the understanding of social norms and social responsibility.

Although dysfunction in social cognition has been recognized as a key feature of FTD for some time, it has only recently become a focus of investigation in ALS (30,31). An updated meta-analysis of cognitive impairment in ALS noted the addition of social cognition deficits as a new integral component of the cognitive profile of PALS (10). PALS demonstrated an altered response to emotionally charged stimuli, regarding pictures as being more positive and exciting than controls (32), and rated the faces of strangers as more approachable (33). PALS also show a reduced capacity to recognize emotional expressions, particularly negative emotions (34–37), which has been supported by neuroimaging (38), but not consistently found (28,39), and may be more likely in those with ALS-FTD (36). There is some interaction with memory processes, wherein healthy adults demonstrated enhancement of memory when information had an emotional component, but PALS did not show a similar benefit (39).

PALS have been also shown to have difficulty on tests of ToM in which the thoughts and beliefs of another are inferred. Fundamental to this process is the understanding that other people may have thoughts or beliefs that are different to one's own. ToM can refer to the ability to infer a person's emotional state (*affective* ToM) or the ability to infer a person's thoughts (*cognitive* ToM). The *faux pas* test is a commonly used measure of ToM. Individuals are read a short story or shown a comic strip, in which one of the characters says something they should not have, for example:

> Sally is a three-year-old girl with a round face and short blonde hair. She was at her Aunt Carol's house. The doorbell rang and her Aunt Carol answered it. It was Mary, a neighbour. 'Hi,' Aunt Carol said, 'Nice of you to stop by.' Mary said, 'Hello,' then looked at Sally and said, 'Oh, I don't think I've met this little boy. What's your name?' (40).

Despite demonstrating intact comprehension of the story a third of patients have been shown to be impaired at detecting the *faux pas* (41). Similarly, Cavallo et al. (42) presented comic strips of social (e.g. a person preparing a romantic dinner) and non-social (e.g. a person changing a light bulb in order to read) situations, and asked them to interpret the intentions of the characters. PALS performed worse than healthy controls in interpreting the social cartoons, but not the non-social cartoons indicating a specific difficulty in social understanding.

A fundamental process of ToM is the interpretation of the direction of eye gaze. This has been assessed using cartoon figures in the Judgement of Preference Task (Fig. 8.2) and shown to be impaired in ALS (35). Van der Hulst et al. (43) extended these findings to demonstrate that 36% of patients showed a deficit in affective ToM (which picture does the face love?) while 27% of patients showed a cognitive ToM deficit (which picture is the face thinking of?)

Debate continues as to the source of social cognitive impairments in pwALS. Cavallo et al. (42) and Meier et al. (41) found social cognitive deficits to be independent of executive function, while more thorough examinations have found strong connections between the two (28,44).

Language

Language dysfunction has also recently become a focus of attention in ALS and may have been previously masked by difficulties with measurement and dissociation from dysarthria. Language dysfunction may be even more common than executive dysfunction in ALS (45,46). In a study of 51 ALS patients, Taylor et al. used an extensive battery of tests including naming, semantics, and grammar, and revealed language impairment in 43%, while executive dysfunction was found in 31%. Of note, is that there was some interaction between these two functions and analyses indicated that scores on the executive tests accounted for 44% of the variance in the language tests. Conversely this indicates that much of language deficit was independent of executive dysfunction.

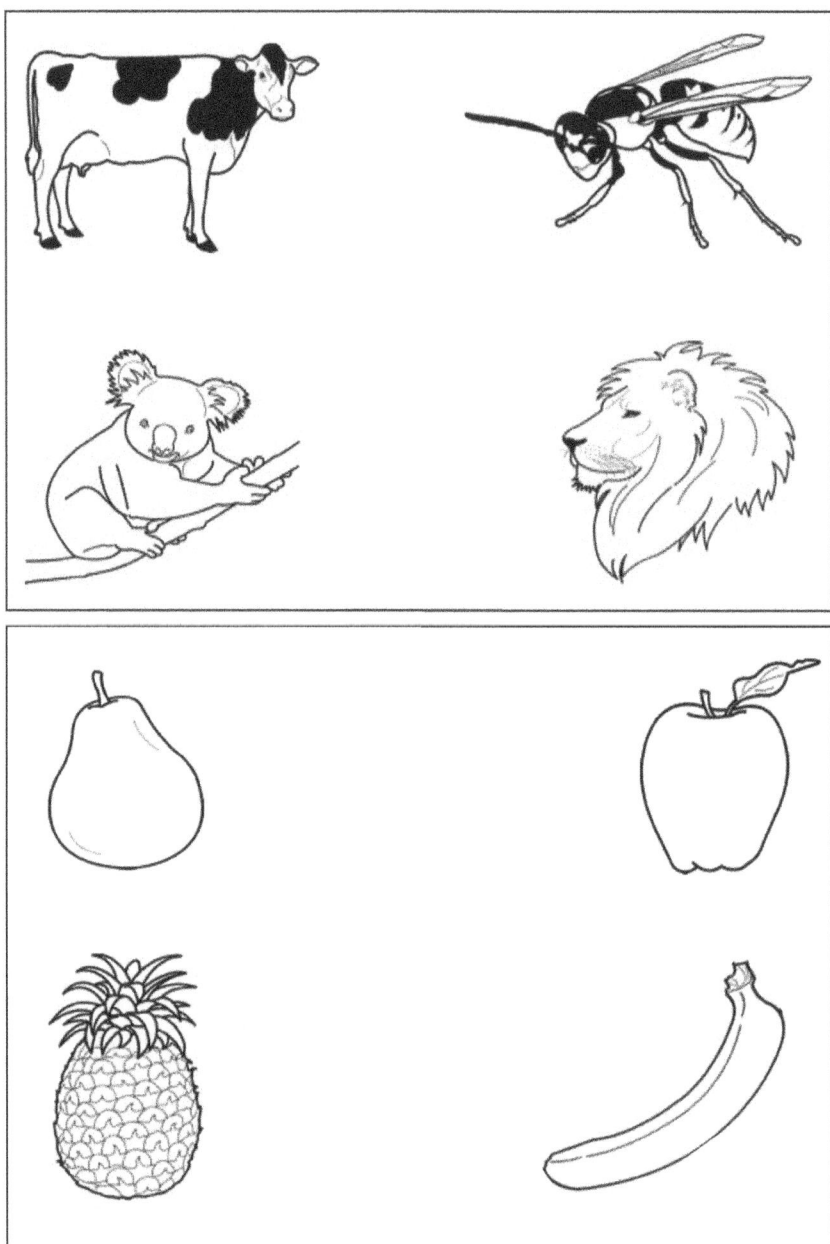

Fig. 8.2 Judgement of preference task.
'Which picture do you like best?'

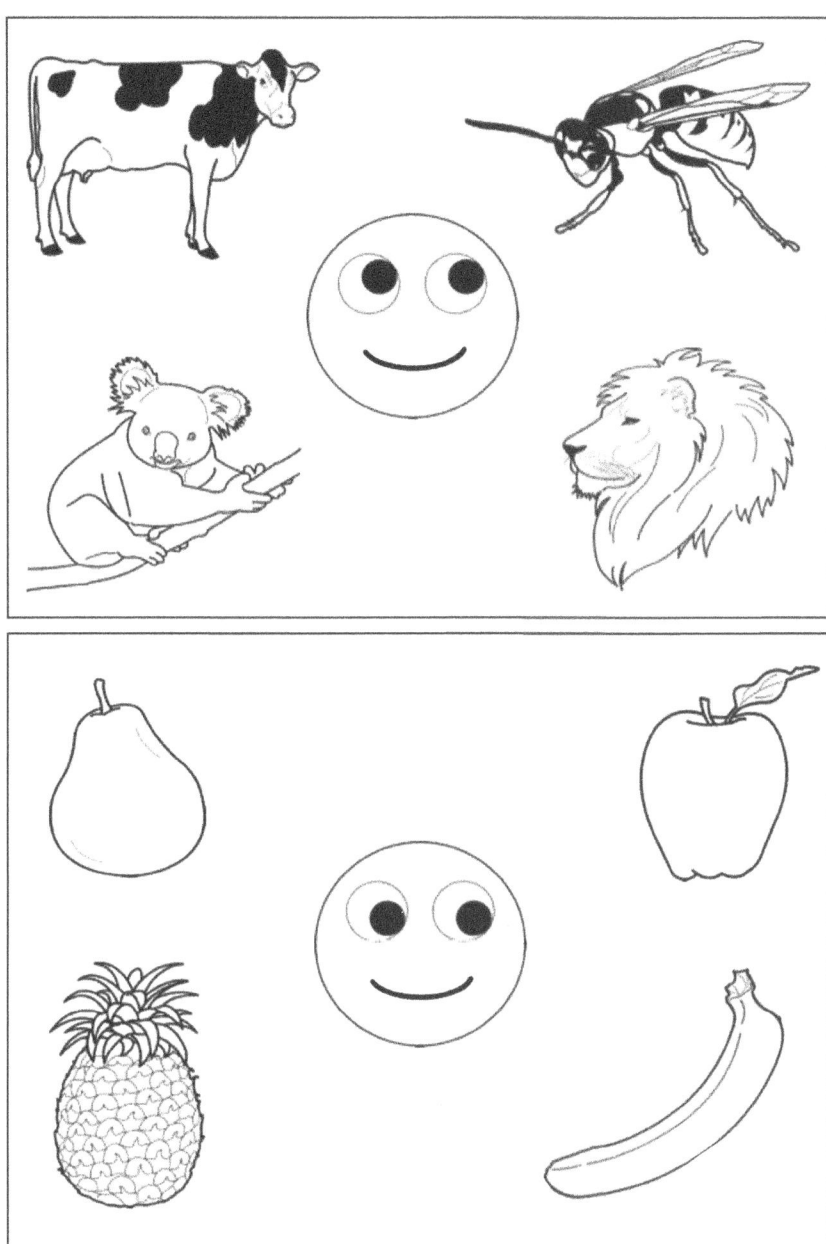

Fig. 8.2 (continued)
'Which picture does the face like best?'

One of the most ground-breaking findings is the association between language and motor actions in that ALS patients are worse at processing verbs and actions, compared with nouns (47,48). This verb–noun dissociation has been attributed to the role of the motor cortex in language, where verbs associated with specific body parts (e.g. chew-mouth) are related to corresponding areas of the motor cortex.

Impaired performance has also been observed in patients' grammar abilities (49,50), naming of objects (13,24), and most recently semantic knowledge (51) demonstrating deficits in both expression and reception. In the latter, ALS patients were less impaired than ALS-FTD and patients with semantic dementia, on tests of naming, comprehension, and semantic association. This has led to the suggestion that these patterns may be reflective of subclinical presentations of language-variants of FTD in ALS.

Memory

Memory functions refer to our ability to encode, store, and retrieve information, and are the most widely studied in psychology. In PALS, research has focused on the *type* of information being processed (verbal and visual information):

- the capacity for consolidation (immediate memory compared to delayed memory);
- whether the retrieval of information is by direct recall (e.g. being asked to recall a list of previously learned words) or recognition (e.g. being given a list of words and asked to identify which you were asked to learn).

Memory has been found to be largely intact by many researchers, although impairments have been found by some (22,52). Some have shown impaired delayed recall and recognition (53) and a recent meta-analysis reported small effect sizes for tests of delayed verbal memory (10). Memory deficits may be partly explained by dysfunction of other cognitive domains, such as problems in attention, mediated by reduced executive functioning. However, Machts et al. (53) found that executive functioning explains only 20.5% of the variability in memory performance in PALS, leaving a significant proportion of the variance unexplained.

Visuoperceptual and spatial functions

Visuoperceptual and spatial functions refer to a range of skills in identifying, locating, and manipulating objects in space. These abilities allow us to perform routine activities, such as recognizing items in the kitchen and where they are stored or navigating through a shop. In FTD, visuospatial changes are rarely reported and when described appear to be mediated by higher-order executive dysfunction such as poor attention to the stimuli or poor organization of the test material, rather than due to simple perceptual difficulties. Studies that have examined these abilities in PALS have generally found that patients perform within normal ranges (10).

Behaviour in PALS

Behavioural change can range from mild and specific symptoms, such as impulsivity or apathy to more global and frank personality change found in bvFTD. The diagnosis of bvFTD is based on the presence of changes in five core domains (behavioural disinhibition, apathy, loss of sympathy/empathy, perseverative and stereotyped behavior, and hyperorality and dietary changes) (3). All of these can be found in ALS, either in isolation or in groups of symptoms. These changes are typically established through an interview with a caregiver or by questionnaire. A systematic review of studies examining behaviour in people with ALS-FTD demonstrated that the most commonly reported changes were in perseveration (40%), apathy (29%), and disinhibition (26%) (54). A person's insight into these difficulties is typically affected in ALS-FTD, but it appears to be less affected in non-demented patients (55).

Disinhibition describes a reduction in an individual's ability to inhibit thoughts or desires that may be seen as socially inappropriate. For example, making rude, offensive, or sexual comments or jokes; violating social norms, such as inappropriate physical contact with strangers; or making decisions that are careless or impulsive, such as buying things without regard of the consequences. Caregivers have reported increases in disinhibited behaviour following the onset of ALS (56,57). However, Grossman et al. (56) also noted that these may occur prior to the onset of weakness, suggesting that behavioural features may predate the development of motor symptoms in some.

Apathy, demotivation, or inertia is the most commonly reported behavioural feature in non-demented ALS (21,56,58,59). A person may appear to lose drive, interest, or motivation. Similarly, a person may require prompting to initiate or maintain common daily tasks, such as self-care. Symptoms of apathy must be dissociated from inactivity due to physical disability and from depression. The latter is associated with negative thinking and emotion, while apathy is a more neutral emotional state. It has been suggested that apathy is multidimensional and Radakovic and colleagues have developed the Dimensional Apathy Scale for people with ALS, which measures initiation, emotional, and executive apathy (60). PALS appear to have pronounced initiation apathy, which consists of reduced motivation for the instigation of self-directed thinking or behaviour, and which may share common underlying mechanisms with deficits in cognition (61).

ALS patients may also show a loss of sympathy and empathy. This behaviour can manifest in a diminished response to the needs and feelings of others, or a decreased interest in socializing and being close to others. These may appear as egocentric behavior, or self-centredness and selfishness that have been reported as prevalent (44). PALS may also demonstrate perseveration, or stereotyped and compulsive behaviours, with simple repetitive movements (e.g., clapping, tapping, or rocking), or more complex behaviours (e.g., such as hoarding, counting, cleaning rituals). Changes in diet or eating behaviours include cravings for sweet foods or carbohydrates, or continuing to eat despite being full. These changes are dissociated from changes in intake resulting from bulbar symptoms and are found as a spectrum of changes in ALS increasing in those with cognitive impairment (62). The combination of an eating disturbance, such as food cramming, together with executive dysfunction causing impulsivity and perseveration, can be particularly hazardous for patients with bulbar dysfunction with a risk of aspiration.

A further change common in ALS is emotional lability. Described as pathological laughing, crying, and smiling (63), emotional lability can be highly variable and is estimated to affect 10-71% of patients (44, 63, 64). Patients may laugh, cry, or grimace at an inappropriate time or place. Emotional lability may be caused by several pathological reasons including dysfunction of the frontal lobes and poor executive functioning (65). It can be present at early stages of the disease and is thought to be more common in patients with bulbar dysfunction (64,66). Although common in ALS, emotional lability is not specific to the disease or to FTD, and as such is not part of the diagnostic criteria.

The relationship between cognitive and behavioural dysfunction

The distinction between changes in behaviour and cognition is somewhat artificial given that cognitive processes, or their loss, must underlie all behaviours. However, when discussing cognitive change, researchers describe processes that are measureable, such as by tests of memory, object naming, problem solving, etc. It is well recognized that patients with bvFTD early in the course of the disease may show abnormal behaviours, but maintain normal performance on standard tests of cognition and executive functioning. This dissociation between behavioural change and seemingly intact cognition is primarily due to the limitations of standard cognitive testing. Novel, experimental methods of assessing social cognition have revealed deficits in FTD patients with normal cognitive functioning by standard testing. Demonstrating a relationship between cognitive deficits and the abnormal behaviours in ALS has been somewhat elusive. A relationship has been shown between verbal fluency and behavioural symptoms (67,68), in particular apathy (21,56), and between emotional lability and errors made on the Wisconsin Card Sorting Test (65). In a group of patients with ToM dysfunction, there was also evidence of reduced empathy, high levels of apathy, and increased behavioural dysfunction (43). It is also probable that the behaviour change of loss of sympathy and empathy is most likely due to underling deficits in social cognition.

Cognitive and behaviour change during the course of the disease

A number of studies have attempted to monitor the course of cognitive and behavioural change over time in PALS with repeated assessments, although the findings of these studies are often invalidated by high attrition rates, which results in only a small group of patients (those with the less aggressive disease) being tested at later time points. Two studies (69,70) reported no difference in cognitive performance and behaviour over time, while Robinson et al. (71) found no significant change in their group analyses, although analyses of individuals revealed that 36.84% of patients showed progression of abnormal cognitive performance over 6 months. Several studies found mixed results where performance on some cognitive tasks worsened (e.g. word finding), some remained stable (e.g. verbal fluency), while others even improved (e.g. visuospatial), the latter most likely due to practice effects of repeat testing (72–74). In a large-scale study of 186 patients, Elamin et al. (75) revealed that executive dysfunction at initial assessment was associated with higher rates of attrition due to disability or death, and more rapid motor functional decline (particularly bulbar), whereas those who showed no cognitive impairment at baseline demonstrated a tendency to remain cognitively intact.

Studies investigating the relationship between cognitive and behaviour change and physical symptoms of the disease have produced mixed results, with many studies finding little to no relationship (5,21,57,59,76–78). However associations between cognitive functioning and respiratory function in PALS has been reported (79) with memory and fluency performance significantly worse in patients with respiratory failure (80). These deficits were partially corrected by non-invasive ventilation (79). Further associations have been found between verbal fluency and functional status (64), and symptom duration and rate of progression (73). Several studies have reported an association between cognitive impairment and bulbar symptoms or onset although not consistently (5,11). In a sample of 175 patients, Sterling et al. (81) reported that dysarthria was significantly associated with executive functioning, even after controlling for motor speed. More recently, in the large USA study of 286 patients, Murphy et al. (6) showed that behavioural (but not cognitive) symptoms were significantly associated with functional status, respiratory function, region of onset, and emotional lability.

Diagnosis of cognitive and behaviour dysfunction in PALS

Consensus criteria (82), which are currently under revision, recommend the classification of patients based on their cognitive and behavioural profile. Non-demented ALS patients with cognitive impairment are termed ALSci (cognitive impairment), while those with behavioural impairment are categorized as ALSbi (behavioural impairment). These patients do not meet criteria for ALS-FTD. At present, patients classified as ALSci must demonstrate cognitive impairment in at least two distinct tests of executive functioning, whereas patients classified as ALSbi must present with two non-overlapping behavioural features. The consensus criteria are currently being updated to include newly described deficits in language and social cognition, in addition to other non-motor symptoms, and to include those who show both cognitive and behavioural symptoms. In terms of ALS-FTD given that bvFTD is the most common type of FTD in ALS, a diagnosis can be made on the basis of the most recent criteria (3), which specifies the need for a progressive deterioration of cognition and/or behaviour, marked by the presence of three symptoms from Table 8.1. There is also the more recent diagnostic criteria for the other two progressive aphasia variants of FTD which can be used (83).

The impact of cognitive and behavioural change

Cognitive and behavioural symptoms appear to contribute uniquely to patients' and caregivers' quality of life, mood, and burden (see Chapter 9). Patients' quality of life has been shown to be related to subjective cognitive lapses (84). However, it may be behavioural symptoms, and not cognition, that most impacts caregiver burden (58,85), quality of life and depression (58), and relationship intimacy (86). In a survey of the caregivers of PALS, Lillo, Mioshi, and Hodges (87) found that 48% of caregivers experienced high levels of burden, and that abnormal behaviour and caregiver stress, not physical symptoms, significantly predicted this. A recent study of 84 patients and

Table 8.1 Criteria for diagnosis of bvFTD

Possible bvFTD

1 **Early behavioural disinhibition marked by *one* of the following:**
   a. Socially inappropriate behaviour
   b. Loss of manners or decorum
   c. Impulsive, rash or careless actions

2 **Early apathy or inertia marked by *one* of the following:**
   a. Apathy
   b. Inertia

3 **Early loss of sympathy or empathy marked by *one* of the following:**
   a. Diminished response to other people's needs and feelings
   b. Diminished social interest, interrelatedness or personal warmth

4 **Early perseverative, stereotyped or compulsive/ritualistic behaviour marked by *one* of the following:**
   a. Simple repetitive movements
   b. Complex, compulsive, or ritualistic behaviours
   c. Stereotypy of speech

5 **Hyperorality and dietary changes marked by *one* of the following:**
   a. Altered food preferences
   b. Binge eating, increased consumption of alcohol or cigarettes
   c. Oral exploration or consumption of inedible objects

6 **Neuropsychological profile: executive/generation deficits with relative sparing of memory and visuospatial functions marked by the presence of *all* of the following:**
   a. Deficits in executive tasks
   b. Relative sparing of episodic memory
   c. Relative sparing of visuospatial skills

Probable bvFTD

Meets criteria for possible bvFTD in addition to:
   a. Significant functional decline
   b. Imaging results demonstrating frontal and/or anterior temporal lobe atrophy, hypoperfusion, or hypometabolism

Definite bvFTD

Meets criteria for possible or probably bvFTD in addition to:
   a. Histopathological evidence of FTLD on biopsy or at post-mortem
   b. Presence of known pathogenic mutation

Adapted from *Brain*, 134(Pt 9), Rascovsky, K., Hodges, J.R., Knopman, D., et al., Sensitivity of revised diagnostic criteria for the behavioural variant of frontotemporal dementia, pp. 2456–77, Copyright (2011), with permission from Oxford University Press.

caregivers demonstrated that the caregiver burden was significantly associated with patients' behaviour, even after controlling for functional severity (85).

Behavioural change (most notably apathy) and executive dysfunction are negative prognostic indicators in PALS, with significant reduction in survival time of approximately 1 year (88–91). Whether this is due to a more aggressive disease course, differing clinical pathways or failure to adhere to interventions is unclear. In 2005, Olney et al. (92) found that PALS and comorbid bvFTD were less compliant with respiratory and nutritional interventions. Rates of non-compliance in ALS-FTD patients were twice that of those with ALS without comorbid dementia. Additionally, Chio et al. (89) found that while PALS with and without behavioural symptoms showed similar rates of nutritional and respiratory intervention uptake, patients with behavioural symptoms survived for shorter periods, suggesting poor treatment compliance. Furthermore, using a medication scheduling task, it was shown that PALS were significantly less able to safely schedule a day's medication use, due to poorer ability to schedule pills at the correct time and due to significantly more errors and omissions (15). These studies highlight the potential impact that cognitive impairment can have on intervention compliance.

Assessment of cognitive and behavioural dysfunction in PALS

The importance of assessment

Cognitive and behavioural symptoms are common in PALS and can impact carergiver and patients' psychological well-being, impair patients' ability to engage with interventions, and have a negative prognostic effect on survival. Despite this increased understanding of the spectrum of cognitive and behavioural problems in ALS, the cognitive status of many patients attending local clinics remains unknown (93). This is due to:

+ limited resources from clinical neuropsychology services;
+ previous sparse availability of assessment tools appropriate for use with ALS patients with physical disability;
+ a focus on physical symptoms and away from the acknowledgement of the impact of these changes on patients, families and care pathways.

Recently published UK health guidelines on the assessment and management of patients with MND/ALS have emphasized the need for timely assessment of cognitive and behavioural symptoms as part of a multidisciplinary team (94). These guidelines highlight the impact that cognitive and behavioural status can have on issues of capacity, patient management, and care planning. The guideline advises tailoring the multidisciplinary team's assessment to the person's needs, including adjustment if the person has cognitive or behaviour changes. It also advises that these issues should be taken into account when engaging in advance care planning for those with cognitive problems and should be considered before decisions are made on use of gastrostomy or non-invasive ventilation.

New screening tools for cognition and behaviour specifically for ALS have now been developed that permit rapid identification of those patients who may be experiencing these changes. These tools can be used within clinics by non-neuropsychologists and are designed for screening patients to identify those who may benefit from full neuropsychological assessment and subsequent intervention based on those findings. A full neuropsychological assessment undertaken by a neuropsychologist can determine the presence of cognitive or behaviour change, the severity of that impairment, the specific type of impairment, and the impact of these deficits on the person's life. These assessments may be particularly important in patients with suspected low or high intelligence, education, or comorbid conditions including depression or developmental language delay, all of which may affect performance on screening tools, and need expert assessment and interpretation. Furthermore, the neuropsychologist can provide a detailed profile of both the patients' cognitive strengths and weaknesses. Identification of the patients' strengths may be important to provide guidance on the use of compensatory strategies. The neuropsychologist can help with educating the patient, carergiver, and clinicians on the type and impact of the changes, and can provide a tailored intervention programme where needed.

In some instances patients may not be able to undertake extensive neuropsychological assessment or travel to facilities with neuropsychology services, in which case screening tools become a vital source of information. These can be undertaken by members of the multidisciplinary team with appropriate training, although given the complex nature of the symptoms it is advisable that the interpretation of these tools should always be supervised by a qualified clinical neuropsychologist.

Assessment of cognition

In assessing the cognitive status of an individual, it is important to contextualize that information within their unique history and consider factors that may be affecting performance. These include demographic factors, such as education, intelligence, age, culture, and ethnicity. The use of standardized appropriate normative data is recommended. Other important factors to consider relate to the extent to which impairment on one type of cognitive domain may affect performance across tests, e.g. poor attention may affect performance on a test of visuoperceptual functions. Many tests will be at risk of producing practice effects with repeated administration, and this can persist for several months. Furthermore, many neuropsychological assessment tools rely on intact motor functioning, reinforcing the importance of using tools specifically designed for ALS. The effect of fatigue and respiratory status, and the importance of conducting the interview in a location free of distractions or disturbances, should also be considered in assessment of ALS patients.

Cognitive screening tools

Edinburgh Cognitive and Behavioural ALS Screen

The ECAS is a multi-domain cognitive and behavioural measure specifically designed for PALS (95). It assesses a range of functions typically impaired in ALS including the newly recognized deficits in language functions and social cognition (termed ALS-specific) and those not typically affected in ALS, but which are common in other disorders of aging such as Alzheimer's disease (termed ALS non-specific) (see Figs 8.2 and 8.3 for a sample of ECAS subtests). ALS-specific tests include measures of executive functioning (oral trails, backward digit span, attention-inhibition, and social cognition), language (naming, comprehension, and spelling), and verbal fluency and they incorporate the verbal fluency index calculation to control for motor speed. ALS non-specific functions assessed are memory and visuospatial functions. Using the ECAS,

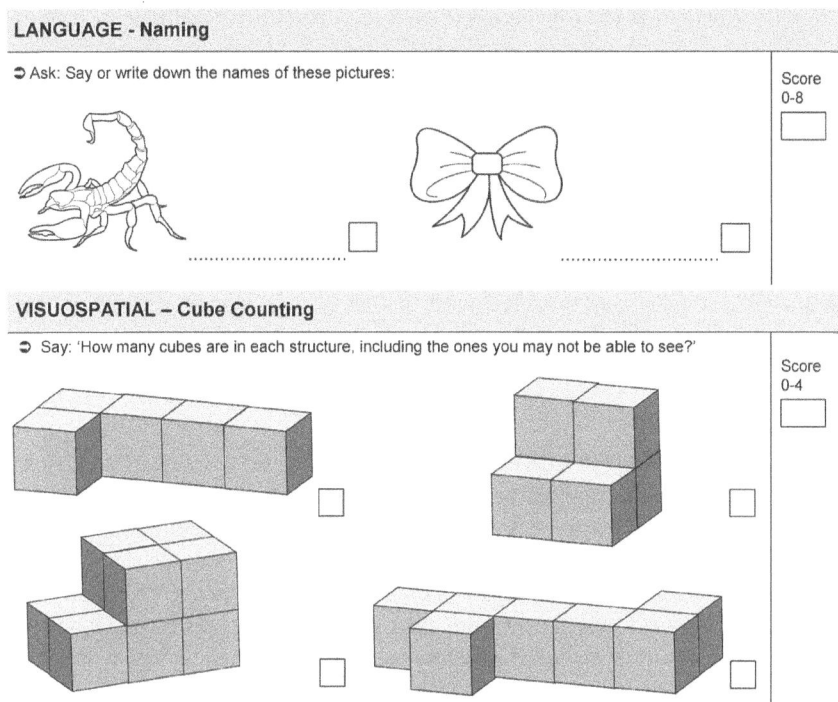

LANGUAGE - Naming

➲ Ask: Say or write down the names of these pictures:

Score
0-8

VISUOSPATIAL – Cube Counting

➲ Say: 'How many cubes are in each structure, including the ones you may not be able to see?'

Score
0-4

Fig. 8.3 Sample of ECAS subtests.

the most prevalent deficits were reported in language functions (35%) followed by executive functions and letter fluency (23% each), which demonstrates the importance of assessment of language functions (95). The ECAS has been validated against a full and extensive neuropsychological battery, and shows good sensitivity (85%) and specificity (85%) to cognitive impairment in non-demented ALS patients (96). Additionally, the ECAS has also been validated in German, Italian, and Chinese, and in an Irish population and shows good convergent validity with general screening tools including the Frontal Assessment Battery and the Montreal Cognitive Assessment (97–101). The ECAS has been translated into a number of other European languages and a North American version is also available. Alternate versions are currently in development, which will allow for repeat testing (102). Given it is multi-domain and can be completed in ~20 minutes, it may be regarded as a brief assessment tool, rather than a simple screening measure, and is used by both neuropsychologists and ALS health professionals, within clinics or in home visits. The ECAS also includes a separate behaviour interview described below.

ALS Cognitive Behavioural Screen

The ALS Cognitive Behavioural Screen (ALS-CBS) is a short cognitive and behavioural screen specifically designed for ALS (103). It is a single domain measure assessing executive functioning and contains eight short cognitive tests. It additionally includes a behaviour questionnaire described below. The ALS-CBS benefits from being brief and can be utilized by any health care professional. While the ALS-CBS is largely independent of motor functioning, it does not adjust for motor speed in verbal fluency although patients are able to speak, write, or use assistive communication devises. It has been validated against a neuropsychological battery and is able to distinguish those with cognitive impairment from those with no cognitive impairment with 85% sensitivity and 71% specificity. The ALS-CBS has been incorporated into the UCSF Screening Exam (6), which includes the Abrahams et al. (14) fluency test adjusted for motor speed. While the ALS-CBS primarily measures executive functioning, and does not directly measure language, memory, or visuospatial functioning, the expanded UCSF Screening Exam includes an expanded ALS-specific behavioural measurement (ALS-FBI) (6,104).

Other cognitive screening tools used in ALS

Data has been recently reported on 70 ALS patients using the mini-ACE (105). This new test is an abbreviated version of the Addenbrookes Cognitive Examination-III, and includes the verbal fluency correction for motor deficits (14). However, the test also includes assessment of visuospatial functions using drawing of a clock face and therefore has limited use in patients with marked upper limb involvement. Finally, the test lacks assessment of executive functioning, an area of specific difficulty in PALS. Details of some other screening assessments are in Table 8.2 (106).

Assessment of behaviour in PALS

As with cognition there are a number of factors to consider when assessing behaviour. Cultural and family context may impact what is normal or abnormal. Determining whether there has been a change in behaviour or personality may be confounded as behavioural symptoms may manifest before physical symptoms. Furthermore, it is important to determine whether the person is depressed or anxious. It is advisable to interview the caregiver in a confidential manner away from the patient and to use measures that have been designed for physical disability. Some measurements used in ALS research are summarized in Table 8.3 (107).

ECAS Behaviour Interview

The behaviour screen of the ECAS is an informant interview undertaken with a clinician that is the only screen to directly address the behavioural diagnostic criteria for bvFTD (3), measuring five behavioural domains. Using the ECAS behaviour interview, behaviour change was reported in 40% of patients with the most frequent being Apathy (95). The behaviour screen is a useful counterpart to the cognitive assessment in this tool. Being a caregiver interview it permits the freedom to explore the frequency, severity, time-line, and qualitative nature of observed behaviours. Furthermore, the behaviour interview includes three separate questions on psychosis, which were included following the finding of these symptoms in individuals with ALS-FTD (108).

Table 8.2 ALS cognitive screening measures and brief assessments

Name (reference)	Time Taken	Description	Strengths and weaknesses
Edinburgh Cognitive and Behavioural ALS Screen (95)	15–20 min	Measures executive functions, social cognition, language, visuospatial functions, and memory.	Measures multiple domains of cognition. Only tool to include social cognition. All tasks adjusted for, or independent of motor disability. Validated in ALS and in several languages. Includes behaviour screen (See Table 8.3). Validated in a non-demented ALS group only to date.
ALS-Cognitive Behavioural Screen (103)	5–0 min	Measures executive functions including fluency and attention.	Very brief and most tasks independent of motor speed. Spanish version available (Turon-Sans et al., 2016). Good accuracy in detecting bvFTD (Woolley, York, et al., 2010). Formally validated in ALS (Woolley, York, et al., 2010). Includes behaviour screen (See Table 8.3). Measures executive functions only and does not include language functions. Fluency task does not adjust for motor speed. Limited ability to detect mild cognitive impairments (Woolley, York, et al., 2010).
Penn State Screen Exam (110)	20 min	Measures executive functions, language, visuospatial, fluency, and memory.	Revised adjusted for motor disability (Flaherty-Craig et al., 2009). Measures multiple areas of cognition. May be useful in detecting language variants of bvFTD. Not formally validated. Originally designed for other neurological disorders. Includes behaviour screen unadjusted for motor impairment.
Montreal Cognitive Assessment (111)	15 min	Measures visuospatial, executive, language, memory, attention, orientation.	Parallel versions allow for repeat testing, and additionally has a 'mini form'. Measures multiple areas of cognition. Has been validated in numerous diseases and available in many languages. Not designed for ALS and relies on intact motor function although adaptations may be possible. No behaviour measurement included.
Frontal Assessment Battery (FAB) (112)	5–10 min	Measures executive functions, fluency, and motor programming.	Well validated for measuring frontal-executive functions. Only measures frontal lobe functions, Not suitable for patients with motor disability. No behaviour screen included

(Continued)

Table 8.2 Continued

Name (reference)	Time Taken	Description	Strengths and weaknesses
UCSF Brief Screening Battery (6)	40 min	A combination of the ALS-CBS, Abrahams' verbal fluency test and an ALS version of the FBI administered to caregiver.	Combines a motor-independent measure of fluency with the ALS-CBS. Includes behaviour measure (ALS-FBI; Table 8.3). Improves predictive ability of ALS-CBS (Murphy et al., 2015). Includes a behaviour screen. Does not include assessment of multiple cognitive domains including language functions.
ALS Brief Cognitive Assessment (91)	~5 min	A 5-item tool measuring executive functioning, fluency, and bvFTD behaviours.	Good accuracy for detecting bvFTD. Extremely brief. Not good at detecting mild cognitive impairment. Only measures executive functions. Does not control or motor speed.

bvFTD = behavioural variant of frontotemporal dementia; ALS-CBS = ALS Cognitive Behavioural Screen; FBI = Frontal Behavioural Inventory; UCSF = University of California, San Francisco.

ALS-Cognitive Behavioural Screen (ALS-CBS)

The behavioural section of the ALS-CBS is a brief 15-item questionnaire for caregivers. Usefully, four additional questions address depression, anxiety, emotional lability, and fatigue. The ALS-CBS was specifically designed for PALS and, as such, the behaviour screen is not dependent on motor function. Like the ECAS, the ALS-CBS benefits from being a joint cognitive and behavioural screen, which provides an overall indication of non-motor symptoms. Currently, the ALS-CBS has demonstrable ability to detect bvFTD, however, has poor predictive ability to differentiate mild behaviour change from bvFTD (103).

FBI-ALS

The Frontal Behavioural Interview has been recently adapted to measure changes in behaviour, frequency of behaviour, and to account for motor disability. An example of this is, 'When you think about those personal hygiene activities that they can complete on their own, does s/he neglect to initiate grooming or personal care activities as compared with their behaviour in the past?' While the FBI-ALS is promising and has recently been used in a large multi-centre research study (6), its validity has not been fully established.

MiND-B

The MiND-B consists of nine questions measuring levels of apathy, disinhibition, and stereotyped behaviour. Research suggests that it is good at differentiating behavioural symptoms in general, although it may lack the ability to differentiate mild from severe behavioural features (105). While it may be useful for detecting general behavioural involvement, it does not allow for detection of specific behavioural features and only queries three behaviour domains.

Table 8.3 ALS behavioural screening instruments

Name (reference)	Time Taken	Description	Strengths and Weaknesses
Edinburgh Cognitive and Behavioural ALS Screen (95)	5–10 min	Assesses 10 behaviour symptoms across five behaviour domains. Based on diagnostic criteria for bvFTD. Information is provided by caregiver.	Specifically designed for PALS. Interview provides opportunity to gather qualitative information about behaviours including frequency, severity, and time course. Based on bvFTD diagnostic criteria and includes cognitive screen. Restricted to diagnostic criteria for bvFTD.
ALS-CBS (103)	5 min	Assesses overall behavioural involvement with 15 questions measuring multiple areas of behaviour. Four additional questions address depression, anxiety, emotional lability, and fatigue. Information is provided by caregiver.	Specifically designed for PALS and research driven. Behaviour screen accounts for symptom severity. Includes cognitive screen. Does not measure specific behaviour domains or all items included in bvFTD diagnostic criteria.
ALS-FTD Q (109)	5–10 min	25 items including apathy, irritability, emotional lability and altered food preference	Specifically designed for PALS based on a systematic review of the literature. Good validity and gives information on frequency and severity and distinguishes between mild and more severe symptoms although not for particular behaviours.
Neuropsychiatric Inventory (NPI) (113)	10 min	Developed for Alzheimer's disease, measures aspects of behaviour and psychiatric symptoms.	Measures frequency, severity, and impact of symptoms. Available in numerous languages. Short form version available (NPI-Q) (Kaufer et al., 2000). Not specific to PALS and not independent of motor disability.
MiND-B (105)	5 min	9-item caregiver questionnaire measuring apathy, disinhibition, and stereotypic behaviours.	Very brief, independent of motor function. Provides clinical cut-offs for presence of behaviour. Unable to differentiate severity of symptoms, i.e. ALSbi to ALS-FTD. Does not accommodate the heterogeneity of behavioural features.
Frontal Behavioural Inventory-ALS (104)	10 min	The 24-item FBI was originally designed to measure behaviours associated with frontal lobe dysfunction. It has been adapted for motor disability in ALS. Information is provided by caregiver.	Instructions explicitly specify *changes* in behaviour not due to physical symptoms. Accounts for frequency of behaviour. No direct measure of symptom severity. Inconclusive results on its predictive ability. No cut-offs for impairment provided.

ALS-CBS: ALS Cognitive Behavioural Screen; ALS FTD Q: ALS and Frontotemporal Dementia Questionnaire; MiND-B: Motor Neuron Disease Behaviour Scale.

ALS-FTD-Q

The ALS-FTD-Q is a 25-item caregiver questionnaire providing an overall behavioural symptomatology score, in addition to assessing the frequency or severity of the symptoms. Questions include the domains of apathy, irritability, disinhibition, emotional lability, and altered food preferences. This scale was developed following a systematic search of behaviour symptoms in PALS. It has good validity and reliability and relates well to other measures of behaviour (109). The cut-offs for this scale provide distinctions between mild behavioural symptoms (ALSbi) and more severe symptoms, although not for a particular behaviour.

Conclusions and future directions

Cognitive and behavioural dysfunction in ALS is common, occurring in up to half of ALS patients. There is a spectrum of cognitive and behavioural involvement with up to 15% of ALS patients presenting with a full blown ALS-FTD syndrome, while ~ 35% show deficits detected through neuropsychological assessment. Most common deficits are found in letter fluency, executive functioning, and language, while social cognition deficits have been recently described. These impairments are found independent of motor disability. In addition, patients may show a behavioural syndrome with changes ranging from mild specific difficulties to fulfilling diagnostic criteria for bvFTD. Changes are most commonly found in apathy, but disinhibition, perseveration, loss of sympathy/empathy, and change in eating behaviour are also described. These symptoms may impact on quality of life for both patient and caregiver, and behaviour abnormalities in particular are related to high caregiver burden.

The importance of assessment is being increasingly recognized and incorporated into new guidelines for management. A distinction is made between brief assessment tools and screening measures useful within clinics for use by the members of the ALS health care team and more extensive neuropsychological assessment by a qualified clinical neuropsychologist. All assessment should be supervised by a clinical neuropsychologist to aid in training of administration and interpretation, and to guide intervention.

Future research will determine the impact of cognitive screening and assessment on care pathways and clinical management. Increased knowledge of the relevance of the different types of presentation (language vs executive functions), how presentations may change over time and their relation to disease course will also aid in our understanding of the disease. Exploration of the impact of these changes on day to day functioning is also vital to improving intervention. It is predicted that the implementation of these newly developed ALS assessment methods will make a valuable contribution to clinical care.

References

1. BaK, T.H. (2010) Motor neuron disease and frontotemporal dementia: One, two, or three diseases?. *Annals of the Indian Academy of Neurology*, **13**, S81–8.

2. Nitrini, R. (2014) Frontotemporal dementia and amyotrophic lateral sclerosis: Revisiting one of the first case reports with neuropathological examination. *Dementia & Neuropsychologia*, **8**(1), 83–6.

3. **Rascovsky, K., Hodges, J.R., Knopman, D.**, et al. (2011) Sensitivity of revised diagnostic criteria for the behavioural variant of frontotemporal dementia. *Brain*, **134**(Pt 9), 2456–77.

4. **Massman, P.J., Sims, J., Cooke, N., Haverkamp, L.J., Appel, V.,** and **Appel, S.H.** (1996) Prevalence and correlates of neuropsychological deficits in amyotrophic lateral sclerosis. *Journal of Neurology, Neurosurgery & Psychiatry*, **61**(5), 450–5.

5. **Ringholz, G.M., Appel, S.H., Bradshaw, M., Cooke, N.A., Mosnik, D.M.,** and **Schulz, P.E.** (2005) Prevalence and patterns of cognitive impairment in sporadic ALS. *Neurology*, **65**(4), 586–90.

6. **Murphy, J., Ahmed, F.,** and **Lomen-Hoerth, C.** (2016) The UCSF screening exam effectively screens cognitive and behavioral impairment in patients with ALS. *Amyotrophic Lateral Sclerosis & Frontotemporal Degeneration*, **16**(1–2), 24–30.

7. **Phukan, J., Elamin, M., Bede, P.,** et al. (2012) The syndrome of cognitive impairment in amyotrophic lateral sclerosis: A population-based study. *Journal of Neurology, Neurosurgery & Psychiatry*, **83**(1), 102–8.

8. **Montuschi, A., Iazzolino, B., Calvo, A.,** et al. (2015) Cognitive correlates in amyotrophic lateral sclerosis: a population-based study in Italy. *Journal of Neurology, Neurosurgery & Psychiatry*, **86**(2), 168–73.

9. **Goldstein, L.H.** and **Abrahams, S.** (2013) Changes in cognition and behaviour in amyotrophic lateral sclerosis: Nature of impairment and implications for assessment. *Lancet Neurology*, **12**(4), 368–80.

10. **Beeldman, E.R.J., Klein Twennaar, M., de Visser, M., Schmand, B.A.,** and **de Haan, R.J.** (2016) The cognitive profile of ALS: A systematic review and meta-analysis update. *Journal of Neurology Neurosurgery and Psychiatry*, **87**(6), 611–19.

11. **Abrahams, S., Goldstein, L.H., Al-Chalabi, A.,** et al. (1997) Relation between cognitive dysfunction and pseudobulbar palsy in amyotrophic lateral sclerosis. *Journal of Neurology, Neurosurgery & Psychiatry*, **62**(5), 464–72.

12. **Abrahams, S., Goldstein, L.H., Kew, J.J.,** et al. (1996) Frontal lobe dysfunction in amyotrophic lateral sclerosis. A PET study. *Brain*, **119**(Pt 6), 2105–20.

13. **Abrahams, S., Goldstein, L.H., Simmons, A.,** et al. (2004) Word retrieval in amyotrophic lateral sclerosis: A functional magnetic resonance imaging study. *Brain*, **127**(Pt 7), 1507–17.

14. **Abrahams, S., Leigh, P.N., Harvey, A., Vythelingum, G.N., Grise, D.,** and **Goldstein, L.H.** Verbal fluency and executive dysfunction in amyotrophic lateral sclerosis (ALS). *Neuropsychologia*, **38**(6), 734–47.

15. **Stukovnik, V., Zidar, J., Podnar, S.,** and **Repovs, G.** (2010) Amyotrophic lateral sclerosis patients show executive impairments on standard neuropsychological measures and an ecologically valid motor-free test of executive functions. *Journal of Clinical & Experimental Neuropsychology*, **32**, 1095–109.

16. **Abrahams, S., Goldstein, L.H., Suckling, J.,** et al. Frontotemporal white matter changes in amyotrophic lateral sclerosis. J Neurol. 2005;**252**(3):321–31.

17. **Libon, D., McMillan, C., Avants, B.,** et al. (2012) Deficits in concept formation in amyotrophic lateral sclerosis. *Neuropsychology*, **26**, 422–9.

18. **Pettit, L.D., Bastin, M.E., Smith, C., Bak, T.H., Gillingwater, T.H.,** and **Abrahams, S.** (2013) Executive deficits, not processing speed relates to abnormalities in distinct prefrontal tracts in amyotrophic lateral sclerosis. *Brain*, **136**(Pt 11), 3290–304.

19. **Pinkhardt, E.H., Jurgens, R., Becker, W.,** et al. (2008) Signs of impaired selective attention in patients with amyotrophic lateral sclerosis. *Journal of Neurology*, **255**(4), 532–8.

20. Volpato, C.P.S.M., Silvoni, S., Segato, N., et al. (2016) Selective attention impairment in amyotrophic lateral sclerosis. *Amyotrophic Lateral Sclerosis and Frontotemporal Degeneration*, **17**(30–4), 236–44.

21. Witgert, M., Salamone, A.R., Strutt, A.M., et al. (2010) Frontal-lobe mediated behavioral dysfunction in amyotrophic lateral sclerosis. *European Journal of Neurology*, **17**(1), 103–10.

22. Christidi, F., Zalonis, I., Smyrnis, N., and Evdokimidis, I. (2012) Selective attention and the three-process memory model for the interpretation of verbal free recall in amyotrophic lateral sclerosis. *Journal of the International Neuropsychological Society*, **18**(5), 809–18.

23. Zalonis, I., Christidi, F., Paraskevas, G., Zabelis, T., Evdokimidis, I., and Kararizou, E. (2012) Can executive cognitive measures differentiate between patients with spinal- and bulbar-onset amyotrophic lateral sclerosis? *Archives of Clinical Neuropsychology*, **27**(3), 348–54.

24. Hanagasi, H.A., Gurvit, I.H., Ermutlu, N., et al. (2002) Cognitive impairment in amyotrophic lateral sclerosis: evidence from neuropsychological investigation and event-related potentials. *Cognitive Brain Research*, **14**(2), 234–44.

25. Lillo, P., Savage, S., Mioshi, E., Kiernan, M.C., and Hodges, J.R. (2012) Amyotrophic lateral sclerosis and frontotemporal dementia: A behavioural and cognitive continuum. *Amyotrophic Lateral Sclerosis*, **13**(1), 102–9.

26. Hammer, A., Vielhaber, S., Rodriguez-Fornells, A., Mohammadi, B., and Muente, T.F. (2011) A neurophysiological analysis of working memory in amyotrophic lateral sclerosis. *Brain Research*, **1421**, 90–9.

27. Libon, D.J., McMillan, C., Avants, B., et al. (2012) Deficits in concept formation in amyotrophic lateral sclerosis. *Neuropsychology*, **26**(4), 422–9.

28. Watermeyer, T.J., Brown, R.G., Sidle, K.C., et al. (2015) Executive dysfunction predicts social cognition impairment in amyotrophic lateral sclerosis. *Journal of Neurology*, **262**(7), 1681–90.

29. Lange, F.V.M., Seer, C., Fürkötter, S., et al. (2016) Impaired set-shifting in amyotrophic lateral sclerosis: An event-related potential study of executive function. *Neuropsychology*, **30**(1), 120–34.

30. Abrahams, S. (2012) Social cognition in amyotrophic lateral sclerosis. *Neurodegenerative Disease Management*, **1**(5), 397–405.

31. Elamin, M., Pender, N., Hardiman, O., and Abrahams, S. (2012) Social cognition in neurodegenerative disorders: a systematic review. *Journal of Neurosurgery, Neuropsychology & Psychiatry*, **83**, 1071–9.

32. Lule, D., Kurt, A., Jurgens, R., et al. (2005) Emotional responding in amyotrophic lateral sclerosis. *Journal of Neurology*, **252**(12), 1517–24.

33. Schmolck, H., Mosnik, D., Schulz, P., Schmolck, H., Mosnik, D., and Schulz, P. (2007) Rating the approachability of faces in ALS. *Neurology*, **69**(24), 2232–5.

34. Crespi, C., Cerami, C., Dodich, A., et al. (2014) Microstructural white matter correlates of emotion recognition impairment in Amyotrophic Lateral Sclerosis. *Cortex*, **53**, 1–8.

35. Girardi, A., MacPherson, S.E., and Abrahams, S. (2011) Deficits in emotional and social cognition in amyotrophic lateral sclerosis. *Neuropsychology*, **25**(1), 53–65.

36. Savage, S.A., Lillo, P., Kumfor, F., Kiernan, M.C., Piguet, O., and Hodges, J.R. (2014) Emotion processing deficits distinguish pure amyotrophic lateral sclerosis from frontotemporal dementia. *Amyotrophic Lateral sclerosis & Frontotemporal Degeneration*, **15**(1–2), 39–46.

37. Zimmerman, E.K., Eslinger, P.J., Simmons, Z., et al. (2007) Emotional perception deficits in amyotrophic lateral sclerosis. *Cognitive & Behavioral Neurology*, **20**(2), 79–82.

38. Palmieri, A., Naccarato, M., Abrahams, S., et al. (2010) Right hemisphere dysfunction and emotional processing in ALS: An fMRI study. *Journal of Neurology*, **257**(12), 1970–8.

39. Papps, B., Abrahams, S., Wicks, P., Leigh, P.N., and Goldstein, L.H. (2005) Changes in memory for emotional material in amyotrophic lateral sclerosis (ALS). *Neuropsychologia*, **43**(8), 1107–14.

40. Stone, V.E., Baron-Cohen, S., and Knight, R.T. (1998) Frontal lobe contributions to theory of mind. *Journal of Cognitive Neurosciences*, **10**(5), 640–56.

41. Meier, S.L., Charleston, A.J., Tippett, L.J., Meier, S.L., Charleston, A.J., and Tippett, L.J. (2010) Cognitive and behavioural deficits associated with the orbitomedial prefrontal cortex in amyotrophic lateral sclerosis. *Brain*, **133**(11), 3444–57.

42. Cavallo, M., Adenzato, M., MacPherson, S.E., Karwig, G., Enrici, I., and Abrahams, S. (2011) Evidence of social understanding impairment in patients with amyotrophic lateral sclerosis. *PLoS One*, **6**(10), e25948.

43. van der Hulst, E.J., Bak, T.H., and Abrahams, S. (2015) Impaired affective and cognitive theory of mind and behavioural change in amyotrophic lateral sclerosis. *Journal of Neurology, Neurosurgery & Psychiatry*, **86**(11), 1208–15.

44. Gibbons, Z.C., Richardson, A., Neary, D., et al. (2008) Behaviour in amyotrophic lateral sclerosis. *Amyotrophic Lateral Sclerosis*, **9**(2), 67–74.

45. Abrahams, S. (2013) Executive dysfunction in ALS is not the whole story. *Journal of Neurology, Neurosurgery & Psychiatry*, **84**(5), 474–5.

46. Taylor, L.J., Brown, R.G., Tsermentseli, S., Al-Chalabi, A., Shaw, C.E., Leigh, P.N., and Goldstein, L.H. (2013) Is language impairment more common than executive dysfunction in amyotrophic lateral sclerosis? *Journal of Neurology, Neurosurgery & Psychiatry*, **84**(5), 494–8.

47. Bak, T.H. and Chandran, S. (2012) What wires together dies together: verbs, actions and neurodegeneration in motor neuron disease. *Cortex*, **48**(7), 936–44.

48. Grossman, M., Anderson, C., Khan, A., Avants, B., Elman, L., and McCluskey, L. (2008) Impaired action knowledge in amyotrophic lateral sclerosis. *Neurology*, **71**(18), 1396–401.

49. Ash, S., Olm, C., McMillan, C.T., et al. (2015) Deficits in sentence expression in amyotrophic lateral sclerosis. *Amyotrophic Lateral sclerosis & Frontotemporal Degeneration*, **16**(1–2), 31–9.

50. Tsermentseli, S., Leigh, P.N., Taylor, L.J., Radunovic, A., Catani, M., & Goldstein, L.H. (2015) Syntactic processing as a marker for cognitive impairment in amyotrophic lateral sclerosis. *Amyotrophic Lateral Sclerosis & Frontotemporal Degeneration*, **17**(1–2), 69–76.

51. Leslie, F.V., Hsieh, S., Caga, J., et al. (2015) Semantic deficits in amyotrophic lateral sclerosis. *Amyotrophic Lateral Sclerosis & Frontotemporal Degeneration*, **16**(1–2), 46–53.

52. Raaphorst, J., van Tol, M.J., de Visser, M., et al. (2015) Prose memory impairment in amyotrophic lateral sclerosis patients is related to hippocampus volume. *European Journal of Neurology*, **22**(3), 547–54.

53. Machts, J., Bittner, V., Kasper, E., et al. (2014) Memory deficits in amyotrophic lateral sclerosis are not exclusively caused by executive dysfunction: a comparative neuropsychological study of amnestic mild cognitive impairment. *BMC Neuroscience*, **15**, 83.

54. Raaphorst, J., Beeldman, E., De Visser, M., De Haan, R.J., and Schmand, B. (2012) A systematic review of behavioural changes in motor neuron disease. *Amyotrophic Lateral Sclerosis*, **13**(6), 493–501.

55. Woolley, S.C., Moore, D.H., Katz, J.S., Woolley, S.C., Moore, D.H., and Katz, J.S. (2010) Insight in ALS: Awareness of behavioral change in patients with and without FTD. *Amyotrophic Lateral Sclerosis*, **11**(1–2), 52–6.

56. Grossman, A.B., Woolley-Levine, S., Bradley, W.G., et al. (2007) Detecting neurobehavioral changes in amyotrophic lateral sclerosis. *Amyotrophic Lateral Sclerosis*, **8**(1), 56–61.

57. Terada, T., Obi, T., Yoshizumi, M., Murai, T., Miyajima, H., and Mizoguchi, K. (2011) Frontal lobe-mediated behavioral changes in amyotrophic lateral sclerosis: are they independent of physical disabilities? *Journal of Neurological Sciences*, **309**(1–2), 136–40.

58. Chio, A., Vignola, A., Mastro, E., et al. (2010) Neurobehavioral symptoms in ALS are negatively related to caregivers' burden and quality of life. *European Journal of Neurology*, **17**, 1298–303.

59. Lillo, P., Mioshi, E., Zoing, M.C., et al. (2011) How common are behavioural changes in amyotrophic lateral sclerosis? *Amyotrophic Lateral Sclerosis*, **12**(1), 45–51.

60. Radakovic, R. and Abrahams, S. (2014) Developing a new apathy measurement scale: Dimensional Apathy Scale. *Psychiatry Research*, **219**(3), 658–63.

61. Radakovic, R., Stephenson, L., Colville, S., Swingler, R., Chandran, S., & Abrahams, S. (2016) Multidimensional apathy in ALS: Validation of the Dimensional Apathy Scale. *Journal of Neurology Neurosurgery and Psychiatry*, **87**(6), 663–9.

62. Ahmed, R.M. Caga, J., Devenney, E., et al. (2016) Cognition and eating behavior in amyotrophic lateral sclerosis: effect on survival. *Journal of Neurology*, **263**(8), 1593–608.

63. Newsom-Davis, I.C., Abrahams, S., Goldstein, L.H., and Leigh PN. (1999) The emotional lability questionnaire: A new measure of emotional lability in amyotrophic lateral sclerosis. *Journal of Neurological Sciences*, **169**(1–2), 22–5.

64. Palmieri, A., Abrahams, S., Sorarù, G., et al. (2009) Emotional lability in MND: Relationship to cognition and psychopathology and impact on caregivers. *Journal of Neurological Sciences*, **278**(1–2), 16–20.

65. McCullagh, S., Moore, M., Gawel, M., and Feinstein, A. (1999) Pathological laughing and crying in amyotrophic lateral sclerosis: An association with prefrontal cognitive dysfunction. *Journal of Neurological Sciences*, **169**(1–2), 43–8.

66. Tortelli, R., Copetti, M., Arcuti, S., et al. (2016) Pseudobulbar affect (PBA) in an incident ALS cohort: results from the Apulia registry (SLAP). *Journal of Neurology*, **263**(2), 316–21.

67. Gordon, P.H., Wang, Y., Doorish, C., et al. (2007) A screening assessment of cognitive impairment in patients with ALS. *Amyotrophic Lateral Sclerosis*, **8**(6), 362–5.

68. Raaphorst, J., Beeldman, E., Schmand, B., et al. (2012) The ALS-FTD-Q: A new screening tool for behavioral disturbances in ALS. *Neurology*, **79**(13), 1377–83.

69. De Silva, D., Hsieh, S., Caga, J., et al. (2016) Motor function and behaviour across the ALS-FTD spectrum. *Acta Neurologica Scandinavica*, **133**(5), 367–72.

70. Kilani, M., Micallef, J., Soubrouillard, C., et al. (2004) A longitudinal study of the evolution of cognitive function and affective state in patients with amyotrophic lateral sclerosis. *Amyotrophic Lateral Sclerosis & Other Motor Neuron Disorders*, **5**(1), 46–54.

71. Robinson, K.M., Lacey, S.C., Grugan, P., Glosser, G., Grossman, M., and McCluskey, L.F. (2006) Cognitive functioning in sporadic amyotrophic lateral sclerosis: A six month longitudinal study. *Journal of Neurology, Neurosurgery & Psychiatry*, **77**(5), 668–70.

72. Abrahams, S., Leigh, P.N., and Goldstein, L.H. (2005) Cognitive change in ALS: A prospective study. *Neurology*, **64**(7), 1222–6.

73. Gordon, P.H., Goetz, R.R., Rabkin, J.G., et al. (2010) A prospective cohort study of neuropsychological test performance in ALS. *Amyotrophic Lateral Sclerosis*, **11**(3), 312–20.

74. Schreiber, H., Gaigalat, T., Wiedemuth-Catrinescu, U., et al. (2005) Cognitive function in bulbar- and spinal-onset amyotrophic lateral sclerosis. A longitudinal study in 52 patients. *Journal of Neurology*, **252**(7), 772–81.

75. Elamin, M., Bede, P., Byrne, S., et al. (2013) Cognitive changes predict functional decline in ALS: A population-based longitudinal study. *Neurology*, **80**, 1590–6.

76. Consonni, M., Iannaccone, S., Cerami, C., et al. (2013) The cognitive and behavioural profile of amyotrophic lateral sclerosis: Application of the consensus criteria. *Behavioural Neurology*, **27**(2), 143–53.

77. Lillo, P., Garcin, B., Hornberger, M., et al. (2010) Neurobehavioral features in frontotemporal dementia with amyotrophic lateral sclerosis. *Archives of Neurology*, **67**(7), 826–30.

78. Woolley, S.C., Zhang, Y., Schuff, N., et al. (2011) Neuroanatomical correlates of apathy in ALS using 4 Tesla diffusion tensor MRI. *Amyotrophic Lateral Sclerosis*, **12**(1), 52–8.

79. Newsom-Davis, I.C., Lyall, R.A., Leigh, P.N., Moxham, J., and Goldstein, L.H. (2001) The effect of non-invasive positive pressure ventilation (NIPPV) on cognitive function in amyotrophic lateral sclerosis (ALS): A prospective study. *Journal of Neurology, Neurosurgery & Psychiatry*, **71**(4), 482–7.

80. Kim, S.M., Lee, K.M., Hong, Y.H., et al. (2007) Relation between cognitive dysfunction and reduced vital capacity in amyotrophic lateral sclerosis. *Journal of Neurology, Neurosurgery & Psychiatry*, **78**(12), 1387–9.

81. Sterling, L.E., Jawaid, A., Salamone, A.R., et al. (2010) Association between dysarthria and cognitive impairment in ALS: A prospective study. *Amyotrophic Lateral Sclerosis*, **11**(1–2), 46–51.

82. Strong, M.J., Grace, G.M., Freedman, M., et al. (2009) Consensus criteria for the diagnosis of frontotemporal cognitive and behavioural syndromes in amyotrophic lateral sclerosis. *Amyotrophic Lateral Sclerosis*, **10**(3), 131–46. [Erratum appears in *Amyotrophic Lateral Sclerosis*, **10**(4), 252].

83. Gorno-Tempini, M.L., Hillis, A.E., Weintraub, S., et al. (2011) Classification of primary progressive aphasia and its variants. *Neurology*, **76**(11), 1006–14.

84. Goldstein, L.H., Atkins, L., and Leigh, P.N. (2002) Correlates of quality of life in people with motor neuron disease (MND). *Amyotrophic Lateral Sclerosis & Other Motor Neuron Disorders*, **3**(3), 123–9.

85. Tremolizzo, L., Pellegrini, A., Susani, E., et al. (2016) Behavioural but not cognitive impairment is a determinant of caregiver burden in amyotrophic lateral sclerosis. *European Neurology*, **75**(3–4), 191–4.

86. Goldstein, L.H., Adamson, M., Jeffrey, L., et al. (1998) The psychological impact of MND on patients and carers. *Journal of Neurological Sciences*, **160**(Suppl. 1), S114–21.

87. Lillo, P., Mioshi, E., & Hodges, J.R. (2012) Caregiver burden in amyotrophic lateral sclerosis is more dependent on patient's behavioral changes than physical disability: a comparative study. *Neurology*, **12**, 156.

88. Caga, J., Turner, M.R., Hsieh, S., et al. (2016) Apathy is associated with poor prognosis in amyotrophic lateral sclerosis. *European Journal of Neurology*, **23**(5), 891–7.

89. **Chio, A., Ilardi, A., Cammarosano, S., Moglia, C., Montuschi, A.,** and **Calvo, A.** (2012) Neurobehavioral dysfunction in ALS has a negative effect on outcome and use of PEG and NIV. *Neurology*, **78**(14), 1085–9.

90. **Elamin, M., Phukan, J. Bede, P.** et al. (2011) Executive dysfunction is a negative prognostic indicator in patients with ALS without dementia. *Neurology*, **76**, 1263–9.

91. **Hu, W.T., Shelnutt, M., Wilson, A.,** et al. (2013) Behavior matters—cognitive predictors of survival in amyotrophic lateral sclerosis. *PLoS One*, **8**(2), e57584.

92. **Olney, R.K., Murphy, J., Forshew, D.,** et al. (2005) The effects of executive and behavioral dysfunction on the course of ALS. *Neurology*, **65**(11), 1774–7.

93. **Abrahams, S.** (2013) ALS, cognition and the clinic. *Amyotrophic Lateral Sclerosis and Frontotemporal Degeneration*, **14**(1), 3–5.

94. **Excellence NIfHaC.** (2016) UK Motor neurone disease: assessment and management, NG521–47. Available at: https://www.nice.org.uk/guidance/NG42.

95. **Abrahams, S., Newton, J., Niven, E., Foley, J.,** and **Bak, T.H.** (2014) Screening for cognition and behaviour changes in ALS. *Amyotrophic Lateral Sclerosis and Frontotemporal Degeneration*, **15**(1–2), 9–14.

96. **Niven, E., Newton, J., Foley, J.,** et al. (2015) Validation of the Edinburgh Cognitive and Behavioural Amyotrophic Lateral Sclerosis Screen (ECAS): A cognitive tool for motor disorders. *Amyotrophic Lateral Sclerosis & Frontotemporal Degeneration*, **16**(3–4), 172–9.

97. **Loose, M., Burkhardt, C., Aho-Ozhan, H.,** et al. (2016) Age and education-matched cut-off scores for the revised German/Swiss-German version of ECAS. *Amyotrophic Lateral Sclerosis & Frontotemporal Degeneration*, **17**(5–6), 374–6.

98. **Lulé, D., Burkhardt, C., Abdulla, S.,** et al. (2015) The Edinburgh Cognitive and Behavioural Amyotrophic Lateral Sclerosis Screen: A cross-sectional comparison of established screening tools in a German-Swiss population. *Amyotrophic Lateral Sclerosis & Frontotemporal Degeneration*, **16**(1–2), 16–23.

99. **Poletti, B., Solca, F, Carelli, L.,** et al. (2016) The validation of the Italian Edinburgh Cognitive and Behavioural ALS Screen (ECAS). *Amyotrophic Lateral Sclerosis & Frontotemporal Degeneration*, **17(7–8), 489–98**.

100. **Ye, S, Ji, Y., Li, C., He, J., Liu, X.,** and **Fan, D.** (2016) The Edinburgh Cognitive and Behavioural ALS Screen in a Chinese Amyotrophic Lateral Sclerosis Population. *PLoS One*, **11**(5), e0155496.

101. **Pinto-Grau, M., Burke, T., Lonergan, K., McHugh, C., Mays, I.,** and **Madden, C.** (2017) Screening for cognitive dysfunction in ALS: validation of the Edinburgh Cognitive and Behavioural ALS Screen (ECAS) using age and education adjusted normative data. *Amyotrophic Lateral Sclerosis & Frontotemporal Degeneration*, **18**, 99–106.

102. **Crockford, C., Kleynhans, M., Wilton, E.,** et al. (2015) Development of parallel versions of the Edinburgh Cognitive and Behavioural ALS Screen (ECAS). *Amyotrophic Lateral Sclerosis & Frontotemporal Degeneration*, **16**, 115–23.

103. **Woolley, S.C., York, M.K., Moore, D.H.,** et al. (2010) Detecting frontotemporal dysfunction in ALS: Utility of the ALS Cognitive Behavioral Screen (ALS-CBS). *Amyotrophic Lateral Sclerosis*, **11**(3), 303–11.

104. **Kertesz, A., Davidson, W.,** and **Fox, H.** (1997) Frontal behavioral inventory: Diagnostic criteria for frontal lobe dementia. *Canadian Journal of Neurological Sciences*, **24**, 29–36.

105. **Hsieh, S., Caga, J., Leslie, F.V.,** et al. (2016) Cognitive and behavioral symptoms in ALSFTD: Detection, differentiation, and progression. *Journal of Geriatric Psychiatry & Neurology*, **29**(1), 3–10.

106. **Turon-Sans, J., Gascon-ayarri, J., Reñé, R.,** et al. Cognitive impairment in ALS patients and validation of the Spanish version of the ALS-CBS test. *Amyotrophic Lateral Sclerosis and Frontotemporal Degeneration*, 2016, **17**, 221–7.

107. **Kaufer, D.I., Cummings, J.L., Ketchel, P.,** et al. Validation of the NPI-Q, a brief clinical form of the neuropsychiatric inventory. *Journal of Neuropsychiatry and Clinical Neuroscience*, 2000 Spring, **12**(2), 233–9.

108. **Snowden, J.S., Rollinson, S., Thompson, J.C.,** et al. (2012) Distinct clinical and pathological characteristics of frontotemporal dementia associated with C9orf72 mutations. *Brain*, **135**, 693–708.

109. **Raaphorst, J., Beeldman, E., Schmand, B.,** et al. (2012) The ALS-FTD-Q: a new screening tool for behavioral disturbances in ALS. *Neurology*, **79**, 1377–83.

110. **Flaherty-Craig, C., Brothers, A., Dearman, B.,** et al. (2009) Penn State screen exam for the detection of frontal and temporal dysfunction syndromes: Application to ALS. *Amyotrophic Lateral Sclerosis*, **10**(2), 107–12.

111. **Nasreddine, Z.S., Phillips, N.A., Bedirian, V.,** et al. (2005) The Montreal Cognitive Assessment, MoCA: A brief screening tool for cognitive impairment. *Journal of the American Geriatric Society*, **53**, 695–9.

112. **Dubois, B., Slachevsky, A., Litvan, I.,** and **Pillon, B.** (2000) The FAB: A frontal assessment battery at bedside. *Neurology*, **55**, 1621–6.

113. **Cummings, J.L., Mega, M., Gray, K., Rosenberg-Thompson, S., Carusi, D.A.,** and **Gornbein, J.** (1994) The neuropsychiatric inventory: comprehensive assessment of psychopathology in dementia. *Neurology*, **44**, 2308–14.

Chapter 9

The impact of cognitive and behavioural change on quality of life of caregivers and patients with ALS and other neurological conditions

Tom Burke, Miriam Galvin, Sinead Maguire, Niall Pender, and Orla Hardiman

Introduction

Patients with amyotrophic lateral sclerosis (ALS), experience cognitive and behavioural impairment that share features with Huntington 's disease (HD), Multiple Sclerosis (MS), Frontotemporal Dementia (FTD), Traumatic Brain Injury (TBI), Stroke, and Parkinson 's disease (PD) (1,2). Lessons can be learned across these conditions about recognition, evaluation and management of cognitive and behavioural change, and the impact of these changes on quality of life (QoL) of patients, caregivers and their families.

ALS is a progressive condition, and cognitive deficits at the early stage of the condition can predict functional decline in patients (3). This is also the case in other forms of neurodegeneration- for example measures of cognitive impairment can be used to predict disease trajectory in dementia populations (4). Like other neurodegenerative diseases, ALS can also present with behavioural changes that are sometimes not recognized by family members or healthcare professionals. These changes reflect the extent of the underlying disease progression (5), and combined with cognitive impairment, lead to a significant change from the premorbid personality. In ALS, these cognitive and behavioural deficits can manifest along a continuum from very mild to severe forms (6), and may change independently of each other, and independently of motor decline (see also Chapter 8), leading to management challenges for clinical teams caring for such patients, and daily difficulties for caregivers and families (7).

Compared to classical neurological symptoms such as weakness or sensory loss, and established neuropsychiatric complications such as depression or anxiety, the impact of cognitive deficits and behavioural change on QoL of patients and their primary caregivers has been relatively under-investigated in ALS (8). While clinical teams often rely on established measures of physical impairment, functional decline, and reduced social participation to quantify the impact of a disease, other variables relevant to QoL such as perceived subjective well-being, life satisfaction, or spiritual fulfilment, are not routinely measured (9).

The impact of cognitive and behavioural impairment on QoL in ALS is accordingly complex and multi-dimensional. Cognitive domains such as executive function, social cognition, memory, attention, language/communication, combined with behavioural changes such as apathy, disinhibition, or aggression, can impact the perceived QoL in a patient or caregiver in a multitude of ways (10).

In general, cognitive and behavioural changes in the neurodegenerations also have real-world implications for people, not least of which is their impact on personal and domestic activities of daily living (ADLs) (11). Such impairments in the context of relative preservation of motor function can of themselves impact heavily on an individual's ability to pursue gainful employment. Indeed, a decline in ability to engage with the requirements of a job can sometimes be the first harbinger of a neurodegenerative condition—a factor that has until recently been under-recognized in ALS. The ensuing loss of employment can then represent one of the first assaults on an individual's autonomy, independence, and overall QoL (12). As the impairment progresses, there can be a profound impact on day-to-day activities. It is helpful to consider a few examples of the consequences of specific types of cognitive impairment in neurodegenerative disorders:

Visuo-spatial impairment is the most significant predictor of decline in ability to dress, bathe, use the telephone, or retain mobility (13). A decline in these abilities is often seen early in the course of posterior variants of Alzheimer's disease (Posterior Cortical Atrophy) or with Parkinsonian conditions.

A decline in *attention* impacts on an individual's capability for awareness of basic personal ADLs such as washing and independent toileting, enjoyment from social relationships, and may even create a health and safety risk in navigating new environments, identifying risk and monitoring behavioural errors (14).

Language impairment (a feature in left lateralized frontotemporal dementia) is associated with poor communication, both verbally and with the use of communication aids (15).

Memory impairment, can lead to confusion, getting lost in familiar places, and potentially hazardous situations (e.g. a gas stove may have been ignited and forgotten about, a failure to take prescribed medication or adhere to strict medical regimes). Such impairment often leads to the need for 1:1 supervision as the disease progresses (16).

Speed of information processing can have a serious impact on a patient's daily functioning. Many patients struggle to follow conversations, quickly make decisions, or even understand their favourite television programmes (17). Due to these limitations, many patients begin to avoid social gatherings due to their inability to keep up with rapid social communication. This is often compounded by difficulties with social cognition, which can impact on their ability to understand the intentions and emotional needs of others, as well as produce socially appropriate affection and emotion (18).

As all aspects of cognitive dysfunction impact on adherence to treatment plans (19), performance on cognitive testing can provide valuable insights into the patient's daily functioning and enable clinical teams to make suitable arrangements for care and management (20, 21). Discussing treatment options early in the course of the disease may reduce health-related stress for patients and their caregivers as the disease progresses (22).

Cognitive and behavioural change in ALS and FTD

In recent years, there has been an increasing awareness of the relationship between ALS and FTD (23). This overlap has been strengthened by recent studies that focus on the cognitive and behavioural continuum in ALS (See Chapter 8). On-going genetic discoveries, such as the C9*orf*72 variant (24), have contributed to our understanding of these conditions. Taken together, it is now clear that recognition of cognitive and behavioural impairment is an essential component in the management of patients with ALS (25), as up to 13% of ALS patients are known to present with a comorbid FTD (26). Due to the triad of physical, cognitive, and behavioural features associated with ALS-FTD, greater caregiver burden and lower QoL have been recognized in patients with both ALS and FTD (27). The most commonly reported cognitive deficit in population-based ALS research is executive dysfunction (in up to 25%), followed by non-executive cognitive deficits, i.e. language, memory, visual impairment (14%), with the remainder remaining relatively intact (28).

Selective cognitive impairment in the form of verbal fluency deficits, most likely indicating executive dysfunction, appears relatively early in the course of the disease, and language functions may become more vulnerable as the disease progresses (29). Planning, organizing information, problem solving, shifting attention, inhibiting behaviour, and negotiating social norms are all examples of executive dysfunction in ALS (30). Within ALS, higher levels of cognitive and behavioural impairment specific to executive dysfunction indicate a more rapid disease progression (31).

Behavioural change can appear early and can precede more classic ALS symptoms (32). The most prominent behavioural change in ALS is apathy, present in up to 60% of ALS patients, followed by disinhibited and dysexecutive behaviours such as impulsivity (33). These neuropsychiatric symptoms have been shown to impact greatly on family caregivers and should be addressed early in the diagnosis and management of ALS (34). Recent findings suggest that patients with ALS who do not fulfil diagnostic criteria for ALS-FTD may also exhibit subtle neuropsychiatric and cognitive changes, which have been shown to negatively impact caregiver relationships (35).

FTD is characterized by a number of different sub-phenotypes (36-38), the most common of which is the behavioural variant (bvFTD). At the onset of bvFTD, behavioural changes dominate. These behavioural changes are associated with prominent personality changes, and early decline in interpersonal conduct (disinhibition). Impairment in regulation of personal conduct, emotional blunting, and loss of insight may occur early in the condition (39). Alongside these behavioural changes, patients often present with severe executive impairment.

As bvFTD advances, patients develop progressive disturbance of executive functions, loss of initiative, reduced mental flexibility, and poor organization (40). Language can be impaired, but not to the same extent as other FTD variants (41). Behavioural alterations such as pacing and repetitive stereotyped behaviours may also develop. More severe cognitive impairment and behavioural change at baseline tends to be associated with greater caregiver burden (42).

The impact of cognitive and behaviour change on patient QoL in ALS and FTD

In ALS, cognitive and behavioural deficits may present before the onset of motor symptoms, and there is an increasing recognition of the importance of categorizing a broad spectrum of cognitive impairments. However, there is a dearth of studies investigating the specific role of cognitive impairment on QoL (43). As has been shown in the case of other neurological conditions, quantifying the detrimental impact that cognitive and behavioural changes have on an individual's functional ability, lifestyle, and social interactions are of value as there is growing recognition that cognitive and behavioural changes are likely to negatively impact self-esteem, personal relationships, threaten social support, and consequently reduce QoL (44).

To date, there has been an absence of longitudinal research that assesses the degree to which QoL is influenced by changes in cognitive dysfunction and behavioural change (45). Cognitive deficits are conceived as a cumulative loss of function supported by specific systems, and the impact of heterogeneous losses is difficult to study. In ALS, cognitive deficits are rarely static and are often influenced by the natural history of disease (46). Longitudinal studies of cognition in ALS indicate that selective cognitive impairment, in the form of verbal fluency deficits, indicating executive dysfunction, appears very early in the course of the disease, and language functions become more vulnerable as the disease progresses. However, performance on cognitive testing close to the time of diagnosis of ALS is not predictive of burden or QoL. Within cross-sectional studies, QoL scores correlate positively with the existence of confiding and emotional support and correlate negatively with the presence of self-rated everyday cognitive difficulties, as described above.

A lack of insight in patients with ALS is associated with impaired executive skills such as decision-making (47). This represents a substantial clinical problem, with numerous studies documenting the negative impact of reduced insight. In a study comparing patients with ALS and those with ALS-FTD, patients with ALS–FTD had a worse compliance for the use of ventilatory support measures and nutritional supplements. Impaired deficit awareness has increasingly been recognized as a multifaceted neuropsychological problem (48). This is often assessed within the ALS literature, by relying on patients' subjective reports of difficulties and experiences in daily life, or disease related change using discrepancies between patients' self-report and that of a significant other (49).

Lessons from other neurological conditions

Recent work in ALS and ALS-FTD suggest that it is possible to identify those patients and caregivers most likely to remain burdened using data routinely collected, although more detailed work is required. Literature from other conditions highlights the importance of assessing and managing cognitive and behavioural changes. A detailed understanding of patients' cognitive and behavioural profiles can help inform individualized care-plans, which can in turn have a positive effect on patient and caregiver QoL. We have reviewed the literature regarding both static conditions (traumatic brain injury) and progressive disorders, to gain further insight into how best to measure, evaluate, and manage the effects of cognitive and behavioural change in ALS, in the context of rapidly progressive and ultimately fatal disability.

Traumatic brain injury

Traumatic Brain Injury (TBI) occurs suddenly and unexpectedly, and has lifelong implications. In this respect, the implications are not dissimilar to ALS, which often presents abruptly in otherwise healthy individuals in mid-life. As a result of the broad cognitive dysfunction following a TBI, substantial negative consequences in the QoL of both the patient and their family have been reported. Parents, siblings, spouses, or children might inadvertently become caregivers (50). The patient may experience significant limitations in the ability to engage in productive employment or social situations. Independent living can be challenging in many instances. While limits to self-awareness might mitigate the understanding of lifestyle and functional changes, patients and their families may also require intense input from acute and post-acute rehabilitation services to maintain QoL (51).

Many studies on TBI report that informants or caregivers rate the QoL of the patient lower than the patient's own self-report, as has also been described in some ALS studies (52). Potential explanatory factors for this discrepancy may be caregiver depression, caregiver burden, and gradual change of the patient's life goals into areas where more control can be exerted. The discrepancy may also be caused by the fact that some patients lack insight into their symptoms or that those patients may be unaware of lost functions, activities, and social relationships (53). However, some studies also suggest that patients rely on social comparison to rate their QoL and that patients might rate themselves high in relation to other patients who are perceived to have a great number of deficits rather than in relation to their former selves (54). These factors could also pertain to some patients with ALS, as they reflect on both their accruing losses, while also recognizing some aspects of their preserved function, although to our knowledge, no studies have formally assessed this as a coping strategy in ALS/FTD.

In TBI, the physical and cognitive impairments produced by the injury are frequently associated with serious functional limitations, thus resembling ALS. Persons with TBI may experience frustration, and a sense of lack of control that exacerbates their difficulties and lowers their QoL (55). Use of transportation and the freedom to interact with people and pursue one's interests are often restricted due to loss of driving privileges, related cognitive impairment, or mobility issues (56). Communication problems are characteristic of many persons with TBI (57). Implemented interventions with TBI patients can benefit from using QoL-based outcome measures in conjunction with conventional measures, such as TBI severity; such an approach can also be of utility in ALS.

Brain tumour

There has been growing interest in the link between cognitive impairment and QoL in brain tumour patients, as subtle cognitive deficits are being identified. The diagnosis, management, and treatment of brain tumours have a major impact on patients' QoL. Most brain tumours are ultimately fatal, and for long survivors, cognitive deficits can prevent return to premorbid autonomy and occupation. Moreover, cognitive symptomatology may enhance the burden of other symptoms. These factors also apply to ALS.

Considering the impact of cognitive deficits on QoL in this cohort, patients also experience secondary symptoms including (but not limited to) motor deficits, personality changes, aphasia, or visual field defects. These additional symptoms can further impact on patient QoL. Tumour hemispheric laterality, size, and location, have also been reported to be contributory factors associated with lower QoL. This appears to be a consequence of greater cognitive impairment and behavioural change, associated with larger and more aggressive tumours in frontotemporal regions.

A multidimensional approach has been recommended when investigating the impact of cognitive and behavioural change on QoL of patients with brain tumours. Measures of well-being, which reflect psychosocial and cognitive aspects have been shown to be more appropriate to detect the impact on QoL for both the patient and the family, than traditionally isolated functional instruments. Lessons can be drawn from the brain tumour population in supporting ALS patients with severe cognitive and behavioural change.

Stroke

Stroke is sudden in onset and often leads to long term physical and cognitive deficits. Stroke patients report poorer QoL in the presence of memory and thinking difficulties (58). Ischaemic stroke patients have reported communication difficulties resulting in lower QoL (59). Infarct volume, aphasia, impaired motor function, and impaired cognitive function were independently linked with poorer QoL (60). Cognitive impairment (particularly problems with visual perception and construction), increasing age, and functional dependence, further predicted a reduced QoL. The combination of cognitive impairment, communication impairment, and asymmetric motor impairment that occurs in stroke can parallel the multi-domain changes that are characteristic of ALS.

The impact of cognitive impairment on QoL was investigated in 129 patients with ischaemic stroke (64 men; mean age 63.2±14.6 years). Infarct volume, aphasia, impaired motor function, disability relating to ADLs, disturbed global functional health and impaired cognitive function were significantly associated with poorer QoL (61). In another study of 1572 stroke patients, mean age 69 years (±12 years), cognitive impairment was present in 38%. Cognitive impairment was significantly related to lower functional outcomes and lower QoL. Attention and visuospatial ability were again the cognitive domains most closely associated with QoL (62). While ALS patients do not generally exhibit visuospatial impairment, the QoL implication of communication impairment associated with stroke can help to inform those associated with ALS.

Alzheimer's disease

QoL studies in AD recognize the importance of the patient-caregiver dyad, and are of value when considering the impact of cognitive and behavioural change in ALS. As has been described in TBI and ALS, patients with early AD generally report higher QoL than their informants. This disagreement is sometimes associated with the presence of anosognosia, which can also be a feature of FTD associated with ALS. Several other factors, such as dementia severity, memory impairment, and impairments in ADLs have also been reported to have a significant impact on QoL in AD.

Research on determinants of QoL for patients with AD, and interventions to increase QoL are current priorities in dementia care. In a recent study of AD patient and caregiver dyads, and an additional comparison group of 22 dyads without cognitive impairment, correlations of patient reported QoL with patient depression scores were significant, alongside satisfaction with life scale reports (63). Caregiver QoL was correlated with the Neuropsychiatric Inventory total score, distress, and patient MMSE. Patient QoL ratings were higher than caregiver ratings. Both patient- and caregiver-rated QoL scores were lower in patients with cognitive impairment than in the comparison group without cognitive impairment. 164 patients-caregiver dyads were recruited to investigate the role of anosognosia on QoL. The results showed that lower depression scores and greater anosognosia explained 33% and 10% of the variance in QoL, respectively. That is, greater anosognosia was associated with higher perceived QoL in the patient. Conversely, anosognosia was associated with greater caregiver burden and a greater discrepancy between patient and caregiver ratings of QoL.

The role of formal versus informal healthcare settings has been widely researched in AD, compared to ALS and other related neurodegenerative conditions. For example, total QoL score has been shown to be higher (i.e. better QoL) for patients living at home than for institutionalized patients. These types of studies have not yet been performed in ALS.

Impaired ADLs predicted lower QoL in the later stages of cognitive impairment, or more severe AD. Behavioural disturbances, especially agitation, appeared to be negatively related to proxy-rated QoL in AD. There appeared to be a negative relation between QoL, ADLs, and cognition, although this is not confirmed in all studies. In longitudinal studies, depressive symptoms were negatively related to QoL, and cognition was positively related to self-rated QoL. Dependency and depressive symptoms were negatively related to proxy-rated QoL.

Parkinson's disease

Parkinson's Disease (PD) shares similarities with ALS as an age-related neurodegeneration with a combination of motor and cognitive domains. Cognitive, behavioural, and sleep disturbances are associated with reduced QoL in PD (64). Non-motor symptoms have been shown to be more important for reduced health-related QoL than motor symptoms. Fatigue, depression, sensory complaints, and gait disturbances emerge as relevant symptoms and should be given corresponding attention in the management of patients with early PD. However, few studies have interrogated the trajectory of cognitive decline in PD, and the relationship between poor cognitive performance and QoL.

A recent study (65) compared 3 groups of people with PD: those with a mild cognitive impairment (PD-MCI), those with a dementia like syndrome (PDD), and those with no cognitive abnormalities (PD-NCA). QoL and disability were measured in 3 groups of participants with PD (PD-NCA, n = 54; PD-MCI, n = 48; and PDD, n = 25). Caregivers (n = 102) were assessed using the Zarit Burden Inventory. Patient QoL and caregiver burden were similar in the groups without dementia, but were significantly different than those with PDD. By contrast, disability was progressively greater as cognition declined across the 3 groups. The presence of dementia significantly increases caregiver burden and decreases QoL. However, mild levels of cognitive impairment are correlated with an increase in physical disability and overall functional impairment progresses in tandem with cognitive decline. Unlike ALS, depression and functional ability predict QoL in patients with PD.

Huntington's disease

In HD, the influence of cognitive and behavioural symptoms on patients' QoL determined the strongest associations with patient self-reported QoL (66). As is the case in ALS, the role of cognitive and behavioural change on QoL is understudied within HD literature, as QoL based research tends to focus on the impact of predictive genetic testing (67). These studies are likely to be of relevance in future QoL studies in ALS, as testing for known genes is increasingly available in specialist clinics. However, the relationship between gene carrier status and likelihood of developing disease is less certain in ALS than in HD, and the impact of this uncertainty on QoL will require more detailed analyses.

In HD, executive dysfunction, as reflected in everyday behaviour, has been associated with lower patient QoL (68). Patient QoL is also associated with cognitive performance MMSE score, age, and time since motor symptom onset. Neuropsychiatric symptoms are not directly related to QoL in HD.

In a more comprehensive study of cognition, behaviour, and QoL in 20 genetically confirmed HD patients, QoL was significantly lower for patients who exhibited greater apathy and showed more evidence of executive dysfunction in their everyday behaviour as assessed by the FrSBe (69).

Multiple sclerosis

MS differs from ALS in that it is a chronic disorder that is characterized by uncertainty. While ALS patients and their families are aware that the disease is invariably fatal, until recently patients with Relapsing Remitting MS faced an uncertain future potentially punctuated by intermittent relapses, but with no method of predicting the likelihood of long term disability. With the advent of new therapies, the outcome of MS is much improved, and future QoL studies will be of interest in determining the impact of reducing uncertainty on patients and caregivers (70).

To date, QoL studies in MS have focussed primarily on disability. In one study, speech difficulties accounted for emotional distress, loneliness, and isolation, with limitations in communication with family and friends resulting in lower QoL (71). By contrast, physical symptomatology has not been consistently reported as a predictor of low QoL in ALS. In MS, a significant relationship was found between both memory impairment and executive dysfunction, and QoL (72). In the early stages of MS, patients with a recent diagnosis tend to report significantly lower scores on both physical and mental aspects of QoL compared with matched controls. A longitudinal study of MS patients considered the role of cognitive and behavioural dysfunction in MS patients with a sample of 65 newly diagnosed MS patients followed up over a 7-year period (73). Self-reported QoL at baseline was severely reduced in MS patients compared with healthy controls. The independent predictors for QoL composite scores at follow-up were the baseline depression score and the memory impairment. Among the MS patients who did not work at the time of the follow-up assessment, 72.7% were cognitively impaired. Occupational status and its change over time was significantly associated with cognitive deterioration. Memory dysfunction related cognitive impairment in the early stages of MS was correlated with a decreased level in health perception and lower QoL, independent of fatigue, depression, and physical disability, which are widely reported in MS.

Summary of perspectives from other neurologic conditions

Research within other neurologic conditions offers valuable insights, which can in turn enhance our understanding of QoL in ALS. Cognitive and behavioural change have a profoundly negative impact on the QoL of patient and caregiver, regardless of whether symptomatology is sudden onset (e.g. TBI), or progressive over time (e.g. PD). The presence and prevalence of motor symptoms does not appear to be a significant predictor of patient-caregiver burden, as seen within HD and MS. Often it is the functional impact of cognitive difficulties, which impacts patients' QoL, and behavioural change within the patient that negatively impacts caregivers' QoL, as reported within the Stroke and Brain Tumour literature. The negative impact of cognitive and behavioural change on QoL in these neurologic conditions resonates with the findings of ALS research, and clinical practice. Literature from other conditions suggest that the assessment of cognitive and behavioural change, followed by clinical tailoring of individualized or group-based interventions, can enhance and maintain QoL, which may prevent subsequent distress in caregivers, and can reduce behavioural disturbances in patients.

Quality of life from the patient-caregiver dyad perspective

Caregivers: 'The Unseen Patient'

The heterogeneity of caregiver-patient relationships adds an additional dimension to understanding the complexities associated with the impact of cognitive and behavioural change in neurological conditions on QoL (74). In general, relationship strain has been correlated to several factors including the premorbid relationship quality of patients and caregivers, as described in detail in Chapter 16. Loss of intimacy, reduced social contacts, and the extent of change caused by the disease increase tension, worry, and stressful situations for both patient and caregiver (75).

Family members are increasingly being asked to perform complex tasks similar to those carried out by paid health or social service providers, often at great cost to their own well-being and great benefit to their relatives and society as a whole (76). Caregiving presents difficult, sometimes intractable problems, and although we have learned a great deal about how to describe and characterize the challenges of caregiving, assess its impact on family members, and identify promising intervention approaches, yet more needs to be done. Understanding caregiving processes and stages across the disease trajectories may enable us to develop stage-appropriate preventive intervention strategies that may protect the caregiver from adverse outcomes.

Caregiver burden is a multidimensional construct and encompasses both objective and subjective aspects. Cognitive, behavioural, and neuropsychiatric symptoms are significant factors that contribute to caregiver burden, and negatively impact QoL. ALS caregivers with high QoL and low psychological morbidity (i.e. anxiety/depression) are those with a positive problem orientation (viewing problems as opportunities rather than threats) and those whose behavioural response style is rational rather than impulsive, careless, or characterized by avoidance (see Chapter 7). There is also evolving evidence that caregivers' psychological status may also influence the mental and physical outcome of patients.

In general, the various dimensions of caregiver burden are exemplified in ALS, which can develop at any stage of life, is often characterized by an insidious onset and rapid decline, and demonstrates great variability in cognitive and behavioural phenotypes. These factors render the multidimensional determinants of caregiving uniquely complex in ALS compared to other neurodegenerative diseases.

Existing data suggests that behavioural change is of great importance as a mediator of caregiver burden and QoL in ALS caregivers (27). The influence of cognitive change poses a significant burden to both patients and their caregivers. However, the presence of cognitive/behavioural changes in ALS patients is often under-recognized by healthcare professionals, and the burden of care associated with these changes is not consistently addressed in current clinical practice (77). Moreover, the relentless disease progression typically seen in ALS exemplifies how the factors maintaining and precipitating strain and caregiver burden, changing care activities, roles, and relationship dynamics vary alongside the disease trajectory. Relatively little is known about transitions into, and out of, the caregiving role. It is therefore necessary to develop methods by which burden and strain in patients and caregivers can be assessed and predicted to ensure that adequate supports and referral pathways exist.

In ALS, caregiver burden and reduced caregiver QoL are modulated by patients' cognitive and behavioural status, but do not significantly impact patient survival (27). Highly stressed caregivers show remarkable signs of recovery after the death of their loved one, suggesting that much of the work of dealing with loss occurs before the death. However, during the illness, caregivers are at high risk of developing stress, anxiety, and depression. Anxiety and depression in caregivers have been repeatedly shown to independently affect their QoL. Identifying predictors of anxiety and depression in people with ALS is also important because affective state may be amenable to psychopharmacologic and psychotherapeutic interventions, as depression may negatively impact QoL. The concordance between caregiver and patient distress tends to be high. Caregiver mental status can in turn have a great influence on patients (78). Attention to the mental health needs of caregivers may not only relieve caregivers' distress, but also alleviate patient distress, and improve QoL.

Interventions for cognitive and behavioural impairment to improve QoL for patients and caregivers

Interventions to address cognitive and behavioural impairments in ALS and other neurodegenerative diseases aim to improve QoL for patients and caregivers. Despite new insights into the psychological issues of patients with neurodegenerative diseases and their caregivers, few studies have investigated possible protective factors against burden, or controlled trials to enhance QoL. In addition to a patient's reaction to their diagnosis, there are a variety of responses experienced by caregivers and the wider family unit (79). As well as providing care to patients, clinicians should provide appropriate support to the caregivers at the time of diagnosis, during the course of the illness, and post-bereavement.

Interventions can directly and indirectly assist in the management of cognitive and behaviour impairments and contribute to QoL (80). These include provision of training and support to family caregivers, interventions to maintain ADL functioning, limiting sources of conflict and frustration though redirecting and refocusing the patient, and empowerment of caregivers to change or moderate their interaction with the patient. In addition, interventions for caregivers should focus on psychosocial and existential factors such as loss, guilt, resilience, and hope.

Individualized psychotherapeutic and psycho-educational interventions

Psychotherapy includes individual or group-based psychodynamic, behavioural, and cognitive-behavioural therapy. Psycho-education is the structured presentation of information about cognitive impairment, expected caring issues, stress management, and techniques to manage the patients' behaviour (81). Psycho-educational interventions for caregivers may improve the symptoms of the patient also, perhaps by training the caregiver to redirect the patient to avoid escalation of problem behaviour. This can be done on a 1:1 basis, or can be complimented by sharing experiences in group-based settings (82).

Many caregivers and family members recount anecdotal evidence noting the therapeutic effect of individualized or group-based music sessions (83). Beneficial effects have been reported in the areas of behaviour, speech, motor integration, and rhythmic movement with neurodegenerative cohorts (84). Counselling and support have been shown to significantly delay nursing home placement for persons with AD, improving mood and caregiver QoL (85).

Mindfulness Based Stress Reduction, which can be administered in an individual or group setting, has been shown to promote a person's ability to cope with the experience and management of negative emotions, mitigating the effects of disease burden, and promoting psychological adaptation (86). Considering both patients and caregivers, people who practice mindfulness have been shown to be more capable of responding to stressful situations without an automatic or otherwise maladaptive reaction, i.e. avoidant coping strategies. Mindfulness has been shown to be a protective factor against caregiver burden in ALS (87, 88) (See Chapters 4 and 5).

In TBI, as in other groups, problem-focused coping strategies are reportedly more successful than emotion-focused strategies (89). In MS, knowledge of disease related difficulties (fatigue, communication, pain, and depression) may help in prioritizing treatments, and assist in maintaining an optimal QoL (90). Traditional rehabilitation approaches to dysarthria focus on speech impairment and intelligibility (91).

In stroke, outcome studies have shown that rehabilitation programs are effective in improving long-term functional status and in decreasing institutionalization. There is a growing interest in post-stroke care as a means of identifying alternative or compensatory mechanisms that could lead to improved function beyond the expected neural recovery. Compensatory mechanisms to improve post-stroke recovery include psychological adaptations such as self-care self-efficacy, which is defined as the confidence a person has in his or her ability to perform relevant self-care activities (92).

Group based support services

Problem solving and reasoning skills of caregivers are an important determinant of caregiver well-being (93). Developing group interventions to enhance or teach caregivers new methods of problem solving are beneficial. Support groups provide the opportunity to share personal feelings and concerns, encourage mutuality and validation, and overcome feelings of social isolation (94). Respite offers substitute care to provide planned, temporary relief to the caregiver, through group day care, in-home respite, or institutional respite, vacation or emergency respite. Group based psychoeducational programs for family caregivers that target specific problem areas are more effective than other intervention modalities (95).

Cognitive-Behavioural Therapy (CBT) and Peer Support/Counselling group therapy (PSC) aim to improve mood and QoL and to decrease uncertainty in illness (96). This is a useful intervention, though should be facilitated by a healthcare professional.

Cognitive stimulation group

Treatment guidelines have been highly critical of cognitive stimulation/training interventions in AD, in view of the risk that cognitive gains may be achieved at the expense of reduced wellbeing and adverse effects. However, treatments for cognitive decline are showing some promise in PD and may influence QoL. In a recent study, a rehabilitation program of 6 weeks including both motor and cognitive training was undertaken with 20 PD patients in the early stages of the illness, who experienced mild cognitive deficits, but not dementia. At the end of the scheduled sessions, the patients showed a significant improvement in verbal fluency, logic memory, and on the Raven's matrices tests, when compared with baseline (97). Improved QoL scores for participants of cognitive stimulation therapy were associated with better mood that was mediated by improvements in cognition (98).

In a group-based intervention for AD patients, higher QoL was significantly correlated with lower levels of dependency and depression (99). Improvement in QoL was associated with being female, reduced depression, and increased cognitive function. These results suggest that although QoL in dementia appears to be independent of level of cognitive function, interventions aimed at improving cognitive function can have a direct effect on QoL.

Multidisciplinary and multicomponent approaches

Multicomponent interventions combine elements from different interventional approaches. Caregivers who possess more cognitive-behavioural resources are more likely to adjust to their caregiving role with fewer emotional difficulties. Combined with psycho-educational support and mindfulness, patients and their caregivers are likely to experience a greater psychological wellbeing and QoL.

Currently, the best treatment available to patients with neurodegenerative conditions is optimal supportive care. In recent years, multidisciplinary clinics have been developed to provide symptomatic and palliative care to patients with ALS. Greater patient numbers in multidisciplinary clinics (MDCs) leads to an accumulation of resources and clinical expertise that facilitates the management of this relatively rare, progressive disease (100).

MDC care has been shown to improve the mental health and QoL in patients with ALS. Such care has also been shown to improve median patient survival times, and has considerable importance here in relation to cognitive and behavioural changes (101). Identification of cognitive decline and behavioural changes in a MDC can lead to a rapid implementation of psychologically tailored interventions for behaviour change (102). Furthermore, MDCs can offer both formal and informal opportunities for caregivers of patients with ALS, and other neurological conditions, to engage is help-seeking behaviour if required. Of patients who attend an MDC, QoL is elevated in the domains of Social Functioning and Mental Health when compared to those who do not attend, and is independent of the presence of mechanical aids and appliances (103). Accessing appropriate services and support can make a crucial difference. Studies among patients with dementia in general, show that behavioural problems are significant predictors of exhaustion leading to caregivers' mental and physical health problem (104).

QoL assessment facilitating intervention

QoL assessments can be used to identify and prioritize problems and issues of clinical relevance, facilitate communication, screen for potential problems (psychological and social issues can be overlooked unless specifically asked about), facilitate shared clinical decision-making, monitor changes or response to treatment, and train new staff (105). Furthermore, assessing QoL in patient (and caregiver) cohorts can have a positive therapeutic effect due to greater introspection into positive aspects of one's life. Indeed, assessment of individualized QoL may be seen itself as an intervention, with the potential to influence the QoL of that individual through self-evaluation and reflection, and/or their appraisal of QoL as the respondent identifies life domains of importance to them (106).

QoL does not necessarily diminish as neurodegeneration worsens, but continues to be strongly influenced by the patient's mood and interaction with their environment. The routine use of QoL as an outcome measure for people with dementia in care homes is indicated to identify the benefits of clinical interventions and treatments, and to assess the impact of the disease process on individuals through the course of the illness.

Behavioural impairment and suggested interventions

Given the prevalence of cognitive and behavioural impairment in the neurodegenerations, and particularly in ALS, FTD, and TBI, adjustments to roles and responsibilities, interaction styles, and to activities of daily living may be beneficial in reducing caregiver burden and increasing QoL (107). Reconfiguring existing roles within the family could reduce frustration or irritation if cognitive impairment is a prominent feature. If the patient is experiencing executive dysfunction and not able to reliably make decisions, they should still participate in less demanding ways.

Informally observing patterns of behaviour, and noting recurring negative changes, may identify patterns of restlessness and fatigue. Some patients have been reported to become excessively tired by the end of the day and react with anger when demands upon them become overwhelming. Creating a predictable, structured schedule and a calm environment is helpful. The spouse caregiver is often the 'target' of the patient's irritability and may need breaks and respite from caregiving responsibilities. When lack of empathy is present in a patient, the primary intervention is education and support to the family about the nature of ALS-FTD related change (108). This symptom of behavioural change can be confusing and frustrating without proper psycho-education. If new onset behaviours include sensitivity to external stimuli when engaging in activities of daily living. then caregivers should aim to sit in more private and secluded sections of restaurants and waiting rooms to reduce overstimulation (109). Table 9.1 summarizes useful strategies.

For care planning, it is crucial to consider the additional complication of dealing with patients' physical symptoms. Patients should be supervised in tasks that could incur injury such as walking, transferring, and eating. Recommendations to enhance safety must include an assurance that all family members understand that cognitive and behavioural changes are part of the condition.

Caring for the caregiver

Effective caregiving requires that caregivers themselves receive practical and emotional support. Identification of caregiver needs allows for the better management of those needs, leading to a reduction of overall burden and greater caregiver empowerment, while considering that patients' and caregivers' perspectives might differ from those of the health professionals involved in their care.

Routine cognitive-behavioural screening can identify patients who require full neuropsychological examination, and identify caregivers in need of early, targeted interventions. A patient's behavioural impairment can affect interpersonal and social relationships, reducing closeness, communication, and sharing viewpoints. ALS

Table 9.1 Commonly reported strategies for managing cognitive and behavioural change in ALS/FTD (110)

1	Explain clearly that cognitive and behavioural changes are part of the condition.
2	Give a clear structure to the patient's day and make it as predictable as possible. To keep a routine is very important for the patient to be able to initiate and engage with daily activities.
3	Give the patient enough time to make decisions and offer limited choices and closed-ended questions. The 'little and often' rule applies. Give the patient small amounts of information regularly, rather than overloading them with too much detail or content.
4	Encourage the patient to make lists to help organize activities that may need to be done during the day.
5	Avoid distractors in the room to help with concentration.
6	Encourage the patient to use calendars, memory aids, or phone alarms to help him remember appointments or recall to take the medication.
7	Simplify communication to enhance patient's comprehension: speak clearly using a simple and straightforward language, break sentences into short phrases containing not too much information, and slow down when speaking.
8	In patients with increased irritability, look for triggers or predictors that may prompt bursts of anger (tiredness, hunger, etc.) and try to prevent them. In cases of anger outburst, remain calm and avoid arguments, acknowledging the patient's irritability. It is also important to eliminate environmental stimuli that may be annoying for the patient such as loud noise, inadequate temperatures, etc.
9	Avoid surprises that may create confusion or agitation and keep the environment calm and controlled. If visitors are expected, make sure that the patient is aware of this. If large gatherings provoke agitation or irritability in the patient, avoid them.
10	Patient contact with the public may need to be supervised. It is recommendable that the patient frequents places where people are aware of the condition. Sometimes, to gain understanding from the public when visiting crowded places such as waiting rooms or restaurants, families are suggested to bring a small business-size card, which clarifies that the patients suffers from a medical condition that affects behaviour.

Source: data from Research Motor Neurone, Best Practice Guidelines for Health Care Professionals, Copyright (2017). Available at: http://mnd.ie/wp/wp-content/uploads/2017/01/Best-Practice-Guidelines-for-HCPs.pdf (accessed 24 July 2017).

caregivers should be educated as to the nature of the condition, including the likelihood that patients may change their behaviour over time, and to be able to face the modification of their interpersonal relationship. To address the complex needs of caregivers, a detailed appraisal of the cognitive, behavioural, and motor disability of the patient should be accompanied by detailed analysis of the psychological, emotional status, and capacity for resilience of the caregiver. Consideration of the possible positive aspects of caregiving is also important, as support and interventions for caregivers should also enhance the positive aspects of their role that could reinforce their well-being and reduce the impact of caregiving in stress and burden.

Conclusions

Cognitive, and especially behavioural, changes significantly impact the QoL of patients with neurological diseases and of their caregivers. This is congruent with other areas of medicine where memory difficulties, poor concentration, and impaired problem solving are important predictors of low QoL. In the neurodegenerative conditions, cognitive and behavioural impairment can present at different stages of a disease, and can manifest in varying forms, depending on the region of brain involvement and the nature of the underlying pathology. Similarly, patterns of behavioural change are a function of the neurological pathways that are affected by the illness, and can range from extreme apathy to disruptive disinhibition, and accordingly require different types of tailored intervention. While a range of interventions have been described that can help to support the QoL of patients and caregivers, there is no 'one size fits all', and there is an urgent need for further research into the longer-term impact of cognitive and behavioural changes on QoL of patients and caregivers, such that an evidence base for effective targeted interventions can be generated.

References

1. Arciniegas, D.B., Held, K., and Wagner P. (2002) Cognitive impairment following traumatic brain injury. *Current Treatment Options in Neurology*, **4**(1), 43–57.

2. Duff, K., Paulsen, J.S., Beglinger, L.J., et al. (2010) 'Frontal' behaviors before the diagnosis of Huntington's disease and their relationship to markers of disease progression: evidence of early lack of awareness. *Journal of Neuropsychiatry and Clinical Neurosciences*, **22**(2), 196–207.

3. Elamin, M., Bede, P., Byrne, S., et al. (2013) Cognitive changes predict functional decline in ALS: A population-based longitudinal study. *Neurology*, **80**(17), 1590–7.

4. Elamin, M., Phukan, J., Bede, P., et al. (2011) Executive dysfunction is a negative prognostic indicator in patients with ALS without dementia. *Neurology*, **76**(14), 1263–9.

5. Zhou, J., Greicius, M.D., Gennatas, E.D., et al. (2010) Divergent network connectivity changes in behavioural variant frontotemporal dementia and Alzheimer's disease. *Brain*, **133**(5), 1352–67.

6. Lillo, P., Savage, S., Mioshi, E., Kiernan, M.C., and Hodges, J.R. (2012) Amyotrophic lateral sclerosis and frontotemporal dementia: a behavioural and cognitive continuum. *Amyotrophic Lateral Sclerosis*, **13**(1), 102–9.

7. Wilson, C.M., Grace, G.M., Munoz, D.G., He, B.P., and Strong, M.J. (2001) Cognitive impairment in sporadic ALS: A pathologic continuum underlying a multisystem disorder. *Neurology*, **57**(4), 651–7.

8. Jenkinson, C., Peters, M., and Bromberg, M.B. (eds) (2011) *Quality of Life Measurement in Neurodegenerative and Related Conditions*. Cambridge: Cambridge University Press.

9. Halpern, A.S. (1993) Quality of life as a conceptual framework for evaluating transition outcomes. *Exceptional Children*, **59**(6), 486–98.

10. Li, J., Bentzen, S.M., Li, J., Renschler, M., and Mehta, M.P. (2008) Relationship between neurocognitive function and quality of life after whole-brain radiotherapy in patients with brain metastasis. *International Journal of Radiation Oncology, Biology, and Physics*, **71**(1), 64–70.

11. **Doody, R.S., Gavrilova, S.I., Sano, M.,** et al. (2008) Effect of dimebon on cognition, activities of daily living, behaviour, and global function in patients with mild-to-moderate Alzheimer's disease:A randomized, double-blind, placebo-controlled study. *Lancet,* **372**(9634), 207–15.

12. **Rao, S.M., Leo, G.J., Ellington, L., Nauertz, T., Bernardin, L.,** and **Unverzagt, F.** (1991) Cognitive dysfunction in multiple sclerosis. II. Impact on employment and social functioning. *Neurology,* **41**(5), 692–6.

13. **Simard, M., van Reekum, R.,** and **Myran, D.** (2003) Visuospatial impairment in dementia with Lewy bodies and Alzheimer's disease: a process analysis approach. *International Journal of Geriatric Psychiatry,* **18**(5), 387–91.

14. **Boyle, P.A., Malloy, P.F., Salloway, S., Cahn-Weiner, D.A., Cohen, R.,** and **Cummings, J.L.** (2003) Executive dysfunction and apathy predict functional impairment in Alzheimer disease. *The American Journal of Geriatric Psychiatry,* **11**(2), 214–21.

15. **Sachdev, P.S., Brodaty, H., Valenzuela, M.J.,** et al. (2004) The neuropsychological profile of vascular cognitive impairment in stroke and TIA patients. *Neurology,* **62**(6), 912–9.

16. **Perneczky, R., Pohl, C., Sorg, C.,** et al. (2006) Impairment of activities of daily living requiring memory or complex reasoning as part of the MCI syndrome. *International Journal of Geriatric Psychiatry,* **21**(2), 158–62.

17. **Goldberg, T.E., Koppel, J., Keehlisen, L.,** et al. (2010) Performance-based measures of everyday function in mild cognitive impairment. *American Journal of Psychiatry,* **167**(7), 845–53.

18. **Fratiglioni, L., Hui-Xin, W., Ericsson, K., Maytan, M.,** and **Winblad, B.** (2000) Influence of social network on occurrence of dementia: a community-based longitudinal study. *The Lancet,* **355**(9212), 1315.

19. **Hinkin, C.H., Castellon, S.A., Durvasula, R.S.,** et al. (2002) Medication adherence among HIV+ adults effects of cognitive dysfunction and regimen complexity. *Neurology,* **59**(12), 1944–50.

20. **Dunbar-Jacob. J.** and **Mortimer-Stephens, M.** (2001) Treatment adherence in chronic disease. *Journal of Clinical Epidemiology,* **54**(12), S57–60.

21. **Trahan, E., Pépin, M.,** and **Hopps, S.** (2006) Impaired awareness of deficits and treatment adherence among people with traumatic brain injury or spinal cord injury. *Journal of Head Trauma Rehabilitation,* **21**(3), 226–35.

22. **Farlow, M.R., Miller, M.L.,** and **Pejovic, V.** (2008) Treatment options in Alzheimer's disease: Maximizing benefit, managing expectations. *Dementia and Geriatric Cognitive Disorders,* **25**(5), 408–22.

23. **Burrell, J.R., Halliday, G.M., Kril, J.J.,** et al. (2016) The frontotemporal dementia-motor neuron disease continuum. *Lancet,* **388**(10047), 919–31.

24. **Majounie, E., Renton, A.E., Mok, K.,** et al. (2012) Frequency of the C9orf72 hexanucleotide repeat expansion in patients with amyotrophic lateral sclerosis and frontotemporal dementia: A cross-sectional study. *Lancet Neurology,* **11**(4), 323–30.

25. **Sadowsky, C.H.** and **Galvin, J.E.** (2012) Guidelines for the management of cognitive and behavioral problems in dementia. *Journal of the American Board of Family Medicine,* **25**(3), 350–66.

26. **Phukan, J., Pender, N.P.,** and **Hardiman, O.** (2007) Cognitive impairment in amyotrophic lateral sclerosis. *Lancet Neurology,* **6**(11), 994–1003.

27. Burke, T., Elamin, M., Galvin, M., Hardiman, O., and Pender N. (2015) Caregiver burden in amyotrophic lateral sclerosis: A cross-sectional investigation of predictors. *Journal of Neurology*, **262**(6), 1526–32.

28. Phukan, J., Elamin, M., Bede, P., et al. (2012) The syndrome of cognitive impairment in amyotrophic lateral sclerosis: a population-based study. *Journal of Neurology, Neurosurgery & Psychiatry*, **83**(1), 102–8.

29. Taylor, L.J., Brown, R.G., Tsermentseli, S., et al. (2013) Is language impairment more common than executive dysfunction in amyotrophic lateral sclerosis?. *Journal of Neurology, Neurosurgery & Psychiatry*, **84**(5), 494–8.

30. Abrahams, S., Leigh, P.N., Harvey, A., Vythelingum, G.N., Grise, D., and Goldstein, L.H. (2000) Verbal fluency and executive dysfunction in amyotrophic lateral sclerosis (ALS). *Neuropsychologia*, **38**(6), 734–47.

31. Chio, A., Ilardi, A., Cammarosano, S., Moglia, C., Montuschi, A., and Calvo, A. (2012) Neurobehavioral dysfunction in ALS has a negative effect on outcome and use of PEG and NIV. *Neurology*, **78**(14), 1085–9.

32. Mioshi, E., Caga, J., Lillo, P., et al. (2014) Neuropsychiatric changes precede classic motor symptoms in ALS and do not affect survival. *Neurology*, **82**(2), 149–55.

33. Lillo, P., Mioshi, E., Zoing, M.C., Kiernan, M.C., and Hodges, J.R. (2011) How common are behavioural changes in amyotrophic lateral sclerosis? *Amyotrophic Lateral Sclerosis*, **12**(1), 45–51.

34. Chio, A., Vignola, A., Mastro, E., et al. (2010) Neurobehavioral symptoms in ALS are negatively related to caregivers' burden and quality of life. *European Journal of Neurology*, **17**(10), 1298–303.

35. Lillo, P., Mioshi, E., and Hodges, J.R. (2012) Caregiver burden in amyotrophic lateral sclerosis is more dependent on patients' behavioral changes than physical disability: a comparative study. *BMC Neurology*, **12**(1), 156.

36. Traynor, B.J., Codd, M.B., Corr, B., Forde, C., Frost, E., and Hardiman, O. (1999) Incidence and prevalence of ALS in Ireland, 1995–1997: A population-based study. *Neurology*, **52**(3), 504–9.

37. Ratnavalli, E., Brayne, C., Dawson, K., and Hodges, J.R. (2002) The prevalence of frontotemporal dementia. *Neurology*, **58**(11), 1615–21.

38. Banks, S.J. and Weintraub, S. (2008) Neuropsychiatric symptoms in behavioral variant frontotemporal dementia and primary progressive aphasia. *Journal of Geriatric Psychiatry and Neurology*, **21**(2), 133–41.

39. Lough, S., Kipps, C.M., Treise, C., Watson, P., Blair, J.R., and Hodges, J.R. (2006) Social reasoning, emotion and empathy in frontotemporal dementia. *Neuropsychologia*, **44**(6), 950–8.

40. Lough, S., Gregory, C., and Hodges, J.R. (2001) Dissociation of social cognition and executive function in frontal variant frontotemporal dementia. *Neurocase*, **7**(2), 123–30.

41. Blair, M., Marczinski, C.A., Davis-Faroque, N., and Kertesz, A. (2007) A longitudinal study of language decline in Alzheimer's disease and frontotemporal dementia. *Journal of the International Neuropsychological Society*, **13**(02), 237–45.

42. Diehl-Schmid, J., Schmidt, E.M., Nunnemann, S., et al. (2013) Caregiver burden and needs in frontotemporal dementia. *Journal of Geriatric Psychiatry and Neurology*, **26**(4), 221–9.

43. Gauthier, A., Vignola, A., Calvo, A., et al. (2007) A longitudinal study on quality of life and depression in ALS patient–caregiver couples. *Neurology*, **68**(12), 923–6.

44. Goldstein, L.H., Atkins, L., Landau, S., Brown, R.G., and Leigh, P.N. (2006) Longitudinal predictors of psychological distress and self-esteem in people with ALS. *Neurology*, **67**(9), 1652–8.

45. Courtens, A.M., Stevens, F.C., Crebolder, H.F., and Philipsen H. (1996) Longitudinal study on quality of life and social support in cancer patients. *Cancer Nursing*, **19**(3), 162–9.

46. Kilani, M., Micallef, J., Soubrouillard, C., et al. (2004) A longitudinal study of the evolution of cognitive function and affective state in patients with amyotrophic lateral sclerosis. *Amyotrophic Lateral Sclerosis and Other Motor Neuron Disorders*, **5B**(1), 46–54.

47. Goldstein, L.H. and Abrahams, S. (2013) Changes in cognition and behaviour in amyotrophic lateral sclerosis: nature of impairment and implications for assessment. *Lancet Neurology*, **12**(4), 368–80.

48. Hoerold, D., Pender, N.P., and Robertson, I.H. (2013) Metacognitive and online error awareness deficits after prefrontal cortex lesions. *Neuropsychologia*, **51**(3), 385–91.

49. Grehl, T., Rupp, M., Budde, P., Tegenthoff, M., and Fangerau, H. (2011) Depression and QOL in patients with ALS: How do self-ratings and ratings by relatives differ? *Quality of Life Research* **20**(4), 569–74.

50. Degeneffe, C.E., Gagne, L.M., and Tucker, M. (2013) Family systems changes following traumatic brain injury: Adult sibling perspectives. *Journal of Applied Rehabilitation Counseling*, **44**(3):32.

51. Ylvisaker, M., Adelson, P.D., Braga, L.W., et al. (2005) Rehabilitation and ongoing support after pediatric TBI: twenty years of progress. *Journal of Head Trauma Rehabilitation*, **20**(1), 95–109.

52. Clarke, S., Hickey, A., O'Boyle, C., and Hardiman, O. (2001) Assessing individual quality of life in amyotrophic lateral sclerosis. *Quality of Life Research*, **10**(2), 149–58.

53. Flashman, L.A. and McAllister, T.W. (2002). Lack of awareness and its impact in traumatic brain injury. *NeuroRehabilitation*, **17**(4), 285–96.

54. Franz, M., Meyer, T., Reber, T., and Gallhofer, B. (2000) The importance of social comparisons for high levels of subjective quality of life in chronic schizophrenic patients. *Quality of Life Research*, **9**(5), 481–9.

55. Delmonico, R.L., Hanley-Peterson, P., and Englander, J. (1998) Group psychotherapy for persons with traumatic brain injury: management of frustration and substance abuse. *The Journal of Head Trauma Rehabilitation*, **13**(6), 10–22.

56. Griffen, J.A., Rapport, L.J., Bryer, R.C., Bieliauskas, L.A., and Burt, C. (2011) Awareness of deficits and on-road driving performance. *Clinical Neuropsychologist*, (7), 1158–78.

57. Dahlberg, C., Hawley, L., Morey, C., Newman, J., Cusick, C.P., and Harrison-Felix, C. (2006) Social communication skills in persons with post-acute traumatic brain injury: Three perspectives. *Brain Injury*, **20**(4), 425–35.

58. Baumann, M., Couffignal, S., Le Bihan, E., and Chau N. (2012) Life satisfaction two-years after stroke onset: The effects of gender, sex occupational status, memory function and quality of life among stroke patients (Newsqol) and their family caregivers (Whoqol-bref) in Luxembourg. *BMC Neurology*, **12**(1), 105.

59. Nys, G.M., Van Zandvoort, M.J., Van Der Worp, H.B., et al. (2006) Early cognitive impairment predicts long-term depressive symptoms and quality of life after stroke. *Journal of the Neurological Sciences*, **247**(2), 149–56.

60. **Benejam, B., Sahuquillo, J., Poca, M.A.,** et al. (2009) Quality of life and neurobehavioral changes in survivors of malignant middle cerebral artery infarction. *Journal of Neurology*, **256**(7), 1126.

61. **Kwa, V.I., Limburg, M.,** and **Haan, R.J.** (1996) The role of cognitive impairment in the quality of life after ischaemic stroke. *Journal of Neurology*, **243**(8), 599–604.

62. **Logsdon, R.G., Gibbons, L.E., McCurry, S.M.,** and **Teri, L.** (2002) Assessing quality of life in older adults with cognitive impairment. *Psychosomatic Medicine*, **64**(3), 510–9.

63. **Shin, I.S., Carter, M., Masterman, D., Fairbanks, L.,** and **Cummings, J.L.** (2005) Neuropsychiatric symptoms and quality of life in Alzheimer disease. *American Journal of Geriatric Psychiatry*, **13**(6), 469–74.

64. **Herlofson, K.** and **Larsen, J.P.** (2003) The influence of fatigue on health-related quality of life in patients with Parkinson's disease. *Acta Neurologica Scandinavica*, (1), 1–6.

65. **Leroi, I., McDonald, K., Pantula, H.,** and **Harbishettar, V.** (2012) Cognitive impairment in Parkinson disease: impact on quality of life, disability, and caregiver burden. *Journal of Geriatric Psychiatry and Neurology*, **25**(4):208–14.

66. **Mitchell, A.J., Kemp, S., Benito-León, J.,** and **Reuber, M.** (2010) The influence of cognitive impairment on health-related quality of life in neurological disease. *Acta Neuropsychiatrica*, **22**(1), 2–13

67. **Paulsen, J.S., Nance, M., Kim, J.I.,** et al. (2013) A review of quality of life after predictive testing for and earlier identification of neurodegenerative diseases. *Progress in Neurobiology*, **110**, 2–8.

68. **Banaszkiewicz, K., Sitek, E.J., Rudzińska, M., Sołtan, W., Sławek, J.,** and **Szczudlik, A.** (2012) Huntington's disease from the patient, caregiver and physician's perspectives: three sides of the same coin? *Journal of Neural Transmission*, **119**(11), 1361–5.

69. **Eddy, C.M.** and **Rickards, H.E.** (2013) Impact of cognitive and behavioural changes on quality of life in Huntington's disease. *Basal Ganglia*, **3**(2), 123–6.

70. **O'Doherty, L.J., Hickey, A.,** and **Hardiman, O.** (2010) Measuring life quality, physical function and psychological well-being in neurological illness. *Amyotrophic Lateral Sclerosis*, **11**(5), 461–8.

71. **Klugman, T.M.** and **Ross, E.** (2002) Perceptions of the impact of speech, language, swallowing, and hearing difficulties on quality of life of a group of South African persons with multiple sclerosis. *Folia Phoniatrica et Logopaedica*, **54**(4), 201–21.

72. **Cutajar, R., Ferriani, E., Scandellari, C.,** et al. (2000) Cognitive function and quality of life in multiple sclerosis patients. *Journal of Neurovirology*, **6**(2), S186.

73. **Ruet, A., Deloire, M., Hamel, D., Ouallet, J.C., Petry, K.,** and **Brochet, B.** (2013) Cognitive impairment, health-related quality of life and vocational status at early stages of multiple sclerosis: A 7-year longitudinal study. *Journal of Neurology*, **260**(3), 776–84.

74. **Logsdon, R.G., Gibbons, L.E., McCurry, S.M.,** and **Teri, L.** (1999) Quality of life in Alzheimer's disease: Patient and caregiver reports. *Journal of Mental Health and Aging*, **5**, 21–32.

75. **Rodrigue, J.R.** and **Baz, M.A.** (2007) Waiting for lung transplantation: Quality of life, mood, caregiving strain and benefit, and social intimacy of spouses. *Clinical Transplantation*, **21**(6), 722–7.

76. **Bień, B., Wojszel, B.,** and **Sikorska-Simmons, E.** (2007) Rural and urban caregivers for older adults in Poland: perceptions of positive and negative impact of caregiving. *International Journal of Aging and Human Development*, **65**(3), 185–202.

77. **Galvin, M., Corr, B., Madden, C.,** et al. (2016) Caregiving in ALS–a mixed methods approach to the study of Burden. *BMC Palliative Care*, **15**(1), 81.

78. **Perlick, D.A., Rosenheck, R.R., Clarkin, J.F., Raue, P.,** and **Sirey J.** (2001) Impact of family burden and patient symptom status on clinical outcome in bipolar affective disorder. *Journal of Nervous and Mental Disease*, **189**(1), 31–7.

79. **Aminzadeh, F., Byszewski, A., Molnar, F.J.,** and **Eisner, M.** (2007) Emotional impact of dementia diagnosis: exploring persons with dementia and caregivers' perspectives. *Aging and Mental Health*, **11**(3), 281–90.

80. **Lechner, S.C., Antoni, M.H., Lydston, D.,** et al. (2003) Cognitive–behavioral interventions improve quality of life in women with AIDS. *Journal of Psychosomatic Research*, **54**(3), 253–61.

81. **Martín-Carrasco, M., Martín, M.F., Valero, C.P.,** et al. (2009) Effectiveness of a psycho-educational intervention program in the reduction of caregiver burden in Alzheimer's disease patients' caregivers. *International Journal of Geriatric Psychiatry*, **24**(5), 489–99.

82. **Pinquart, M.** and **Sörensen S.** (2006) Helping caregivers of persons with dementia: which interventions work and how large are their effects?. *International Psychogeriatrics*, **18**(04), 577–95.

83. **Choi, A.N., Lee, M.S., Cheong, K.J.,** and **Lee, J.S.** (2009) Effects of group music intervention on behavioral and psychological symptoms in patients with dementia: A pilot-controlled trial. *International Journal of Neuroscience*, **119**(4), 471–81.

84. **Lin, Y., Chu, H., Yang, C.Y.,** et al. (2011) Effectiveness of group music intervention against agitated behavior in elderly persons with dementia. *International Journal of Geriatric Psychiatry*, **26**(7), 670–8.

85. **Mittelman, M.S., Ferris, S.H., Shulman, E., Steinberg, G.,** and **Levin, B.** (1996) A family intervention to delay nursing home placement of patients with Alzheimer disease: A randomized controlled trial. *Journal of the American Medical Association*, **276**(21), 1725–31.

86. **Larouche, E., Hudon, C.,** and **Goulet, S.** (2015) Potential benefits of mindfulness-based interventions in mild cognitive impairment and Alzheimer's disease: An interdisciplinary perspective. *Behavioural Brain Research*, **276**, 199–212.

87. **Pagnini, F., Phillips, D., Bosma, C.M., Reece, A.,** and **Langer, E.** (2016) Mindfulness as a protective factor for the burden of caregivers of amyotrophic lateral sclerosis patients. *Journal of clinical psychology*, **72**(1), 101–11.

88. **Pagnini, F., Marconi, A., Tagliaferri, A., Manzoni, G.M., Gatto, R., Fabiani, V.,** et al. (2017) Meditation training for people with amyotrophic lateral sclerosis: A randomised clinical trial. *Eur J Neurol*. **24**, 578–86.

89. **Ashworth, F., Gracey, F.,** and **Gilbert, P.** (2011) Compassion focused therapy after traumatic brain injury: Theoretical foundations and a case illustration. *Brain Impairment*, **12**(02), 128–39.

90. **O'Brien, A.R., Chiaravalloti, N., Goverover, Y.,** and **DeLuca, J.** (2008) Evidenced-based cognitive rehabilitation for persons with multiple sclerosis: A review of the literature. *Archives of Physical Medicine and Rehabilitation*, **89**(4), 761–9.

91. **Sellars, C., Hughes, T.,** and **Langhorne, P.** (2002) Speech and language therapy for dysarthria due to nonprogressive brain damage: A systematic Cochrane review. *Clinical Rehabilitation*, **16**(1), 61–8.

92. **Robinson-Smith, G., Johnston, M.V.,** and **Allen, J.** (2000) Self-care self-efficacy, quality of life, and depression after stroke. *Archives of Physical Medicine and Rehabilitation*, **81**(4), 460–4.

93. **Murphy, V., Felgoise, S.H., Walsh, S.M.,** and **Simmons, Z.** (2009) Problem solving skills predict quality of life and psychological morbidity in ALS caregivers. *Amyotrophic Lateral Sclerosis*, **10**(3), 147–53.

94. **Dowrick, C., Dunn, G., Ayuso-Mateos, J.L., Dalgard, O.S., Page, H., Lehtinen, V.,** et al. (2000) Problem solving treatment and group psychoeducation for depression: Multicentre randomised controlled trial. *British Medical Journal,* **321**(7274), 1450.

95. **Acton, G.J.** and **Kang, J.** (2001) Interventions to reduce the burden of caregiving for an adult with dementia: A meta-analysis §. *Research in Nursing & Health,* **24**(5), 349–60.

96. **Ng, L., Amatya, B.,** and **Khan, F.** (2013) Outcomes of a peer support program in multiple sclerosis in an Australian community cohort: A prospective study. *Journal of Neurodegenerative Diseases,* **2013,** 429171

97. **Sinforiani, E., Banchieri, L., Zucchella, C., Pacchetti, C.,** and **Sandrini, G.** (2004) Cognitive rehabilitation in Parkinson's disease. *Archives of Gerontology and Geriatrics,* **38,** 387–91.

98. **Hindle, J.V., Petrelli, A., Clare, L.,** and **Kalbe, E.** (2013) Nonpharmacological enhancement of cognitive function in Parkinson's disease: A systematic review. *Movement Disorders,* **28**(8), 1034–49.

99. **Woods, B., Thorgrimsen, L., Spector, A., Royan, L.,** and **Orrell, M.** (2006) Improved quality of life and cognitive stimulation therapy in dementia. *Aging and Mental Health,* **10**(3), 219–26.

100. **Hutchinson, M., Galvin, R., Sweeney, B., Lynch, T., Murphy, R.,** and **Redmond, J.** (2004) Effect of a multidisciplinary clinic on survival in amyotrophic lateral sclerosis. *Journal of Neurology, Neurosurgery & Psychiatry,* **75**(8):1208–9.

101. **Rooney, J., Byrne, S., Heverin, M.,** et al. (2015) A multidisciplinary clinic approach improves survival in ALS: A comparative study of ALS in Ireland and Northern Ireland. *Journal of Neurology, Neurosurgery & Psychiatry,* **86**(5), 496–501.

102. **Abrahams, S., Newton, J., Niven, E., Foley, J.,** and **Bak, T.H.** (2014) Screening for cognition and behaviour changes in ALS. *Amyotrophic Lateral Sclerosis and Frontotemporal Degeneration,* **15**(1–2), 9–14.

103. **Seto, E., Leonard, K.J., Cafazzo, J.A., Masino, C., Barnsley, J.,** and **Ross, H.J.** (2011). Self-care and quality of life of heart failure patients at a multidisciplinary heart function clinic. *Journal of Cardiovascular Nursing,* **26**(5), 377–85.

104. **Zoccolella, S., Beghi, E., Palagano, G.,** et al. (2007) ALS multidisciplinary clinic and survival. *Journal of Neurology,* **254**(8), 1107–12.

105. **Fayers, PM.** and **Machin, D.** (2013) Quality of life: The assessment, analysis and interpretation of patient-reported outcomes. Oxford: John Wiley & Sons.

106. **Higginson, I.J.** and **Carr, A.J.** (2001) Using quality of life measures in the clinical setting. *British Medical Journal,* **322**(7297), 1297.

107. **Elliott, T.R., Shewchuk, R.M.,** and **Richards, J.S.** (2001) Family caregiver social problem-solving abilities and adjustment during the inital year of the caregiving role. *Journal of Counseling Psychology,* **48**(2), 223.

108. **Olney, R.K., Murphy, J., Forshew, D.B.,** et al. (2005) The effects of executive and behavioral dysfunction on the course of ALS. *Neurology,* **65**(11), 1774–7.

109. **Merrilees, J., Klapper, J., Murphy, J., Lomen-Hoerth, C.,** and **Miller, B.L.** (2010) Cognitive and behavioral challenges in caring for patients with frontotemporal dementia and amyotrophic lateral sclerosis. *Amyotrophic Lateral Sclerosis,* **11**(3), 298–302.

110. **Research Motor Neurone.** Best Practice Guidelines for Health Care Professionals. http://mnd.ie/wp/wp-content/uploads/2017/01/Best-Practice-Guidelines-for-HCPs.pdf (accessed February 2017).

Chapter 10

Neglected needs: Sexuality, intimacy, anger

Anna Marconi

Emotions in ALS

Recent psychological studies of patients with ALS have mostly concentrated on behavioural changes connected to frontotemporal dementia (FTD) (1) (see also Chapters 8 and 9). Anxiety and depression have been studied in both patients and caregivers (2,3) (see Chapter 2). Most existing studies also assess anxiety and depression as pathological reactions to this disease, but the distinction between an adjustment reaction and a psychological illness is often not clear.

Only a few studies of ALS have examined in-depth the topic of physiological emotional responses to the specific illness. In the ALS literature, patients are sometimes described as positive people with a good quality of life (QoL) despite physical limitations (4). This description, however, is overly simplistic, and ignores the fear, anger, sense of guilt, hopelessness, and other emotions that people often experience during the course of the disease. Although patients with adequate adaptive mechanisms and psychosocial adjustments may appear positive at times, there are other times in which they are terrified or angry. These emotional responses are not necessarily related to a psychopathological disorder and can be considered, especially in the early stages, a physiological response to the diagnosis. To understand this, one must realize that ALS progression results in a series of major physical losses. The experience of loss is very painful, especially in early stages of the disease, when psychological adjustments have not been made (4). Although each patient reacts in a personal way, the most common emotions during these initial stages are caused by feelings of loss and are perceived as intolerable. Patients very often experience the diagnosis as a catastrophe and they fear the eventual loss of goals; these worries become more realistic with the progression of the disease and the unrelenting physical losses. An informed patient knows that there are no curative therapies and this notion may lead to a mental state comparable to a total collapse of life expectations, and thus to a feeling of hopelessness.

Patients must be given time to process their loss, with the associated grief and suffering, before health care professionals begin their work of marshalling psychological resources. This time allows them to reorganize their lives and to react to the disease. The clinical team must avoid mistaking a normal emotional reaction for a psychopathological condition. Loss is psychologically linked to grief and grief is a common reaction to a chronic illness (5).

The diagnosis of ALS generally has a traumatic impact because of the immediate connection to the concept of death. One of the main theories on the grieving process, conceptualized by Elisabeth Kübler-Ross (6), identified different emotional stages that are also useful in the understanding of reactions to chronic diseases (7). The author's theory recognizes a progression across five stages:

+ denial or shock;
+ anger;
+ bargaining;
+ depression;
+ acceptance.

The shock takes place when the loss occurs, which often is in the presence of the health care professional during the communication of the diagnosis. The initial response of denial can be seen as a reaction to the diagnosis, in which the patient's mind does not want to accept the disease and reacts by avoiding thoughts of the illness, and the current and future need for care that is linked to it. Denial is often a temporary protection, useful in providing the patient time to identify psychological adjustment mechanisms. It may reduce the pain in the early stages of the illness, but may have negative consequences if it leads to the postponement of medical treatment (4). For example, if an ALS patient denies her/his respiratory difficulties and avoids the recommended use of non-invasive ventilation, survival may be shortened.

The stage of anger occurs as awareness of the disease grows. A study by Palmieri et al. (8) observed high levels of anger in the ALS population. Anger, fury, and resentment are feelings that originate from thoughts about loss of independences, directed toward the patient's own future and those of his/her loved ones. Anger can result when the affected individual identifies the factors obstructing the attainment of personal goals, which of course leads to the perception of ALS as the main target of such anger (9). When angry, patients may think 'why me?' and focus on the goals that will not be accomplished because of the disease. The anger of the patient can be difficult to face, especially for caregivers who often are the targets of this emotion. This is particularly challenging for caregivers of those with ALS, who often find themselves having to rearrange their aspirations, lifestyle, and employment, leading caregiver psychological distress (10).

The next stage is bargaining, which occurs when the patient tries to negotiate some time by identifying life events as that they wish to witness or achieve. For example, the patient may attempt to negotiate longer survival with God or other forces, in order to be present at the birth of their grandchild or to take part in their child's wedding. This is a way to keep hope alive. The negotiations may involve with both supernatural and concrete entities. In particular, someone may choose to undergo invasive procedures. An example might be a 53-year-old woman with a 3-year history of ALS who chooses to undergo a tracheostomy and support by mechanical ventilation with the goal of participating in her daughter's wedding, scheduled for the following year. This family event may be perceived by her as an important reason to live, and thus may provide the motivation to accept tracheostomy and ventilator.

Kubler-Ross recognizes two types of depression: reactive depression and preparatory grief. In this model, reactive depression in ALS can occur when the patient experiences the feeling of loss. This can be very strong and, as in other degenerative illnesses, can represent the loss of physical functioning and independence, work abilities, social relations, social role, and body image. Loss can be also the loss of hope, which may be caused by loss of autonomy, and can lead to depression and to suicidal ideation (11,12). Preparatory grief is related to future loss. Together with some possible psychological pain, it can lead to the growth of emotional affinity between patients and their loved ones (13). It has been described as a way to prepare for the loss of all of the affective aspects of life and to move on to acceptance. In ALS, however, total acceptance is very difficult to achieve, and it is inappropriate to expect in the early stages. Acceptance is possible as the last stage of the grieving process, but may not be reached by all ALS patients. While not the equivalent of optimism and peace, it can be an asset. In ALS, acceptance can be identified when the person reorganizes her/his own life and experiences the illness, without trying to change it, and without protesting or trying to run away from it. Only some patients, particularly those who are well assisted and supported, reach acceptance. Social support, emotional closeness, and spirituality (1,14) are factors that can help the patient enter this dimension, which is characterized by a coexistence with the disease and the resulting disability.

It's important to identify and study the emotional reactions to the diagnosis in order to facilitate the coping process and to help the entire family. Caregivers and relatives may be helped in supporting the patient by understanding their emotional reactions. The effect that continuous anger can have on a caregiver who is also dealing with a progressive disease can be devastating. Providing a meaning to these emotional expressions and being able to frame them in the context of evolving stages may help with coping.

It is also important to understand when a physiological emotional reaction evolves into real psychological suffering. Even mild depression may reduce a person's motivation to access medical care and follow treatment plans, and so should be treated (15). The optimal treatment of depression in patients with chronic conditions often involves a combination of cognitive and supportive psychotherapies that incorporate awareness of the grief and loss that are consequences of the disease process (16,17). Recently, meditation training, based on the Mindfulness-based Stress Reduction (MBSR) protocol and specifically adapted for people with ALS and for their relatives, has been used with the aim of improving their QoL and psychological well-being (10) (see Chapter 5). Additional studies reveal that meditation training and mindfulness appear to improve QoL, favours acceptance of the disease, improves breathing and sleep quality, and favourably impact upon relationships between patients and their families and caregivers (18,19).

Sexual taboo and the role of intimacy

Clinicians may underestimate or avoid discussion of intimate feelings, which they may consider to be of secondary importance relative to medical issues or about which they may consider themselves inadequately trained. Sexual activity is rarely addressed by physicians, even though many individuals with motor neuron disease and their partners consider it to be important (20). Consistent with this, it has been noted that sexuality is the most neglected need in people with disabilities and in those with chronic diseases (21), and is still a taboo subject for many. Both patients and physicians may be uncomfortable discussing sexuality, but it is an important area to address in the care of those with ALS.

The percentage of patients with ALS that are sexually active is high. In a sample of 24 patients with ALS, we found that 50% were sexually active. Sexual function is usually not directly affected by disease progression (22). Our ongoing research in Italy at Centro Clinico NEMO confirms what Wasner and colleagues (20) wrote in the first paper on this topic. Even if there is a reduction in sexual desire, the majority of people with ALS continue to be sexually active and to consider this activity to be satisfactory. There are a number of reasons for the reduction of sexual desire and of sexual intercourse. Patients identify direct physical consequences of ALS, such as fatigue, pain, and weakness (23). Ventilators and gastrostomy tubes can be barriers for spontaneous sexual activity (24). Changes in physical appearance and the perception of this transformation can have a strong psychological impact and, in some cases, may be a source of distress that results in a decrease in libido. Furthermore, while patients perceive a change in their bodies, their partners remain the same, providing additional discomfort for patients, who may feel unattractive. The imbalance between the caring-role of the partner and the care-receiver role of the patient also can have consequences for their intimacy and sexual relationship (25). The complexity of the situation is perhaps best illustrated by a Case Report:

Case 1: Sexuality

Mr E (not his real initial) is a 38-year-old man diagnosed with ALS 1 year previously, who brought to the psychologist's attention his sexuality question. He is a successful professional who has always been passionate about his job. He has been married for 8 years and he defines his marital relationship as his main resource, in which he shares future projects and passions. For years, he and his wife have had a passionate relationship, spending much time together and having satisfying sexual intercourse regularly. Mr E highlights how, following the diagnosis of ALS and the development of weakness, intimate behaviours have begun to decrease. He thinks a lot about the changes in his marital relationship and he perceives this as an additional stress factor. Initially, he thought that the major cause of these changes was physical. Mr E continues to desire an intimate relationship with his wife, but he feels that his weakness prevents it. Sometimes he feels rejected or ignored by his wife, who has been arranging for them to move to a different home and has changed her job in order to better manage his changed condition. Mr E. recognizes how all of these factors, in addition to the frequent presence in his house of strangers or relatives to provide assistance, force him to continually change his sexual routine. What Mr E has realized over time is that these intimate moments represent times of sharing with his wife. He also recognizes his wife's need to reorganize herself in her new role, not only as a partner, but also as a caregiver. Mr E rearranges his expectations, giving space and time to his wife to rebuild their life, and then telling her of his strong desire to be close to her. That leads to an improvement in their relationship.

As the case of Mr E shows, sexual problems are not always associated with decreasing satisfaction in the overall relationship (25) and do not necessarily indicate a break-up of that.

Sexuality must also be considered in terms of communication and intimacy between the partners, going beyond the concept of sexual intercourse (26). Intimacy is hard to define, but is closely connected to communication. Karen Prager (27) considers two basic concepts of intimacy—intimate interaction and intimate relationship. Intimate interaction can be defined as a dyadic exchange, verbal or non-verbal, when one or both partners share something private or personal with the other one. An intimate relationship is the presence of ongoing, frequently occurring interactions between the partners. In Prager's opinion, a relationship is intimate when it includes three characteristics: affection, trust, and cohesiveness, which result in togetherness, and sharing time and activities (28). However, sexuality can be just one of many ways to be intimate in a relationship. What helps patients feel alive and happy, facilitating their ability to cope with the disease, cannot be restricted to sexual intercourse, but also must include satisfaction in the desire for intimacy (29), especially if that involves tenderness and emotional availability.

Tenderness as a resource for couples

The quality of pre-existing relationships may influence not only each couple's ability to adapt to the disease (25, 30) but the marital satisfaction in general.

Communication and self-disclosure seem to be the main factors that contribute to maintaining emotional closeness and intimacy within a marriage (31). With the passage of time, the ability for emotional disclosure often grows and helps the partners in promoting the sharing of feelings; this happens spontaneously, especially during difficult periods of the illness. Women, in particular, appear to suffer when communication is poor, and seem to feel the most profound intimacy when their partner has understood and validated their own disclosure (32). This is illustrated by the following Case:

Case 2: Intimacy

A 48-year-old woman, diagnosed with ALS 3 years ago, gave us a good explanation of the importance of intimate behaviour during a psychological interview. Ms A (not her real initial) has been married for 25 years, and lives with her husband and children. She is a bright woman with a good understanding of her disease. During the counselling sessions she meditates on how the relationship with her husband has changed: 'Since the disease onset, things have changed: while I claimed my right to live, he had a negative attitude. Our sexual activity failed to continue when the diagnosis was given. This has been my own death: he would touch me only to assess my symptoms, not to actually be with me'. Ms. A's husband has completely identified himself with the caregiver role, mainly providing his wife with assistance. In time, he found himself overwhelmed by his wife's physical needs, ignoring the emotional ones. Ms A emphasizes how his displays of affection represents a moment of comprehension and reassurance, sometimes more significant than the attention given to the assistance necessary for her survival. At present, Ms A uses a wheelchair, mechanical ventilation, and a feeding tube, but she still maintains her dream of intimacy: 'I dreamt about sexual intercourse and I woke up feeling as good as if I had actually gone back to a normal life'.

Clinical experience informs us that the need for closeness exists independently of physical difficulties. In ALS patients, tenderness seems to be the best method to satisfy the need to feel alive and cared for. Even with the physical impairment caused by ALS, there are no physical barriers for hugs and tenderness. Couples may develop a new concept of sexuality and intimacy, and if they had good intimacy pre-illness, they may maintain it during the disease (33). In a study of the cancer population (34), two perspectives were considered in couples' re-elaboration of intimacy: 'alternative sexual practices' redefining sexual intimacy, and couple communication and relational context.

In 2015 we launched a study (24 ALS patients and partners) to try to understand how the physical deterioration caused by ALS can affect couples' intimacy and how sexuality can influence QoL (unpublished data). We used the Partnership Questionnaire (PFB; Partnerschaftsfragebogen) (35) to assess the quality of the couples' relationship. PFB is a 30-item instrument and consist of three subscales: Quarrelling, Tenderness feelings, and Togetherness/communication. These can be combined to create a total score of marital satisfaction. Scores of 54 and below designate low levels of satisfaction, scores between 55 and 72 correspond to medium levels, and scores of 73 and above indicate high levels. The PFB distinguishes between happy and distressed couples in order to evaluate couples' intimacy satisfaction. A semi-structured interview, named PERALS (PERsonality in ALS), was also used as an in-depth clinical interview on sexuality habits (36). We selected the sexuality part of the original questionnaire, composed of three domains (aggressiveness, sexuality, and obsessiveness). The questionnaire permits a binary response (Y/N). One point is given to each affirmative response and no points for each negative answer. We also used the open question aimed at understanding the changes in the sexual sphere of the couple. To date, data has been collected on 24 patients (19 males, mean age 58.3 years, mean time since diagnosis 2.5 years, mean ALSFRS score 25 +/-11) and 23 caregivers (five males, mean age 56.9 years). The average length of marriage was 29 years. Regarding the sexual sphere, 50% of the couples reported that they did not have sexual relations, whereas 50% reported that they still were active sexuality. A total of 54% of the patients and 50% of the caregivers declared themselves satisfied with their sexual life. From the PERALS clinical interview item ('is your dissatisfaction due to issues related to your sexual potential?') it emerged that dissatisfaction was not connected to physical or functional problems. Physical symptomatology, on average, was not related to QoL, which remained moderate both in patients and caregivers. In the first correlations analyses it emerged that the level of functional impairment measured through ALSFRS was not correlated with QoL as perceived by both partners (patients and caregivers) nor did it affect the cohesiveness perception in the couple. Rather, QoL seemed mostly influenced by other aspects, such as social elements, and by the perception that patients had of their own existential well-being (37). These results underscore the importance of additional research into the relationship and couple dimension. PFB scales revealed that both patients and caregivers reported a medium level of marital satisfaction. In both opinions, the conjugal atmosphere was positive and levels in quarrelling were low. The patients' scores in intimacy, and in marital harmony and cohesion were slightly higher than the caregivers' scores. Despite these differences, these results show good levels of marital relationships.

Preliminary results obtained with multivariate correlation analysis of patients' responses revealed, an inverse correlation between 'quarrelling' and QoL, and between 'quarrelling' and physical wellness. A comparison between the two subgroup means showed that quarrelling scores were lower, and togetherness and tenderness scores were higher in patients who maintained sexual intercourse, in comparison with patients who did not (see Fig. 10.1). The partners' scores showed equivalent levels in the same categories. For caregivers, positive correlations between QoL and all of the PFB dimensions were found. Significant correlations emerged between marital satisfaction, and existential well-being and physical wellness. The Quarrelling scores negatively correlated with the caregiver's QoL. As these results confirm, the dimensions associated with affection are the most important ones for the caregivers. Tenderness and togetherness are positively correlated with QoL perception. Although these are preliminary results and our sample is not necessarily representative of the general ALS and caregiver population, our data confirm the literature that defines personal and relational resources as the most useful tool to cope with a chronic disease. People in marriages may build a vision of hope together and their shared marital commitment could represent a protective factor against patients' hateful feelings that may negatively impact their well-being (9). Good conjugal intimacy, both as physical and communicative, and combined with the absence of quarrelling, could guarantee the strength necessary to confront the difficulties imposed by ALS to preserve QoL in general.

How to deal with sexuality in clinical practice

If we consider sexuality as a central aspect of the human being, as the World Health Organization recommends (38,39), and as an essential element of a couple's QoL in ALS (29), providing counselling and proper information is necessary. In our clinical experience we have found that health care professionals are often surprised when patients ask about intimacy. It is frequently seen as not significant by physicians or they may be embarrassed by the subject. However, in the multidisciplinary treatment of ALS, it is important to go beyond the biological aspects and to seek to enhance the value of all of the aspects of a person's life that impact the quality of that life and that are important for each person (7). Unfortunately, many clinicians are not properly trained or knowledgeable about their non-medical concerns, and they may even feel that providing emotional support for families is a source of stress (40). Medical education must include information on the emotional aspects of diseases and their consequence impact on the patient, the patient's family, and the clinicians involved in the treatment (16). Communication skills are fundamental not only for disclosing bad news, but also during conversations with patients on their feelings and psychosocial concerns. Being able to discuss 'negative issues', such as anxieties, uncertainties, fears, losses, and sadness that usually accompany severe illnesses is generally helpful, despite the pressure commonly exerted by families and friends for the patient to always 'keep a positive out-look' (41).

Listening actively to an individual experience, supporting the patient and their partner through the promotion of mutual communication and encouraging emotional expressions such as tenderness are important clinical prescriptions. The

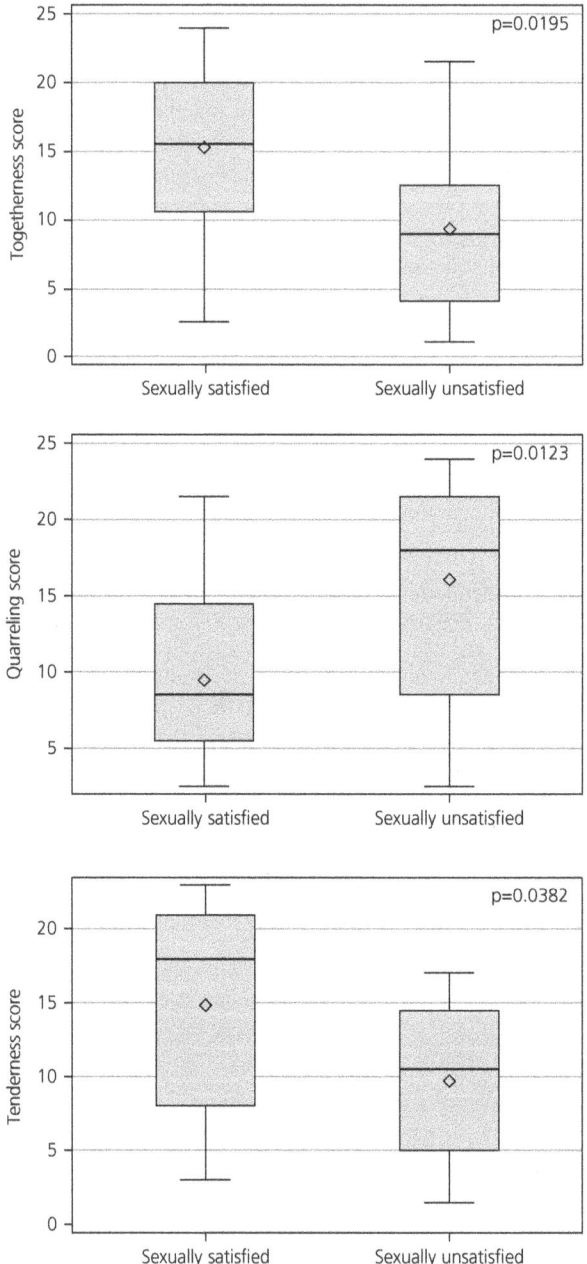

Fig. 10.1 Comparison between the PFB subscales score in sexually satisfied and unsatisfied ALS patients.

'Stepped Skills Model' (42) that has been developed for cancer and palliative care identifies a specialist in each team who develops the necessary skills to discuss topics such as sexuality and intimacy, and who then can lead the team in meditating on these matters during the course of the disease. The PLISSIT (permission, limited information, specific suggestions, and intensive therapy) model has been found to be useful in preparing nurses to address patients' sexual matters (43,44) and to recognize patients' sexual needs in order to identify services or professionals to whom they can be referred. Health care providers must be encouraged to facilitate sexual expression in all patients, irrespective of their level of physical impairment (45).

In summary, we believe that there are four main points for health care professionals to consider when addressing intimacy in ALS:

1. *Provide a non-judgmental setting*: clinicians must remain neutral, regardless of personal opinions and values.

2. *Change perspective*: just as patients change their concepts of QoL and of sexuality, health care providers must change their own perspectives.

3. *Do not be afraid to ask patients about their sexuality and about sexual relationships*: if couples feel there is a problem in this area, this is the time to intervene. Health care providers must be open-minded and able to accept patients' emotions.

4. *Encourage attention and tenderness*: encouraging the reawakening of hugs, caresses, and kisses may facilitate the discovery of new ways to be together and of new ways for couples to share intimacy.

Although couples will probably have to change their way of being together because of the physical limits, they can still enjoy an intimate relationship.

References

1. **Matuz, T., Birbaumer, N., Hautzinger, M.,** and **Kubler, A.** (2010) Coping with amyotrophic lateral sclerosis: an integrative view. *Journal of Neurology, Neurosurgery, & Psychiatry*, **81**(8), 893–8.

2. **Lomen-Hoerth, C., Anderson, T.,** and **Miller, B.** (2002) The overlap of amyotrophic lateral sclerosis and frontotemporal dementia. *Neurology*, **59**(7), 1077–9.

3. **Lulé, D., Hacker, S., Ludolph, A., Birbaumer, N.,** and **Kubler, A.** (2008) Depression and quality of life in patients with amyotrophic lateral sclerosis. *Deutsches Ärzteblatt international Bundesärztekammer; Kassenärztliche Bundesvereinigung (Germany)*, **105**(23), 397–403.

4. **Matuz, T., Birbaumer, N., Hautzinger, M.,** and **Kübler A.** (2015) Psychosocial adjustment to ALS: A longitudinal study. *Frontiers in Psychology*, **6**, 1197.

5. **Sidell, N.L.** (1997) Adult adjustment to chronic illness: a review of the literature. *Health & Social Work*, **22**(1), 5–11.

6. **Kubler-Ross, E.** (1976) *La morte e il morire* (trad. ital). Assisi: La cittadella; 1976.

7. **Engel, G.L.** (1977) The need for a new medical model: A challenge for biomedicine. *Science*, **196**(4286), 129–36.

8. **Palmieri, A., Naccarato, M., Abrahams, S.,** et al. (2010) Right hemisphere dysfunction and emotional processing in ALS: An fMRI study. *Journal of Neurology*, **257**(12), 1970–8.

9. Oster, C. and **Pagnini, F.** (2012) Resentment, hate, and hope in amyotrophic lateral sclerosis. *Frontiers in Psychology*, **3**, 530.

10. **Marconi, A., Gragnano, G., Lunetta, C.,** et al. (2015) The experience of meditation for people with amyotrophic lateral sclerosis and their caregivers—a qualitative analysis. *Psychology, Health & Medicine*, **20**, 1–7.

11. **Racine, M., Choinière, M.,** and **Nielson, W.R.** (2014) Predictors of suicidal ideation in chronic pain patients: An exploratory study. *Clinical Journal of Pain*, **30**(5), 371–8.

12. **Ratcliffe, G.E., Enns, M.W., Belik, S.L.,** and **Sareen, J.** (2008) Chronic pain conditions and suicidal ideation and suicide attempts: An epidemiologic perspective. *Clinical Journal of Pain*, **24**(3), 204–10.

13. **Parkes, C.M.** (1998) Coping with loss: Bereavement in adult life. *British Medical Journal*, **316**(7134), 856–9.

14. **Pagnini, F., Lunetta, C., Rossi, G.,** et al. (2011) Existential well-being and spirituality of individuals with amyotrophic lateral sclerosis is related to psychological well-being of their caregivers. *Amyotrophic Lateral Sclerosis*, **12**(2), 105–8.

15. **Breitbart, W.** (1995) Identifying patients at risk for, and treatment of major psychiatric complications of cancer. *Supportive Care in Cancer*, **3**(1), 45–60.

16. **Turner, J.** and **Kelly, B.** (2000) Emotional dimensions of chronic disease. *Western Journal of Medicine*, **172**(2), 124–8.

17. **Diaz, J.L., Sancho, J., Barreto, P., Banuls, P., Renovell, M.,** and **Servera, E.** (2014) Effect of a short-term psychological intervention on the anxiety and depression of amyotrophic lateral sclerosis patients. *Journal of Health Psychology*, **21**(7), 1426–35.

18. **Pagnini, F., Di Credico, C., Gatto, R.,** et al. (2014) Meditation training for people with amyotrophic lateral sclerosis and their caregivers. *Journal of Alternative and Complementary Medicine*, **20**(4), 272–5.

19. **Pagnini, F., Phillips, D., Bosma, M.C., Reece, A.,** and **Langer, E.** (2014) Mindfulness, physical impairment and psychological well-being in people with amyotrophic lateral sclerosis. *Psychology & Health*, **30**(5), 1–27.

20. **Wasner, M., Bold, U., Vollmer, T.C.,** and **Borasio, G.D.** (2004) Sexuality in patients with amyotrophic lateral sclerosis and their partners. *Journal of Neurology*, **251**(4), 445–8.

21. **Howlett, C., Swain, M., Fitzmaurice, N., Mountford, K.,** and **Love, P.** (1997) Sexuality: The neglected component in palliative care. *International Journal of Palliative Nursing*, **3**(4), 218–21.

22. **Shaw, C.** (2006) Amyotrophic lateral sclerosis/motor neuron disease. In: **Oliver, D., Borasio, G.D.,** and **Walsh, D.** (eds) *Palliative Care in Amyotrophic Lateral Sclerosis: From Diagnosis to Bereavement*, pp. 1–18. Oxford: Oxford University Press.

23. **Taylor, B.** (2014) Sexuality, intimacy and motor neuron disease: Matters of concern. *British Journal of Neuroscience Nursing*, **10**(5), 242–51.

24. **Kaub-Wittemer, D., Steinbüchel, Nv., Wasner, M., Laier-Groeneveld, G.,** and **Borasio, G.D.** (2003) Quality of life and psychosocial issues in ventilated patients with amyotrophic lateral sclerosis and their caregivers. *Journal of Pain and Symptom Management*, **26**(4), 890–6.

25. **Taylor, B.** (2014) Experiences of sexuality and intimacy in terminal illness: A phenomenological study. *Palliative Medicine*, **28**(5), 438–47.

26. **Redelman, M.J.** (2008) Is there a place for sexuality in the holistic care of patients in the palliative care phase of life? *American Journal of Hospital Palliative Care*, **25**(5), 366–71.

27. **Prager, J.K.** (1995) *The Psychology of Intimacy*. New York, NY: Guilford Press.

28. **Beach, S.R.H., Sandeen, E.E.,** and **O'Leary, K.D.** (1990) *Depression in Marriage: A Model for Etiology and Treatment*. New York, NY: Guilford Press.

29. **Simmons, Z., Felgoise, F.H., Bremer, B.A.,** et al. (2006) The ALSSQOL balancing physical and nonphysical factors in assessing quality of life in ALS. *Neurology*, **67**(9), 1659–64.

30. **Atkins, L., Brwon, R.G., Leigh, P.N.,** and **Goldstein, L.H.** (2010) Marital relationships in amyotrophic lateral sclerosis. *Amyotrophic Lateral Sclerosis*, **11**(4), 344–50.

31. **Lawrence, E., Pederson, A., Bunde, M.,** et al. (2008) Objective ratings of relationship skills across multiple domains as predictors of marital satisfaction trajectories. *Journal of Social and Personal Relationships*, **25**(3), 445–66.

32. **Mitchell, A.E., Castellani, A.M., Herrington, R.L., Joseph, J.I., Doss, B.D.,** and **Snyder, D.K.** (2008) Predictors of intimacy in couples' discussions of relationship injuries: An observational study. *Journal of Family Psychology*, **22**(1), 21–9.

33. **Goldstein, L.H., Atkins, L., Landau, S., Brown, R.G.,** and **Leigh, P.N.** (2006) Longitudinal predictors of psychological distress and selfesteem in people with ALS. *Neurology*, **67**(9), 1652–8.

34. **Gilbert, E., Ussher, J.M.,** and **Perz, J.** (2010) Renegotiating sexuality and intimacy in the context of cancer: The experiences of carers. *Archives of Sexual Behaviour*, **39**(4), 998–1009.

35. **Hahlweg, K.** (1996) *Fragebogen zür Partnerschaftsdiagnostik*. Göttingen: Hogrefe.

36. **Marconi, A., Meloni, G., Fossati, F.,** et al. (2012) Aggressiveness, sexuality, and obsessiveness in late stages of ALS patients and their effects on caregivers. *Amyotrophic Lateral Sclerosis*, **13**(5), 452–8.

37. **Simmons, Z., Bremer, B.A., Robbins, R.A., Walsh, S.M.,** and **Fisher, S.** (2000) Measuring quality of life in patients with amyotrophic lateral sclerosis: Validation of instruments. *Neurology*, **54**(7), 343.

38. **World Health Organization [Internet].** (2002) *Working Definition of Sexuality*. Geneva: WHO. Available at: http://www.who.int/reproductivehealth/topics/gender_rights/sexual_health/en/ (accessed 24 July 2017).

39. **World Health Organization.** (2004) Sexual health—A new focus for WHO. *Progress in Reproductive Health Research*, **67**(3), 1–8.

40. **Schaerer, R.** (1993) Suffering of the doctor linked with the death of patients. *Palliative Medicine*, **7**(2), 27–37.

41. **Spiegel, D.** (1999) Healing words: Emotional expression and disease outcome. *Journal of the American Medical Association*, **281**(14), 1328–9.

42. **De Vocht, H., Hordern, A., Notter, J.,** and **van de Wiel, H.** (2011) Stepped skills: A team approach towards communication about sexuality and intimacy in cancer and palliative care. *Australasian Medical Journal*, **4**(11), 610–19.

43. **Ayaz, S.** and **Kubilay, G.** (2009) Effectiveness of the PLISSIT model for solving the sexual problems of patients with stomas. *Journal of Clinical Nursing*, **18**(1), 89–98.

44. **Taylor, B.** and **Davis, S.** (2006) Using the extended PLISSIT model to address sexual healthcare needs. *Nursing Standards*, **21**(11), 35–40.

45. **O'Dea, S.M., Shuttleworth, R.P.,** and **Wedgwood, N.** (2012) Disability, doctors and sexuality: Do healthcare providers influence the sexual wellbeing of people living with a neuromuscular disorder? *Sex and Disability*, **30**(2), 171–85.

Chapter 11

'They embrace you virtually': The internet as a tool for social support for people with ALS

Paul Wicks

Introduction

A diagnosis of ALS leaves patients and their family members in a state of shock, disarray, and grief. Patients must come to terms with powerful emotions like loss of control, fears for the future, and the sense of being a burden to one's caregivers. Against this background there are also practical issues to contend with such as the pattern of losses each patient faces in walking, dressing, feeding, or communication. Throughout the course of the disease there are many questions. *Why me? What is going to happen next? What are researchers doing about this illness? Is there anything I could be doing to improve my outcomes?* While healthcare professionals have a wealth of expertise and empathy to offer, few of them will have ever been in the patient's position and the amount of contact time each patient gets with a neurologist or allied healthcare professional each year may be short.

For those that seek it out, the Internet can provide a diverse array of information and networks that patients and caregivers can tap into, though as we shall see, there are some important caveats too. Throughout this chapter we will explore a brief history of online tools for people with ALS, consider the potential benefits as well as the risks, and share a resource of recommended links that professionals can recommend to patients and caregivers. Many professionals harbour significant concerns about patients using the Internet, based in part on warnings from their professional bodies about the quality of information online, their potential liability from participating in social media, and experience with patients who want to discuss controversial theories or therapy approaches based on information they have gleaned online (1). For some professionals, there may be an element of paternalism at work, based on the long-standing (but now defunct) tradition that only those with professional medical training could access and assess medical information.

However, because patients increasingly share their lives through social media, control their bank accounts online, and are dependent on their mobile devices for communicating, demands to 'stay off the Internet' are likely to be fruitless. Patients recognize that much as the printed word can be as accurate as a medical textbook or as spurious as a tabloid newspaper, it's not the medium, but the message that matters.

Because widespread use of the Internet is still relatively new, with little grant funding available to study it directly, there is a dearth of evidence on the quality of online information sources or the potential benefits and harms of participating online, particularly higher-quality studies such as randomized controlled trials or even well-conducted observational trials (2). Consequently, much of the content in this chapter is derived from the author's 15 years of experience as a developer, participant, caregiver, and advocate in the online health space, but necessarily relies on a much narrower evidence base than is desirable.

Note: Because the Internet can change rapidly please note that all web addresses were correct at the time of publication, but may have changed since then or ceased operating; try searching for the resource by name if the URL provided here returns an error message.

Information seeking in ALS

Before they come to be diagnosed with the condition, most people are relatively unfamiliar with ALS. In a 2014 YouGov/Huffington Post survey of 1,000 US adults, only 21% of respondents said they were 'very familiar' with the disease (3). Public perceptions are highly shaped by well-known figures like Stephen Hawking (4), films such as 'The Theory of Everything' (5) fundraising initiatives such as the ALS Ice Bucket Challenge (6), and high-profile individuals seeking to end their own lives through euthanasia (such as Diane Pretty), which can provide a skewed picture of the disease. As a professional, we might think back to how we first learned about ALS, from textbooks, the clinic, or instruction from mentors; highly curated and expertly produced information designed in a learning environment for those to whom the alarming symptoms and stark prognosis would not personally apply.

Today, 72% of Internet users report having searched online for health information within the past year, with the majority of these (77%) starting at a search engine such as Google or Bing (7). As an experiment, go to your web browser now and enter the search terms *you* might use if you were one of your patients searching for information about ALS, its prognosis, and its treatment. What do you find? Does anything surprise you? Scare you? Impress you?

Today we find that a newly symptomatic person is quite likely to have 'Googled' early symptoms such as 'muscle twitching' or 'slurred speech' and found themselves reading a suggested diagnosis of ALS in the midst of some blunt and alarming statistics on prognosis (8). What they will find depends on the search engine used, where they live, and the precise search term entered, but in an analysis of Google search terms Chen and Turner found that estimates of survival were returned immediately and without filter, giving a range of estimates from 24-60 months, but with some erroneous outliers ('a normal lifespan'). Therefore the outlook of even undiagnosed patients is increasingly being shaped by the nature and availability of online information.

Fortunately, ALS is rare, but many otherwise healthy people who search online because of benign muscle twitches and spasms may also inadvertently stumble upon ALS information and suffer health anxiety as a result of exhaustive searching. Ironically, health professionals are particularly likely to present to neurology outpatient clinics with worries about ALS that frequently turn out to be benign fasciculations (9).

Online patient communities such as ALSForums.com have specific sub-sections for those trying to self-diagnose and provide detailed '*read this first!*' threads that under-line the correct diagnosis process. They also convey just how irritating it can be for those diagnosed with ALS to have to reassure and empathize with otherwise healthy individuals with a muscle twitch in their calf following exercise.

Information-seeking preferences

O'Brien identified three sets of information-seeking preferences that can be held by patients and their caregivers (10), which can differ from one another and even change over time.

'Active seekers' want to know everything about ALS. They search extensively, they may set up automatic search programs or subscribe to medical journals, and may well end up more informed about the latest developments in clinical trials than their own clinicians. The barriers to being an active seeker differ dramatically from even the recent past when those who wanted to learn more about the condition might have to request photocopies from their local library, while those who wanted to avoid informa-tion could do so. With the rise of patient advocacy and the availability of online tools, active seekers are increasingly shaping the research field through advocacy, fundrais-ing, advising pharmaceutical companies, and sitting on advisory boards from grant bodies to the FDA. After a relatively short period of time active seekers can have a robust understanding of many features of ALS—the likely rate of progression, the epi-demiological risk factors, the clinical trials, and the measurement tools. Once they hit this plateau they can become frustrated, and outlets such as ALSTDI (where they can stay up to date on the latest research), ALS Untangled (where they can ask research-ers to investigate alternative therapies), and scientific webinars hosted by ALSA and NEALS can help them to become active participants in the research community.

'Selective seekers' carefully curate the information they receive, picking and choos-ing information as they need it from trusted providers or via proxies like their car-egivers who act as an information buffer or shield (10). Importantly, they accept information timed to the problems in front of them; they don't want to know every-thing about respiratory failure or feeding tubes right at the point of diagnosis. Given the overwhelming nature of the diagnosis this is quite a reasonable position to take, but tensions can exist between a patient that wants to be protected from upsetting information and caregivers, clinicians, or even friends trying to be helpful who give them more information than they can deal with at the time. In the worst-case scenario, planning for important disease milestones such as loss of mobility can come too late, which combined with long lead times for housing modifications or assistive equip-ment could leave these individuals disadvantaged. Real-world meetings with other patients in more advanced states of disease might be overwhelming for this group and they can become frustrated in the off-hand way that professionals, or even other patients may disclose information about prognosis, symptoms, and the consequences of advanced disease. This group may benefit most from being 'signposted' to resources which they can engage with at their own pace, or via an information proxy, rather than being presented with information directly. When there is a critical window in which relevant information about potential interventions such as a wheelchair, home modifications, or a feeding tube must be made, it is worth engaging actively with the patient's caregivers to understand the best way to deliver this information and from whom it should come. They may feel anger and resentment to even the most sensitive and empathetic clinician, particularly in earlier stages.

The third group are 'information avoiders', who don't want to hear any more about ALS until they actively request it themselves. These patients may be in denial that they have ALS and seek information confirming their potential to have an ALS mimic disease. Because this group may be unlikely to actively search for or accept information that could benefit them they could still be offered hard copies of literature and contact details for professional associations so that in the event of a crisis they have the opportunity to be supported.

As described in earlier guidance for ALS professionals (11), both information avoiders and selective seekers may benefit from setting 'information boundaries' with friends and relatives. The patient's best efforts to control the pace at which they learn about their illness may be disrupted by a 'helpful' friend or relative who insists on sending online links, newspaper clippings, or magazine articles of dubious value.

An example message they could be given to distribute over email is below:

> *'Dear Friends & Family,*
>
> *Thank you so much for your support and good wishes since my diagnosis. Many of you have asked how you can help and I'd be grateful if you would consider making a donation to ALS research (e.g. als.net, alsa.org, www.mndassociation.org). I know many of you will want to be helpful by passing on links, magazines, and news articles about ALS or possible cures for ALS to me or my family; however, we've come to the decision as a family that we do not want to hear anything more about ALS until my doctor feels it is necessary.*
>
> *This is one small way in which I am hoping to maximize control over this disease; although I have ALS it does not have me.*
>
> *Thank you for your understanding....'*

Quality of information online

Although many patients under the care of a specialist multidisciplinary team may have a variety of avenues to learn more, a qualitative study of ALS caregivers reported that, for some, the Internet was their *primary* source of information because healthcare professionals provided insufficient information, used technical language, were deemed inaccessible, or showed a lack of empathy (12). By contrast, the humanity and fellowship of an online community of other patients or caregivers provided not just information, but validation and acceptance.

For many patients, the torrent of information ranging from lay-accessible summaries to systematic Cochrane libraries can be overwhelming, like 'drinking from a firehose'. While today the curated information filter seems more difficult to maintain, the quality of information derived from searches is improving. In an initiative to improve the quality of medical information online, Google recently partnered with the Mayo Clinic to provide validated medical information as a prominent search result, with each entry reviewed by an average of 11 physicians (13). Another prominent search hit, Wikipedia, has also evolved in the quality of its medical articles. Initiated as an 'encyclopedia anyone can edit', the site was once notorious for poor-quality information, but efforts by medical professionals and organized quality improvement drives mean that medical information on the site is, for some articles, comparable to the quality of information in medical textbooks (14,15). For example, the Wikipedia page for ALS receives an average of 6,000 views a day from around the world, with occasional spikes related to events in the news such as the 2014 ALS Ice Bucket Challenge (6). Take a look at the Wikipedia page for ALS; is the section on your specialty accurate and up to date? If not, consider learning how to edit Wikipedia and improving it yourself. Wikipedia encourages its readers to **be bold** in improving the information it provides and your edits could reduce fear, uncertainty, and misinformation for thousands of people with just a few minutes of your time.

The internet for social support

For several decades, advocacy, research, and psychosocial support has been provided by patient organizations such as the MND Association (UK), ALS Association (ALSA, USA), or Muscular Dystrophy Association (MDA, USA). These organizations provide information and educational materials to address some of the common questions patients have and maintain a strong network of local branches staffed by volunteers to provide face-to-face support meetings where patients and their caregivers can meet others like them in order to gain both psychosocial and practical support (16). By meeting others who have been through the same experiences and who may be further along in the coping process, patients and caregivers can gain a sense of perspective and hope for the future. Such meetings are also a rich source of problem solving and informal signposting to local resources and sources of emotional and practical support (16). Studies in conditions other than ALS suggest that real-world support groups may offer increased coping ability, the opportunity to express emotions, reductions in depression, and improved medication adherence (17).

Such real-world meetings have limitations, however. Most groups are located in areas with a high population density (particularly cities) and meet only on an occasional basis. Many patients and caregivers report finding it stressful or upsetting to see patients in more advanced states than they are (such as using a wheelchair or a ventilator) or meeting bereaved caregivers who often make up the longer term volunteer members (16). Patients might feel inhibited from discussing sensitive topics such as mood, sexuality, death, or personal hygiene. Those with impaired communication who are difficult to hear or who can only communicate slowly via an assistive communication device may find it difficult to participate and keep up with the flow of conversation. Finally, although the other members might be their fellow patients or caregivers, they may differ on important parameters. For example, an individual with an inherited and rapid form of the disease with a bulbar onset may have relatively little in common with a patient with the slowly progressive 'flail arm' form. Some may be seeking connections with others around non-medical facets of their experience such as faith, parenting, or sexual orientation.

Many people use the Internet to communicate in their daily lives with friends and loved ones, and ALS patients are no different, using email and technologies like Skype for work or to stay in touch with distant family such as grandchildren (18). Over the past 20 years, online support groups have sought to take the support and camaraderie that can arise from local face-to-face meetings and leverage the global, always-on, anonymous, and technologically enhanced capabilities of social networks to benefit a larger number of patients in their own homes. Most systems focus on asynchronous exchange, which allows patients with disabilities to spend as long as they need composing messages, as opposed to synchronous methods such as chatrooms or Skype, which rely upon fast typing skills or functional speech. The use of graphical avatars, nicknames, fun emoticons, and emojis help convey a richness of emotional expression that can help to make up for the facial cues and body language missing from online interactions. However, face-to-face and virtual group participation is not an 'either/or' decision, and many patients participate in both forms of peer support (16).

Although a complete history of online networks in ALS is outside the scope of this chapter (see (19)), online networks such as Braintalk and Bob Broedel's Email digest have functioned in ALS since at least the early 1990's (20). While the number of users that have ever registered on these sites probably only numbers in the tens of thousands, one frequently overlooked factor in measuring the impact of online communities is the high ratio of 'lurkers' (who read and benefit from information shared without contributing themselves) to 'contributors' (who actively participate). A common rule of thumb that has held up to scrutiny states that for every 1 user who posts content, there are 99 reading it (21), and so the reach of such networks is probably far beyond their registered members, particularly for systems that don't require registration to read content.

Benefits of online communities for patients and caregivers

Studies in other conditions such as diabetes have found that participation in an online peer community can have benefits on key outcome measures such as HbA1c levels and secondary outcomes like quality of life (22). However, randomized studies are few and far between in the field as a whole and are absent entirely in ALS. In part this is because of methodological difficulties; it would be impossible to randomize patients to either join an online community or be randomized to some sort of 'placebo' intervention when they could easily join one of the many freely available sites (see Appendix 11.A). Furthermore, online communities are prone to highly skewed patterns of participation, meaning that only a subset of those signing up are likely to become highly engaged and so extract the maximum benefit from taking part (23). The academic-scientific complex is poorly set up to monitor fluid and rapidly developing communities; by the time a grant has been funded, the data collected, and the study published, years may have elapsed in which new forms of social media may have emerged. While we will consider the available evidence from the literature, even the most casual browsing of the recommended resources in Appendix 11.A should quickly persuade readers of the potential value as expressed by active members, anecdotally at least.

An Italian study highlighted the importance of the Internet for informational support for patients and caregivers when their relationship with their physician may be strained (12). One daughter of a patient stated: *'If I had a problem, I never called the hospital. I connected to the internet, looking at what happened to other families.'* Family members reported a lack of empathy and humanity on the part of some healthcare professionals who looked after them, which contrasted with the experience of the daughter when she went online: *'You log in, you read the others' experiences, you write, they respond, they embrace you virtually.'*

In a qualitative analysis of a month's worth of forum posts from an online ALS message board community, researchers found 661 instances of social support in just 499 posts (17). In a typical exchange, a member might request information and receive emotional support and esteem support in addition to the requested information. Looking at the content of each post, the most common form of support was information (42%), signposting to resources (31%), emotional support (15%), and esteem support (11%), with the majority of requests for support occurring in the first year after joining the site. Many participants felt positive about helping others, and it may be empowering for people normally on the receiving end of care to lend their experience to support others in the same position.

In addition to the traditional forms of informational and emotional support, in a qualitative study of 48 patients and 22 caregivers, Locock and Brown identified non-medical forms of support gained from online communities like BUILD-UK in allowing patients to share jokes, photographs, and reflections on their lives outside of ALS (16). As patients become increasingly disabled their real-life social interactions may deteriorate such that their online network comes to occupy more time in their day. However it is also important to remember that online participation may be only one facet of the support a patient receives from family, friends, healthcare professionals, and the wider community.

PatientsLikeMe is an online community founded by a family affected by ALS that offers members traditional social features like a message forum, but also self-reported tracking tools such as the ALSFRS-R and ways to record treatments, symptoms, and side effects in a personal health record (19). In a retrospective survey, which included 218 ALS patients who had used the site for a median of 15 months, reported benefits included learning about a symptom they had experienced, understanding the side effects of treatment, and finding another patient like them (24). Specific to ALS, nearly half of patients (47%) reported that using the site had been helpful in supporting patients to make a decision about receiving a feeding tube. A follow-up study of the PatientsLikeMe platform for patients with epilepsy using a pre/post design found statistically significant improvements in self-efficacy and self-management, but it is unclear whether this would generalize to ALS (25). Future studies are underway to expand upon this work in ALS.

Potential risks and pitfalls of online communities

While the evidence reviewed to date paints a picture that is positive, that is not to say that there aren't some potential concerns with the use of online communities. Such concerns generally fall into four categories; misinformation, scams, representativeness, and becoming 'too close' to the disease.

Misinformation

Fears about misinformation online have abounded in the medical profession since the 1990's, with professionals' first impression of this nascent technology focusing on the relative lack of quality and consistency in health information available (26) (27). While quality is undoubtedly improving, the Internet is an unregulated space, and when patients seek out only what they want to hear they can quickly find themselves reading information that was not written by qualified professionals. Therefore connecting patients with trusted and well-moderated communities, which contain experienced veterans of the condition may serve as a defence mechanism and readily available vetting tool.

Information about ALS online may be out of date, inaccurate, or incomplete, a problem particularly acute for those who do not speak English as their first language, given that the bulk of high-quality information online comes from the US, UK, and Commonwealth countries. Representations of ALS in the mainstream media such as a plot device in a television soap opera or film are better today than they once were, due in part to strong advocacy from patient associations to correct harmful misconceptions.

Scams

Given the prognosis of ALS and the lack of effective treatments, patients may seek out complementary and alternative medicine (CAM) (see Chapter 5), and equally those that sell such products may see in the ALS population a viable market. There are a spectrum of CAM providers ranging from benign, cheap, pleasant interventions such as aromatherapy or massage, which may indeed be helpful, through to nutritional supplements, which may vary in price and are generally ineffective, but do not cause much harm, right up to highly invasive and potentially lethal treatments such as 'stem cell treatments' in offshore clinics (28). Online advertisements are unregulated, targeted to appeal to ALS patients and caregivers desperate for help, and may even appear 'inline' on otherwise trust-worthy websites when hosted through an ad network.

Dr Richard Bedlack has explored this area in more detail than any other researcher and he explains that most patients will try at least one CAM during their illness, with patients hoping it will be curative or at least slow the disease down. Patients are often pressured by well-meaning friends or relatives to try things out (for a full review see (29)). As Internet use expanded rapidly in the early 2000's, ALS patients provided rich pickings for unscrupulous individuals peddling curative 'snake oil' (30), and there was risk of a fault line developing between clinicians and patients who were unsatisfied with the lack of options available through conventional medical channels. Many patients felt ignored or patronized when they asked their doctors for their views on treatments they had heard about on the Internet and so took CAM treatments without telling their doctors.

A potential 'détente' was reached in 2009 when a group of ALS clinicians, researchers, and patient advocates came together to form the 'ALS Untangled' consortium. ALS Untangled has a website and social media channels via which patients and caregivers can submit requests for the team to thoroughly review the available basic science, feasibility, and clinical data of CAM therapies (31). Multiple times a year they produce a freely available summary of their findings and to date have produced over 35 reviews including a table of evidence that ranks each putative CAM treatment on a number of key variables (32). To date, no CAM treatment has received a positive endorsement, but a number of articles have been downloaded tens of thousands of times, suggesting a high degree of interest. Clinicians can also rely upon ALS Untangled to more conclusively answer patients' questions about CAM treatments.

Representativeness

While online communities could have great potential for research in ALS, there are understandable concerns as to the biases of who uses such communities or at least participates. One study found a bias towards higher rates of participation by females (17) despite the slight male bias in the epidemiology of ALS (33), and in another, patients with lower educational levels struggled with internet technologies (18). There are statistical approaches to solving such issues, such as benchmarked weighting, but this only works for quantitative, rather than qualitative research. Those who participate actively in online communities are most likely to be 'active seekers' and cannot be thought to represent every other segment of the community. However, online platforms can facilitate surveys, which gain input from a wider cross-section than just those who post actively. The sheer scale of online surveys permits data collection from hundreds of patients in a matter of weeks, a feat that would be difficult through traditional methods.

Becoming too close to the disease

In some of the qualitative studies conducted in online communities, researchers hinted that spending too much time thinking about ALS, interacting with others, and tracking the minutiae of their disease could actually be counterproductive (16). Locock and Brown state: *'However, problems arise when membership of a support group starts to define one's identity as 'a person with MND, rather than the person I am that happens to have MND'. Most people expressed ambivalence about meeting others, and the sadness and fear this could engender. Whilst many chose to 'summon up the courage', others were not ready to identify themselves as 'a person with MND'. This explains the benefit of choosing not to meet others, to protect oneself from witnessing one's possible future'* (see also Chapter 4). As one member of PatientsLikeMe stated: *'Discussing the symptoms and downfalls of this illness is getting to me. The people on the site are great but I get tired of talking about it when nothing is going to help me find a cure in my lifetime.'*

Future directions for online communities

Although the technology is relatively nascent, the high degree of unmet need among patients and caregivers for information and support means that the ALS community is quite advanced when it comes to forming tight-knit virtual communities. As the growth of social networks like Facebook and Twitter has grown to encapsulate the mainstream, we may see a shift from single-purpose disease communities to subgroups that fit within more generic networks like Facebook. Already, informal groups on Facebook for patients and caregivers have recruited substantive membership by virtue of the platform's superior reach. However, constraints such as using one's real name, the higher risks of privacy leaks, and the advertising-based business model of Facebook (and many other social networks) could erode trust. Conversely, the privately held, but rigorously collected medical data stored in electronic medical records is increasingly being opened up, shared, and linked across multiple platforms (34), so that in the future ALS patients might be able to treat their own health data as portable to multiple platforms that can choose to emphasize different aspects of support such as information, emotional support, advocacy, scientific research, or practical issues such as reviews of assistive equipment or recommendations for local resources.

Online communities such as PatientsLikeMe have enabled thousands of patients to participate in research studies that have improved our understanding of the disease. For example a study identifying barriers to clinical trial participation (35) was used to inform the recent 'Airlie House' development of clinical trial guidelines to maximize patient-centeredness. In another example, an online survey of 343 ALS patients was fielded in a matter of weeks and was able to establish that arm-onset ALS patients were more likely to have their first symptoms in their dominant hand, a finding which was subsequently replicated through clinical review and has informed pathophysiological understanding of the disease (36). The most active of active seekers have even taken research into their own hands, obtaining experimental treatments off-label and aggregating their data online to accelerate clinical trials (37), laying the foundation for 'virtual trials' where patients can take part in research from the comfort of their own homes.

In the future the use of assistive technology such as tablet computers, eye-gaze detectors, brain-computer interfaces, and even virtual reality helmets may increasingly permit patients who had once lost their voice to participate actively in a virtual world and continue to effect change despite their daily challenges (18).

Conclusion

Patients and caregivers have enthusiastically shaped vibrant on-line communities. We are past the point of asking whether the Internet is a 'good thing' or a 'bad thing'—like the printing press, it is a technology and it is up to society to use it productively. Like any human endeavour the Internet is imperfect, but it remains the most scalable and consistently available source of information, support, and true community available to patients. Professionals should consider more systematically engaging with patients online to harness these new tools for improved care and better outcomes.

Appendix 11.A Recommended online support resources

Web Address (registration required?)	Founded	Unique Strengths	Owner	Members
www.alstdi.org/forum/ (registration required to read & post)	2004	Experimental treatments, trials	ALSTDI	20k
www.alsforums.com (registration required to post)	2006	Living with ALS, caregivers, rare subgroups, self-diagnosis, Canada	Patient volunteers	28k
www.patientslikeme.com (registration required to read and post)	2006	Self-tracking tools, research studies	Private company	10k
https://forum.mndassociation.org (registration required to post)	2010	UK local care and advocacy	MND Association	2k
www.facebook.com/groups/alscaregivers/ (FaceBook account required, must request access from moderators)	2011	Non-professional caregivers only (closed group)	Facebook	800
www.facebook.com/groups/783085008445585/ (FaceBook account required to read and post)	2015	ALS patient tips for everyday living (open group)	Facebook	2k

References

1. Bedlack, R.S., Salami, V., and Cudkowicz, M.E. (2009) IPLEX and the telephone game: the difficulty in separating myth from reality on the internet. *Amyotrophic Lateral Sclerosis*, **10**(3), 182–4.

2. Hamm, M.P., Chisholm, A., Shulhan, J., et al. (2013) Social media use among patients and caregivers: a scoping review. *British Medical Journal Open*, **3**(5), e002819–9.

3. Moore, P. (2016) Poll results: Ice bucket challenge (Internet). *YouGov* (cited 2016 Apr 1). Available from: http://www.webcitation.org/6gPq7fcI6 (accessed 24 July 2017).

4. Bradley, W.G. (2010) Commentary on Professor Stephen Hawking's disability advice. *Annals of Neurosciences*, **16**(3), 101–2.

5. Simmons, Z. (2015) The theory of everything: The extraordinary and the ordinary. *Neurology*, **85**(23), 2079–80.

6. Wicks P. (2014) The ALS ice bucket challenge—can a splash of water reinvigorate a field? *Amyotrophic Lateral Sclerosis and Frontotemporal Degenerations*, **15**(7–8), 479–80.

7. Fox, S. and Duggan, M. (2016) Information triage (Internet). Pew Internet. (cited 2016 Mar 31). Available at: http://www.webcitation.org/6gPtUI7qS (accessed 24 July 2017).

8. Chen, Z. and Turner, M.R. (2010) The internet for self-diagnosis and prognostication in ALS. *Amyotrophic Lateral Sclerosis*, **11**(6), 565–7.

9. **Simon, N.G.** and **Kiernan, M.C.** (2013) Fasciculation anxiety syndrome in clinicians. *Journal of Neurology*, **260**(7), 1743–7.

10. **O'Brien MR.** (2004) Information-seeking behaviour among people with motor neurone disease. *British Journal of Nursing*,**13**(16), 964–8.

11. **Bedlack, R.S.** and **Mitsumoto, H.** (2012) *Amyotrophic Lateral Sclerosis: A Patient Care Guide for Clinicians.* New York, NY: Demos Medical Publishing.

12. **Cipolletta, S.** and **Amicucci, L.** (2015) The family experience of living with a person with amyotrophic lateral sclerosis: a qualitative study. *International Journal of Psychology*, **50**(4), 288–94.

13. **Verel D.** (2016) *Google to Reshape How it Provides Health Information, Mayo Clinic Joins as Partner.* Available at: http://www.webcitation.org/6gPthQjbr (accessed 24 July 2017)

14. **Reavley, N.J., Mackinnon, A.J., Morgan, A.J.,** et al. (2012) Quality of information sources about mental disorders: A comparison of Wikipedia with centrally controlled web and printed sources. *Psychological Medicine*, **42**, 1–10.

15. **Kräenbring, J., Penza, T.M., Gutmann, J.,** et al. (2014) Accuracy and completeness of drug information in Wikipedia: A comparison with standard textbooks of pharmacology. *PLoS ONE*, **9**(9), e106930.

16. **Locock, L.** and **Brown, J.B.** (2010) 'All in the same boat?' Patient and carer attitudes to peer support and social comparison in Motor Neurone Disease (MND). *Social Sciences and Medicine*, **71**(8), 1498–505.

17. **Loane, S.S.** and **D'Alessandro, S.** (2013) Communication that changes lives: Social support within an online health community for ALS. *Communication Quarterly*, **61**(2), 236–51.

18. **Londral, A., Pinto, A., Pinto, S., Azevedo, L.,** and **De Carvalho, M.** (2015) Quality of life in amyotrophic lateral sclerosis patients and caregivers: Impact of assistive communication from early stages. *Muscle & Nerve*, **52**(6), 933–41.

19. **Wicks, P.** and **Little, M.** (2013) The virtuous circle of the quantified self: A human computational approach to improved health outcomes. *Handbook of Human Computation*, pp.105–29. New York, NY: Springer.

20. **Feenberg, A.L., Licht, J.M., Kane, K.P., Moran, K.,** and **Smith, R.A.** (1996) The online patient meeting. *Journal of Neurological Sciences*, **139**(Suppl.), 129–31.

21. **van Mierlo, T.** (2014) The 1% rule in four digital health social networks: an observational study. *Journal of Medicine and Internet Research*, **16**(2), e33.

22. **Shaya, F.T., Chirikov, V.V., Howard, D.,** et al. (2014) Effect of social networks intervention in type 2 diabetes: A partial randomised study. *Journal of Epidemiology and Community Health*, **68**(4), 326–32.

23. **Eysenbach, G.** (2005) The law of attrition. *Journal of Medicine and Internet Research*, **7**(1), e11.

24. **Wicks, P., Massagli, M., Frost, J.,** et al. (2010) Sharing health data for better outcomes on PatientsLikeMe. *Journal of Medicine and Internet Research*, **12**(2), e19.

25. **Hixson, J.D., Barnes, D., Parko, K.,** et al. (2015) Patients optimizing epilepsy management via an online community: the POEM Study. *Neurology*, **85**(2), 129–36.

26. **Benigeri, M.** and **Pluye, P.** (2003) Shortcomings of health information on the Internet. *Health Promotion International*, **18**(4), 381–6.

27. **Silberg, W.M., Lundberg, G.D.,** and **Musacchio, R.A.** (1997) Assessing, controlling, and assuring the quality of medical information on the Internet: Caveant lector et viewor—Let

the reader and viewer beware. *Journal of the American Medical Association*, **277**(15), 1244–5.

28. **Chew, S., Khandji, A.G., Montes, J., Mitsumoto, H.,** and **Gordon, P.H.** (2007) Olfactory ensheathing glia injections in Beijing: Misleading patients with ALS. *Amyotrophic Lateral Sclerosis*, **8**(5), 314–6.

29. **Bedlack, R.S., Joyce, N., Carter, G.T., Paganoni, S.,** and **Karam, C.** (2015) Complementary and alternative therapies in amyotrophic lateral sclerosis. *Neurology Clinic*, **33**(4), 909–36.

30. **Kiatpongsan, S.** and **Sipp, D.** (2009) Medicine. Monitoring and regulating offshore stem cell clinics. *Science*, **323**(5921), 1564–5.

31. **Bedlack, R.** and **Hardiman, O.** (2009) ALSUntangled (ALSU): A scientific approach to off-label treatment options for people with ALS using tweets and twitters. *Amyotrophic Lateral Sclerosis*, **10**(3), 129–30.

32. **ALSUntangled Group**. (2015) ALSUntangled: Introducing The table of evidence. *Amyotrophic Lateral Sclerosis and Frontotemporal Degeneration*, **16**(1–2), 142–5.

33. **Wijesekera, L.C.** and **Leigh, P.N.** (2009) Amyotrophic lateral sclerosis. *Orphanet Journal of Rare Diseases*, **4**(3).

34. **Weber, G.M., Mandl, K.D.,** and **Kohane, I.S.** (2014) Finding the missing link for big biomedical data. *Journal of the American Medical Association*, **311**, 2479–80.

35. **Bedlack, R.S., Wicks, P., Heywood, J.,** and **Kasarskis, E.** (2010) Modifiable barriers to enrollment in American ALS research studies. *Amyotrophic Lateral Sclerosis*, **11**(6), 502–7.

36. **Turner, M.R., Wicks, P., Brownstein, C.A.,** et al. (2011) Concordance between site of onset and limb dominance in amyotrophic lateral sclerosis. *Journal of Neurology, Neurosurgery and Psychiatry*, **82**(8), 853–4.

37. **Wicks, P., Vaughan, T.E., Massagli, M.P.,** and **Heywood, J.** (2011) Accelerated clinical discovery using self-reported patient data collected online and a patient-matching algorithm. *Nature Biotechnology*, **29**(5), 411–4.

Chapter 12

Investigating the psychology of assistive device use in ALS: Suggestions for improving adherence and engagement

Christopher D. Graham

Introduction

Although ALS is presently without cure, and no treatment can significantly modify its course, much can be done to improve quality of life (QoL) (1–4). As part of multi-disciplinary care, treatments such as physical therapy, speech and language therapy, and psychological interventions are often employed. These help maintain meaningful functioning and/or alleviate unnecessary suffering, in the hope of preserving QoL. Similarly, assistive devices, such as wheelchairs, augmentative and alternative communication (AAC) devices, and home adaptations are often prescribed to patients as a means of maintaining function in the face of disease progression.

In this chapter, frequently-used assistive devices will be described, alongside evidence supporting their utility. Assistive devices are evolving with developments in computing and medical technology, thus devices involving newer technology (eye-gaze systems, micro-switches, brain computer interfaces) will be outlined. However, despite the effectiveness of assistive devices their use can bring significant psychosocial challenges. Drawing mostly on a small body of qualitative studies, the challenges of assistive technology will be discussed. Psychological, behavioural and technological ways to increase engagement with assistive devices will then be suggested.

Description of assistive device use in ALS

A wide range of assistive devices are applied across the spectrum of functional impairments caused by ALS. These can be broadly classified as aides to maintain mobility, communication ability, or to compensate for other miscellaneous functional impairments.

Mobility

As ALS progresses, it is likely that muscle weakness and spasticity will cause an insidious decline in walking ability. Initially walking sticks or a four-point cane may be sufficient to retain an adequate level of function. Ankle foot orthoses or braces may provide additional stability and reduce the risk of tripping and falling (5,6). However, as lower extremity impairment progresses, rolling walkers (rollators), then wheelchairs and/or powered wheelchairs may become necessary (7). Transferring from or between seated positions (for example, from the wheelchair to a car seat) is another important aspect of mobility, which is often affected by ALS. A slide board can be used to enable such transfers (6).

Communication

Bulbar involvement may result in an insidious decline in communication ability. Alongside this, in some cases, cognitive impairment may involve aphasia. Thus, speech pathology will eventually be present in 80–95% of ALS cases (8). This process often begins with slight and/or intermittent slurring and changes in voice quality (volume, hoarseness), which worsen with fatigue. As movements of the lips, tongue, and pharynx become slower and less responsive, a total loss of speech ability can occur. One may speculate that loss of speech is the most distressing of all ALS symptoms because it represents a significant barrier to maintaining important relationships. Indeed, a qualitative study regarding this topic (9,10) suggested that, among people with ALS, the number one reason for communication was to maintain social closeness with significant others in the face of this life-threatening condition. Consequently, following loss of speech, if alternative methods of communication are not developed then there is the potential for isolation and reduced relationship quality (3,9). In support, a quantitative analyses QoL in people with ALS (N = 338), demonstrated that those with affected speech have a worse QoL than those with normal speech. Here, perhaps indicative of the challenges posed by adjusting to speech impairment, initial impairments in speech had a clear impact on QoL (11).

Given the importance of communication a range of compensatory devices, referred to as augmentative and alternative communication (AAC) devices, have been developed for ALS. Electronic computer-based AAC devices vocalize typed speech or selections made using micro-switches (switches controlled by minimal movements) or via eye-gaze systems. Also, where movement is severely restricted Brain Computer Interfaces—caps which contain electrodes that can detect changes in brain function (e.g. event-related potential)—can be used to make word selections. This group of AAC devices are often referred to as voice output communication aides (12). While these devices can effectively compensate for loss of speech—as is most famously the case with Professor Stephen Hawking—they do present some relatively unique psychological challenges to those who use them. Such challenges include learning to communicate primarily (or perhaps solely) via typed or selected text, and, since devices include a synthetic voice, communicating with voices that are incongruous to one's identity, accent or culture, etc. Thus, although high-tech AAC methods are available, basic communication strategies, such as written communication using a pen and notepad, head-nodding, and letter boards are often used by people with ALS (6,9). Indeed, there are a number of improvised communication strategies that people may develop, such as saying only key words, using confirmation, or relying on partner interpretation of gestures or facial expression (9).

Other aides

Given the breadth of functional impairments caused by ALS, a range of other assistive devices are also used. Environmental controls, such as push button telephones and entertainment systems (that can also be activated by micro-switches, eye-gaze systems or brain–computer interfaces), can be used to ensure comfort and control over the home environment, and enable text messaging or use of webcams. Independence in dressing can be extended by using zipper pulls, button hooks, etc. Independence in bathing and toileting is understandably important for persons with ALS. In response, arm rails and shower seats can facilitate showering, while elevated toilet seats and commodes may facilitate use of the toilet (5).

Satisfaction with assistive devices

Gruis and colleagues (5) investigated the frequency of use of assistive devices alongside patient satisfaction with these. In a telephone survey of 66 patients recruited from an ALS clinic, they observed that the most frequently used assistive devices were:

◆ slip on shoes (i.e. those without laces) (often/always used in 55% of cases);

◆ assistive devices for toileting and showering (e.g. shower seat, 48%; shower bars, 43%; elevated toilet seat, 40%);

◆ transfer boards (46%);

◆ ankle braces (32%);

◆ seating with recliner control (29%);

◆ speaker phone (26%).

Devices used for showering, toileting and mobility were rated most highly for satisfaction and usefulness, whereas those involved in dressing such as button hooks and dressing sticks were rated as less helpful. In a similar survey, regarding wheelchair use in people with ALS, Trail and colleagues (13) noted that most wheelchair-users perceived an improvement in activity levels following uptake of a wheelchair. Unsurprisingly wheelchairs were rated highly for satisfaction. Comfort and manoeuvrability were identified as the two of the most desirable features of wheelchairs (13). One paper (14) assessed interest in brain–computer interfaces amongst 61 people with ALS and the factors which may affect uptake. Here, 84% of the respondents stated that would consider using the requisite electrode cap, with 72% willing to undergo outpatient surgery, and 41% willing to have surgery and a short hospital stay to make the system available. Unsurprisingly, this survey suggested that that people with ALS most value systems that are precise and fast. A later in-depth qualitative study of the perceptions of BCI suggested that pragmatic concerns (social impact of setting-up and managing the system) and usability are key modifiers of acceptance and satisfaction (15).

Impact of assistive devices on quality of life

A small body of research has evaluated the impact of assistive devices on QoL. Londral and colleagues (16) followed a group of participants with ALS, who had been trained to use a tablet-based touchscreen text-to-communication device, over 10 months.

They introduced this communication device at either an early stage (before significant speech impairment was evident) or at the usual later stage (once significant speech impairment was evident). Consistent with the finding that QoL is most affected by the early stages of language impairment (11), researchers observed that those in the early introduction group reported better QoL and psychological well-being at a 10-month follow-up. Qualitatively, they noted that those who had lost the ability to speak or write at follow-up were effective in using AAC devices to communicate.

Lancioni et al. (17), in a case series of five people with ALS, assessed the impact of communication and environmental control system activated by micro-switches on time spent communicating or undertaking a leisure activity. This device enabled users to select and manage communication strategies (e.g. text messages, statements and requests) and leisure activities (music and videos) using micro-switches controlled via minimal movements (e.g. finger or eyelid movements). Use of these devices resulted in increased time spent communicating or engaging in a leisure activity—by up to 80%. Two further case studies support the benefits of micro-switch controlled devices. In one, an improvement in social functioning, as measured by time spent interacting with loved ones, was observed following introduction of a micro-switch enabled messaging and video phone system. This micro-switch was operated by an infra-red light detection unit activated by a slight head-tilt (18). In the other case study, the authors demonstrate how the method of micro-switch control can be changed following losses of function. Here, activation method was changed to a voice-sensitive micro-switch activated by a throat microphone as the person's ability to operate the switch via eye-movements reduced. Importantly, the ability to control the device was maintained following change in activation method (19).

A case study of the impact of brain–computer interface use on functional impairment/QoL in a professional man with ALS, demonstrated encouraging outcomes in the context of significant physical impairment: The user and his family stated that the device had improved his independence in social and occupational functioning (20). A case series also observed improved QoL and life satisfaction (although not mood) in three individuals with ALS, following adoption of an eye-gaze communication system (21).

Psychosocial challenges affecting use of assistive devices

The information presented thus far suggests that assistive devices are needed, widely-used, show good patient satisfaction and can improve functioning and QoL. Nonetheless, uptake of, and adherence to, assistive devices is not optimal. Fullam et al., (2015) (22) noted that compliance with recommendations made for physical function, support, and environmental support—these categories presumably included adherence to assistive devices—was frequent, but not complete.

This poses the question, if these devices can make such a difference, then why might people with ALS decide not to use them? A vast literature suggests that treatment non-adherence—and thus probable adherence to assistive technology—is affected by a number of biological, psychological, and social factors, such as cognitive impairment, self-efficacy, illness beliefs and treatment beliefs. In the specific context of ALS (23), a small body of qualitative literature has begun to shed light on this issue, suggesting that several psychosocial challenges are implicit in the use of assistive devices. Drawing on this I detail the most salient of these challenges, alongside some pragmatic methods (psychological, behavioural, or technological), which may improve engagement with assistive devices.

Cognitive impairment and mood

The insidious decline in mobility and other functioning in ALS necessitates continual change in the types of assistive devices that are used. This is illustrated by the aforementioned change in mobility aides, from sticks to wheelchairs, and from tablet-controlled AAC systems to those using micro-switches or brain–computer interfaces (19). This challenges people with ALS to undertake continual adaptation to maintain optimal functioning, and new skills must be rapidly acquired. While many may be able to engage in this process, the significant proportion of people with ALS who experience cognitive impairment as part of the disease process (24) may find the uptake of new assistive devices difficult. ALS appears to form part of a disease spectrum with fronto-temporal dementia (24,25), thus executive functioning (including flexibility, response inhibition, insight, motivation) may be affected (see Chapters 8 and 9) (26). These cognitive domains are particularly important for initiating, organizing, and monitoring behaviour, thus dysfunction here may affect the acquisition of new skills. In a study assessing the uptake of AAC devices by people with ALS, it was noted that respondents with behavioural impairment (i.e. showing signs of apathy, mental rigidity, and lack of motivation), were least interested in learning to use newer brain–computer interfaces. In addition, those with the greatest levels of general cognitive impairment were most interested—suggesting that reduced insight led to unrealistic judgements of one's own ability to learn to use new technology (27). In addition, a study assessing performance predictors of brain–computer interfaces in people with ALS ($N = 25$), showed that cognitive impairment and behavioural dysfunction affected ability to control these devices (28).

Low mood is also quite prevalent in ALS (see Chapter 2). A cohort study ($N = 964$) found that moderate depression was apparent in 33% of cases, moderately-severe depression was evident in 14% of cases, with 5% of cases reporting severe depression (29). Although this remains unstudied in the context of ALS, as with cognitive impairment, depression may have important repercussions for the uptake of assistive devices. Generalizing from studies that have investigated adherence (albeit to medication) in other diseases (23,30) there is evidence that the presence of depression negatively impacts treatment adherence.

Opportunities for intervention

Where adherence to assistive devices is poor, to the extent that it appears to be limiting QoL, then intervention may be helpful. The first step in this process is to understand which factors might contribute to non-adherence in a given case. Thus, assessment of contextual, neurocognitive and psychological factors may be useful. In clinical psychology, such a multi-component assessment results in a working model of how factors interact to give rise to a given problem—in this case poor adherence or uptake. Such a working model is often referred to as a 'formulation' (31).

If there is a suggestion that cognitive impairment may be a contributing factor, then, following informed consent, cognitive assessment can be undertaken. This can ascertain if cognitive impairment is present, then inform a formulation of non-adherence. Assessment can be done quite rapidly using a brief cognitive screen, such as the Edinburgh Cognitive and Behavioural ALS Screen, which includes assessment of cognitive functioning using standardized neuropsychological tests alongside caregiver accounts of behavioural changes (32). This can help delineate which aspects of cognitive impairment might be affecting assistive device use. Following assessment and/or formulation, some practical interventions can be applied. Depending on the pattern of impairment that is identified, such interventions might include prompting, placement of assistive devices (e.g. where they are often seen), encouragement, and reduction of distraction when using assistive devices (33).

In addition to this, as with cognitive impairment, it may be worthwhile offering assessment for depression or anxiety using a brief screens, such as the Patient Health Questionnaire (PHQ-9) (29,34) or the Generalized Anxiety Disorder Questionnaire (GAD-7) (35). If depression is present, then this can also be used to inform a formulation of non-adherence to assistive devices. Subsequent treatment of low mood and anxiety may feasibly result in (or be partially the result of) improved use of assistive devices.

Identity

Decline in physical functioning and assistive device use can challenge a person's established sense-of-self—their identity. Often people with ALS have experienced good levels of health until the advent of ALS symptoms, which immediately begin to affect physical functioning. This rapid change can bring with it some threats to a person's identity, and unwanted labels for oneself may emerge, as demonstrated by this quote from a 52-year-old man with ALS: 'It [ALS] turned me into an old man overnight because suddenly you're going with a walking stick and then you're with a rollator, now you're in this wheelchair … it's just a robbery of everything' (36).

As illustrated in the preceding quote, such identity issues may be brought to the fore by the impending necessity for assistive devices. A wheelchair can become a symbol of a changed identity—the irreversible loss of one's ability to walk. The resultant difficult thoughts, and feelings may then become barriers to the use of assistive devices. Indeed, avoidance of thoughts and feelings evoked by a wheelchair may lead to slow initial uptake, as expressed by a person recounting their initial responses to using a wheelchair,: '… the wheelchair … I rejected it at the start because I felt I didn't need that kind of thing … I hid it in the shed … I just hated the thought of being wheeled in that …' (37).

Opportunities for intervention

Health care professionals should be aware of the threat that assistive devices may pose to a person's identity—perhaps most acutely at the onset of ALS. A patient and empathic approach to offering assistive devices may be most effective in supporting engagement. As will be described in a forthcoming section, people with ALS may have a strong desire to maintain control over their health care decisions, this desire being understandable in light of the uncontrollable nature of ongoing changes to their physical functioning (37).

Also, given that incongruous accents may dissuade the uptake of AAC devices, synthetic voices that closely match the person's speaking voice should be sought. The most effective approach might involve reconstruction of the person's own speaking voice for use in AAC devices—in this way, important aspects of identity can be preserved. Such technology is becoming available. A voice banking project at the University of Edinburgh, Scotland (12), is recording the voices of people with ALS whose speech is beginning to deteriorate. Then, having collected a bank of donor voices from similar geographical regions (to allow congruent accents), synthesized reconstructed voices can then be developed that closely match that of the person with ALS.

Social context

Assistive devices are used to help maintain independence for as long as possible. Similarly, it is no surprise that people with ALS often desire to be as independent as possible. This desire may be informed by one's social context, such that desiring independence may be affected as much by a fear of becoming a burden on immediate others, as by a desire to maintain independence for one's own purposes (38).

However, the use of assistive devices may involve significant changes to home environments, for example, installing chair-lifts, fitting rails, renovating bathrooms, and moving bedrooms downstairs to facilitate the use of a wheelchair. This may cause significant upheaval in home environments and so these devices can themselves become burdensome at times. In a qualitative study, Foley et al. (38) described a person with ALS who desired home adaptations, but whose partner was less enthusiastic about such changes: '... If we had [build] a [accessible] bedroom ... I'll have my own little bit of independence ... But I have a problem with my wife ... and now it's coming to a head over this ...' (38).

Thus, challenges implicit in the uptake of assistive devices must be seen in their social context, encompassing a person's need to maintain independence, potential fears about becoming a burden, as well as the concerns of immediate family members or those who co-habit. Indeed, Murphy (9,10) in a qualitative study of communication strategies between people with ALS and their partners described the relationship tension, which can emerge when a person with ALS does not develop effective alternative communication strategies (possibly AAC devices). Murphy (9) highlighted a case where, across a number of meetings with the couple, the spouse (of the person with ALS) demonstrated 'more and more upset at her husband's unwillingness to compensate for his communication difficulties'.

Opportunities for intervention

Recommending and fitting assistive devices may open up the opportunity for health care providers to discuss the impact (or perceived impact) of ALS on loved ones and those who co-habit. Here, worries about changes in environments that are shared with others (home, car, etc.) can be discussed. A group discussion may allow for reassurance (i.e. that changes to the home environment are welcomed by all) or enable frank description of the salient concerns of all those affected by home adaptations, etc. Open discussion may allow for a shared understanding of issues and mutual decisions regarding ways forward, while the presence of the physician in the group discussion may help clarify issues not generally discussed within the dyad.

Acceptance and adjustment to assistive technology use

At present, declines in physical functioning are inevitable in ALS; functional impairments are then addressed via use of assistive devices. Thus, where these devices are used, one could consider this to be the result of an understandable resignation on the part of the person with ALS—as described by a 51-year-old woman with ALS: 'I know I can't walk so I have to use a wheelchair. I know I can't stand up so I have to be lifted up and I have to be hoisted into bed ... You don't have a choice. I mean if you are sitting there and you can't get up, what choice have you only to be lifted up' (36).

In this description, one can see that resignation appears to be the result of having no other alternative. The prospect of assistive devices may thus be met with ambivalence given the lack of choice or control. Nonetheless, one could argue that there is a qualitatively different response to the use of assistive devices—one which may display an accepting response to ALS. Although not mutually exclusive to resignation, acceptance generally involves a shift in focus towards doing personally meaningful activity outside of illness (see Table 12.1). In the following quote, you may note that assistive devices are seen as a means to an end, a way to connect with the outside world, and a bridge to personally meaningful activity: 'My laptop is very important to me and brings the outside world in. It is my preferred method of communication as I find talking on the telephone challenging ... I use e-mail, Yahoo messenger, and Skype and regularly stay in contact with friends and family' (39).

Opportunities for intervention

Of course, the division between resignation and acceptance might be considered somewhat artificial—one may demonstrate both at the same time, and it is likely that people with ALS will oscillate between the two over the course of their illness. However, if a general problem with illness acceptance is identified then a number of therapeutic modalities could be used to increase acceptance, such as counselling or cognitive behavioural therapies. A newer type of cognitive behavioural therapy, Acceptance and Commitment Therapy (ACT) (40) may be particularly applicable for improving illness acceptance (see Chapter 7). ACT aims to help a person begin to undertake meaningful activity even in the presence of difficult thoughts and feelings that, as described earlier, might arise as a person begins to use assistive devices. ACT involves the application of aspects of mindfulness practice, with a general focus on meta-cognition (i.e. changing the process of thinking as opposed to the content of thoughts). Though as yet untested in the context of ALS, the successful application of ACT may result in an increase in the use of assistive devices—as an individual may require these to undertake personally meaningful activity (41).

One ACT technique that may be particularly applicable to assistive device use, if applied carefully with empathy and compassion, is the Values Compass (42). In this

Table 12.1 The theorized components of illness acceptance

Components of illness acceptance	Description
Cessation of struggle	Choosing to let go of struggles with (i.e. continually worrying about, ruminating on) issues regarding identity, feared outcomes, etc.
Orientation towards values	Shifting focus away from trying to control disease-related experiences and towards finding ways to pursue personally meaningful activity—even with illness
Willingness	An open/accepting stance towards experiencing unpleasant emotions, thoughts and bodily sensations, when doing so enables valued activities

Source: data from *Journal of Health Psychology*, **14**(8), Karademas, E.C., Tsagaraki, A., Lambrou, N., Illness acceptance, hospitalization stress and subjective health in a sample of chronic patients admitted to hospital, pp. 1243–50, Copyright (2009), SAGE Publications (45); *Pain*, **105**(1), McCracken, L.M., Eccleston, C., Coping or acceptance: What to do about chronic pain?, pp. 197–204, Copyright (2003), Wolters Kluwer Health, Inc. (46); *Social Sciences and Medicine*, **56**(2), Risdon, A., Eccleston, C., Crombez, G., McCracken, L., How can we learn to live with pain? A Q-methodological analysis of the diverse understandings of acceptance of chronic pain, pp. 375–86, Copyright (2003), Elsevier (47); *Behaviour Analyst*, **17**(2), Hayes, S.C., Wilson, K.G., Acceptance and commitment therapy: Altering the verbal support for experiential avoidance, pp. 289–303, Copyright (1994), Association for Behavior Analysis International; Graham, C.D., *Explaining and Changing Adverse Illness Perceptions in People with Muscle Disease*, (2012), Institute of Psychiatry, King's College London (48); *Muscle & Nerve*, **52**(1), Graham, C.D., Simmons, Z., Stuart, S.R., Rose, M.R., The potential of psychological interventions to improve quality of life and mood in muscle disorders, pp. 131–6, Copyright (2015), John Wiley and Sons (49).

exercise participants are asked to first consider what is important to them in various aspects of life, for example social relationships, romantic relationships, work (their values). They are then asked to consider, on a scale of 0 to 10, how often they are taking opportunities to act in ways which are consistent with these values. What can then happen is that participants notice a gap between how they want to act (consistently with their values) and how they do act. The final stage is to think about which activities the participant can do to bring their general behaviour more in line with their values. This final step may involve consideration of new assistive devices or of the need to use existing assistive devices more often. To illustrate, a man with considerable communication difficulties may notice that he really values spending time with his children, but that he does not communicate with them much at present. He may then identify that a desire to avoid thoughts associated with changed identity and loss, and feelings of frustration or embarrassment are barriers to the use of AAC devices. Thus, one way to act in a way consistent with his personal values would be to practice engaging with AAC technology, while opening-up to the difficult thoughts and feelings that come along with this (41).

Maintaining control of one's health care

Soundy and Cordon (43), in a review of literature describing the experiences of people with ALS, note that frustration was often generated by potentially well-meaning attempts by health care providers and others to give help when help was not yet needed or wanted. This extends to the provision of assistive devices—as noted by a person with ALS: 'Three of four months ago the occupational therapist was here and I says how do you see this going and she says 'I see a wheelchair'. I said [swears] no way, absolutely no way ...' (36).

Here, it is possible that the health care professional has introduced an assistive device, without first gently assessing the person's (with ALS) possible responses to the introduction of the device, and the consequences of this introduction. Ironically, therefore, the recommendation to use assistive devices that serve the function of increasing independence, may actually challenge autonomy. Indeed, Foley et al. (36) suggest that a desire to maintain control over health care results from the nature of previous losses in ALS. They suggest that loss of control is the central loss in ALS because progressive declines in functioning cannot be stopped. Thus, since health care is something related to their condition where they do, or rather should, have control to make choices, they may strongly value such control.

Opportunities for intervention

Changes in health care provider behaviour may enable service users to have adequate control over health care decisions. For example, ensuring that the person is given time to consider the use of new assistive devices, ensuring informed consent, discussing the pros and cons of each device, giving choices, etc. The following quote, which is from a person with ALS speaking in reference to their medical treatment, suggests that she feels supported to make decisions as suits her purpose: 'Well I'd listen to advice ... But I mean the plan is going ahead ... I mean I've made my plans ...' (36).

Perceived control over health care may be fostered by a high-quality clinician-patient relationship. Foley et al. (36,44) suggest that where patients trusted their health care provider regarding recommendations for assistive devices, they felt more satisfied with the process of adjusting to the use of assistive devices. This is expressed by a person with ALS who had a positive experience of health care—even in the midst of the difficult thoughts and feelings accompanying the initial stages of wheelchair use: '... the wheelchair ... even though I rejected it at the start because I felt I didn't need that kind of thing ... I hid it in the shed ... I just hated the thought of being wheeled in that but I've no bother now ... It's a process to get to that ... I thought that end of it was very professional the way it was left to me and it wasn't forced on me ... I trusted her [the health care professional] then' (37).

Summary and conclusion

Existing evidence suggests that assistive devices perform their function in ALS—they enable personally meaningful activity and independence. Indeed, once these are adopted, they are generally associated with high frequency of use, satisfaction and improved QoL. New assistive technologies are being developed all the time, and many of these are beginning to address salient concerns, such as incongruous accents in AAC devices, and control of social networking and webcam technology.

However, studies also suggest that assistive devices are not without their psycho-social challenges, and in relation to this, adherence and uptake can be affected. In certain cases assistive devices may become tangible symbols of changed identity and loss. Indeed, adherence to, or uptake of, assistive devices may also be affected by acceptance and resignation, social contexts, cognitive impairment, low mood, and a perceived lack of control over health care.

Limited empirical evidence supports the use of interventions to improve the uptake of assistive devices. However, a number of ways to improve uptake and adherence have been suggested, all of which are open to investigation using clinical trial methodology. First, an assessment and subsequent formulation can be used to guide interventions, enabling one to hypothesize the extent to which uptake is affected by an interaction of biopsychosocial factors. Following this one might intervene by, for example, ensuring adequate control over health care decisions, encouraging a focus on valued activity, or facilitating open discussion with the person's family or co-habitants.

References

1. **Pagnini, F.** (2013) Psychological wellbeing and quality of life in amyotrophic lateral sclerosis: A review. *International Journal of Psychology*, **48**(3), 194–205.

2. **Pagnini, F., Simmons, Z., Corbo, M.,** and **Molinari, E.** (2012) Amyotrophic lateral sclerosis: Time for research on psychological intervention? *Amyotrophic Lateral Sclerosis*, **13**(5), 416–17.

3. **Simmons, Z.** (2005) Management strategies for patients with amyotrophic lateral sclerosis from diagnosis through death. *The Neurologist*, **11**(5), 257–70.

4. **Burns, T.M., Graham, C.D., Rose, M.R.,** and **Simmons, Z.** (2012) Quality of life and measures of quality of life in patients with neuromuscular disorders. *Muscle & Nerve*, **46**(1), 9–25.

5. **Gruis, K.L., Wren, P.A.,** and **Huggins, J.E.** (2011) Amyotrophic lateral sclerosis patients' self-reported satisfaction with assistive technology. *Muscle & Nerve*, **43**(5), 643–7.

6. **Simmons, Z.** (2013) Rehabilitation of motor neuron disease. *Handbook of Clinical Neurology*, **110**, 483–98.

7. **Trail, M., Nelson, N., Van, J.N., Appel, S.H.,** and **Lai, E.C.** (2001) Wheelchair use by patients with amyotrophic lateral sclerosis: A survey of user characteristics and selection preferences. *Archives of Physical Medicine and Rehabilitation*, **82**(1), 98–102.

8. **Beukelman, D., Fager, S.,** and **Nordness, A.** (2011) Communication support for people with ALS. *Neurology Research International*, Article ID 714693.

9. **Murphy, J.** (2004) Communication strategies of people with ALS and their partners. *Amyotrophic Lateral Sclerosis and Other Motor Neuron Disorders*, **5**(2), 121–6.

10. **Murphy, J.** (2004) 'I prefer contact this close': perceptions of AAC by people with motor neurone disease and their communication partners. *Augmentative and Alternative Communication*, **20**(4), 259–71.

11. **Felgoise, S.H., Zaccheo, V., Duff, J.,** and **Simmons, Z.** (2016) Verbal communication impacts quality of life in patients with amyotrophic lateral sclerosis. *Amyotrophic Lateral Sclerosis and Frontotemporal Degeneration*, **17**(3–4), 179–83.

12. **Yamagishi, J., Veaux, C., King, S.,** and **Renals, S.** (2012) Speech synthesis technologies for individuals with vocal disabilities: Voice banking and reconstruction. *Acoustical Science and Technology*, **33**(1), 1–5.

13. Trail, M., Nelson, N., Van, J.N., Appel, S.H., and Lai, E.C. (2001) Wheelchair use by patients with amyotrophic lateral sclerosis: A survey of user characteristics and selection preferences. *Archives of Physical Medicine and Rehabilitation*, **82**(1), 98–102.

14. Huggins, J.E., Wren, P.A., and Gruis, K.L. (2011) What would brain–computer interface users want? Opinions and priorities of potential users with amyotrophic lateral sclerosis. *Amyotrophic Lateral Sclerosis*, **12**(5), 318–24.

15. Blain-Moraes, S., Schaff, R., Gruis, K.L., Huggins, J.E., and Wren, P.A. (2012) Barriers to and mediators of brain–computer interface user acceptance: Focus group findings. *Ergonomics*, **55**(5), 516–25.

16. Londral, A., Pinto, A., Pinto, S., Azevedo, L., and de Carvalho, M. (2015) Quality of life in ALS patients and caregivers: Impact of assistive communication from early stages. *Muscle & Nerve*, **52**(6), 933–41.

17. Lancioni, G.E., Simone, I.L., De Caro, M.F., et al. (2015) Assisting persons with advanced amyotrophic lateral sclerosis in their leisure engagement and communication needs with a basic technology-aided program. *NeuroRehabilitation*, **36**(3), 355–65.

18. Lancioni, G.E., Singh, N.N., O'Reilly, M.F., et al. (2012) Technology-aided programs for assisting communication and leisure engagement of persons with amyotrophic lateral sclerosis: Two single-case studies. *Research in developmental Disabilities*, **33**(5), 1605–14.

19. Lancioni, G.E., Singh, N.N., O'Reilly, M.F., et al. (2014) A voice-sensitive microswitch for a man with amyotrophic lateral sclerosis and pervasive motor impairment. *Disability and Rehabilitation: Assistive Technology*, **9**(3), 260–3.

20. Sellers, E.W., Vaughan, T.M., and Wolpaw, J.R. (2010) A brain–computer interface for long-term independent home use. *Amyotrophic Lateral Sclerosis*, **11**(5), 449–55.

21. Calvo, A., Chiò, A., Castellina, E., et al. (2008) Eye tracking impact on quality-of-life of ALS patients. In: Miesenberger, K., Klaus, J., Zagler, W., and Karshmer, A. (eds) *Computers Helping People with Special Needs*, 11th Proceedings of an International Conference, ICCHP 2008, Linz, Austria, July 9–11, pp. 70–7. Berlin: Springer.

22. Fullam, T., Stephens, H.E., Felgoise, S.H., Blessinger, J.K., Walsh, S., and Simmons, Z. (2015) Compliance with recommendations made in a multidisciplinary ALS clinic. *Amyotrophic Lateral Sclerosis and Frontotemporal Degeneration*, **17**(1–2), 30–7.

23. Kardas, P., Lewek, P., and Matyjaszczyk, M. (2013) Determinants of patient adherence: a review of systematic reviews. *Frontiers in Pharmacology*, **4**, 91.

24. Abrahams, S. (2013) ALS, cognition and the clinic. *Amyotrophic Lateral Sclerosis and Frontotemporal Degeneration*, **14**(1), 3–5.

25. Phukan, J., Pender, N.P., and Hardiman, O. (2007) Cognitive impairment in amyotrophic lateral sclerosis. *Lancet Neurology*, **6**(11), 994–1003.

26. Radakovic, R. and Abrahams, S. (2014) Developing a new apathy measurement scale: dimensional apathy scale. *Psychiatry Research*, **219**(3), 658–63.

27. Geronimo, A., Stephens, H.E., Schiff, S.J., and Simmons, Z. (2013) Acceptance of brain-computer interfaces in amyotrophic lateral sclerosis. *Amyotrophic Lateral Sclerosis and Frontotemporal Degeneration*, **16**(3–4), 258–64.

28. Geronimo, A., Simmons, Z., and Schiff, S.J. (2016) Performance predictors of brain-computer interfaces in patients with amyotrophic lateral sclerosis. *Journal of Neural Engineering*, **13**(2), 026002.

29. Thakore, N.J. and Pioro, E.P. (2016) Depression in ALS in a large self-reporting cohort. *Neurology*, **86**(11), 1031–8.

30. **Gonzalez, J.S., Batchelder, A.W., Psaros, C.,** and **Safren, S.A.** (2011) Depression and HIV/AIDS treatment nonadherence: A review and meta-analysis. *Journal of Acquired Immune Deficiency Syndromes (1999)*, **58**(2), 10.

31. **Dawson, D.** and **Moghaddam, N.** (2015) *Formulation in Action: Applying Psychological Theory to Clinical Practice*. Berlin: Walter de Gruyter.

32. **Abrahams, S., Newton, J., Niven, E., Foley, J.,** and **Bak, T.H.** (2014) Screening for cognition and behaviour changes in ALS. *Amyotrophic Lateral Sclerosis & Frontotemporal Degeneration*, **15**(1–2), 9–14.

33. **Wilson, B.A., Gracey, F.,** and **Evans, J.J.** (2009) *Neuropsychological Rehabilitation: Theory, Models, Therapy and Outcome*. Cambridge: Cambridge University Press.

34. **Kroenke, K., Spitzer, R.L.,** and **Williams, J.B.W.** (2001) The PHQ-9: Validity of a brief depression severity measure. *Journal of General Internal Medicine*, **16**(9), 606–13.

35. **Spitzer, R.L., Kroenke, K., Williams, J.B.,** and **Lowe, B.** (2006) A brief measure for assessing generalized anxiety disorder: The GAD-7. *Archives of Internal Medicine*, **166**(10), 1092–7.

36. **Foley, G., Timonen, V.,** and **Hardiman, O.** (2014) Exerting control and adapting to loss in amyotrophic lateral sclerosis. *Social Science & Medicine*, **101**, 113–19.

37. **Foley, G., Timonen, V.,** and **Hardiman, O.** (2014) Understanding psycho-social processes underpinning engagement with services in motor neurone disease: A qualitative study. *Palliative Medicine*, **28**(4), 318–25.

38. **Foley, G., Timonen, V.,** and **Hardiman, O.** (2016) 'I hate being a burden': The patient perspective on carer burden in amyotrophic lateral sclerosis. *Amyotrophic Lateral Sclerosis and Frontotemporal Degeneration*, **17**(5–6), 351–7.

39. **Pavey, A., Warren, N.,** and **Allen-Collinson, J.** (2015) 'It gives me my freedom': Technology and responding to bodily limitations in motor neuron disease. *Medical Anthropology*, **34**(5), 442–55.

40. **Graham, C.D., Gouick, J., Krahé, C.,** and **Gillanders, D.** (2016) A systematic review of the use of Acceptance and Commitment Therapy (ACT) in chronic disease and long-term conditions. *Clinical Psychology Review*, **46**, 46–58.

41. **Graham, C.D., Simmons, Z., Stuart, S.R.,** and **Rose, M.R.** (2015) The potential of psychological interventions to improve quality of life and mood in muscle disorders. *Muscle & Nerve*, **52**(1), 131–6.

42. **Harris, R.** (2009) *ACT Made Simple: An Easy-to-read Primer on Acceptance and Commitment Therapy*. Oakland, CA: New Harbinger Publications.

43. **Soundy, A.** and **Condon, N.** (2015) Patients experiences of maintaining mental well-being and hope within motor neurone disease: A thematic synthesis. *Frontiers in Psychology*, **6** (online).

44. **Foley, G., Timonen, V., Hardiman, O.** (2012) Patients' perceptions of services and preferences for care in amyotrophic lateral sclerosis: a review. *Amyotrophic Lateral Sclerosis*, **13**(1), 11–24.

45. **Karademas, E.C., Tsagaraki, A.,** and **Lambrou, N.** (2009) Illness acceptance, hospitalization stress and subjective health in a sample of chronic patients admitted to hospital. *Journal of Health Psychology*, **14**(8), 1243–50.

46. **McCracken, L.M.** and **Eccleston, C.** (2003) Coping or acceptance: What to do about chronic pain? *Pain*, **105**(1), 197–204.

47. **Risdon, A., Eccleston, C., Crombez, G.,** and **McCracken, L.** (2003) How can we learn to live with pain? A Q-methodological analysis of the diverse understandings of acceptance of chronic pain. *Social Science & Medicine,* **56**(2), 375–86.

48. **Hayes, S.C.** and **Wilson, K.G.** (1994) Acceptance and commitment therapy: Altering the verbal support for experiential avoidance. *Behavior Analyst,* **17**, 289–303.

49. **Graham, C.D.** (2012) Explaining and Changing Adverse Illness Perceptions in People with Muscle Disease. London: Institute of Psychiatry, King's College London.

Chapter 13

End of life: Wishes, values and symptoms, and their impact on quality of life and well-being

David Oliver

Introduction

The aim of all care for all ALS patients, and their families, should be to maintain and maximize the quality of life (QoL) throughout the disease progression. Thus palliative care should be considered from the time of diagnosis, as palliative care is:

> 'An approach that improves the quality of life of patients and their families facing problems associated with life-threatening illness, through the prevention and relief of suffering, early identification and impeccable assessment and treatment of pain and other problems, physical, psychosocial and spiritual' (1)

The consideration of this holistic approach is essential if the QoL of the patient is to be maximized. Moreover from the time of diagnosis many patients and families fear the deterioration and progression of the disease and fear distress as death approaches. This has been accentuated by many media reports, particularly as a person with ALS is often discussed when euthanasia and assisted dying are being advocated, with particular focus on the fear and distress of death from ALS—although research has shown that death is usually peaceful (2,3).

The support of the patient and family relies on careful assessment and listening to the person's fears and concerns. These may be varied and are often multiple:

- Physical issues—such as breathing problems, pain, distress.
- Psychological issues—the concerns about the disease, of dependency, of dying and death.
- Social aspects—most patients are part of wider families and they fear how their family will cope, in the same way as the family are concerned as to how their loved one will be and how they will cope. This may be seen particularly when there is a known genetic influence on ALS—in familial cases, up to 70% (4) may now know the possible gene mutation and this could then be found in the children and other family members, with the potential for distress and many implications for future life planning.
- Spiritual—the existential aspects of coping with a progressive disease, which may encompass religious beliefs or the deeper thoughts and concerns about life.

All these aspects need to be considered and will change as the person with ALS faces the deterioration caused by the disease, and the concomitant losses in their abilities and changes in lifestyle. Many of these issues may be easier to discuss early in the disease progression, when communication and cognition are less likely to be affected. Many patients with ALS face loss of communication due to speech loss, or at best the communication may be more limited using augmentative communication aids, such as computer systems or eye operated systems (Eye gaze) (5). There is also increasing awareness of the risk of cognitive change with 10–15% of ALS patients developing fronto-temporal dementia and a further 30–40% showing evidence of cognitive change—often frontal lobe changes affecting executive / decision making processes (6).

Thus there is the need to help patients and families discuss their wishes and views about the care they would like to receive at the end of life early in the disease progression, when it is easier and more effective, even though they may find these discussions difficult. There may be a fine balance in allowing these discussions and ensuring that any distress is kept to the minimum. These discussions are complex, but can be so helpful if the person later does lose communication or the ability to make decisions for themselves.

Advance care planning

The aim of advance care planning (ACP) is to ascertain the views and thoughts of patients while they can make these clear so that if they lose the ability to make decisions later—from loss of communication or cognitive change leading to loss of capacity to make decisions—these views are known and can be used to aid decision making, particularly at the end of life (7).

ACP has been defined as:

> 'a voluntary process of discussion and review to help an individual who has capacity to anticipate how their condition may affect them in the future and, if they wish, set on record choices or decisions relating to their care and treatment so that these can be referred to by their carers (whether professional or family carers) in the event that they lose capacity to decide once their illness progresses.' (8)

There are several forms that ACP may take:

- Ascertainment of the person's overall views on life and their feelings about QoL. The Patient Preference Questionnaire (9) has been suggested to allow some of these issues to be known. This includes views on how much information they would wish, family members who could or could not be involved in discussions, people they would like to be present when making decisions, any particular preferences on care or treatment and their views on how decisions could be made—by themselves, including others or leaving this to the doctor and caring team. This was appreciated by all involved—patients, families, and professionals (9).

- An advance statement / Living Will—this may be a general statement about the views on future treatment and management. This may not be specific to ALS and is usually not legally binding, but should be taken into account by anyone making decisions in the best interests of the patient, in conjunction with discussions with family and others who know the patient.

- Advance directive (AD)—this may be specific, such as defining certain treatments that the person does not wish to have—for instance stating that they do not wish to receive cardiopulmonary resuscitation, a tracheostomy for ventilation, or a gastrostomy. If this has been completed correctly the AD may be legally binding and should be adhered to by the caring team.

- Power of attorney—this allows a person to nominate an attorney who would make decisions on their behalf, if they were no longer able to do so. Thus if there is a decision to be made the professionals can ask the attorney for their view and this would be adhered to in the same way that the person's own decision would be adhered to. Power of attorney may be for medical decisions or for social care—such as financial aspects or housing—and again if the person has lost capacity to make the decision the attorney can make this for them.

- Physical Orders for Life-Sustaining Treatment (POLST)—is a form completed by a doctor based on conversations with the patient, and gives specific treatment orders for cardiopulmonary resuscitation, medical interventions, artificial nutrition, and the use of antibiotics (10). The aim is to facilitate discussion on the various treatment options and record these clearly so that any professional involved is aware of these earlier discussion and the views of the patient.

- DNACPR—Do No Attempt Cardiopulmonary Resuscitation (also known as DNR or Do Not Resuscitate)—may be discussed and a form completed so that this is not attempted at the end of life. These discussions may be initiated from the patient or family or from the professional team. Again this allows all to know the person's wishes and act accordingly.

For patients with ALS there is a particular need to consider ACP as there are several major interventions that may be considered during the disease progression—gastrostomy, non-invasive ventilation, tracheostomy ventilation, other active treatment at the end of life—which may need decisions urgently due to the sudden deterioration and distress of the patient. For instance if there has been no discussion and the patient appears for emergency care with severe breathlessness and evidence of respiratory failure the use of tracheostomy ventilation may be considered, even though this may not be the wish of the patient. If there has been earlier discussion these wishes can be known in an ACP and the professionals involved can act more appropriately in accordance with the person's views and wishes. In countries where there is no legally accepted ACP patients may receive treatment they did not wish, and it was found that in an emergency situation a tracheostomy was sometimes arranged even though the person did not wish this (11).

There are many differences in how ACP is viewed in different countries. In some, for instance the USA and UK, it is possible to make a legally binding AD and expect that this will be respected (7). In many countries ACP may have no legal standing, although the expression and recording of a patient's wishes would normally be taken into consideration when decisions are made and the person is unable to be involved (11,12).

In all ACP it is important to stress that if the person is able to make a decision they would be asked and their view would be taken—ACP only is applicable if the person has lost the ability to make the decision. This ability to have the individual's views known can be very important in maintaining QoL as the person feels that they have maintained control, even when their illness progresses to that point that they are no longer able to make decisions themselves. Many people would feel that this is very important for them.

The discussion of ACP may be complex, as patients, their families, and professionals may have differing reasons to be reluctant to discuss these areas. Patients may wish to 'maintain hope' and find it difficult to face the future and discuss the issues of deterioration and dying. Moreover there may be 'magical thinking' where the person worries that talking about dying may lead to it happening very soon. They may also fear causing distress to their families. Families may also find discussion difficult as they have to face the issues of the future and they may be particularly worried about upsetting the patient. Professionals are also concerned about causing distress and loss of hope for the patient, and neurologists admit that talking about ALS and ACP are very difficult issues, for which they have had little training (13).

Careful discussion, with full information, is necessary so that all can be aware of the issues and the importance of ensuring that someone's views and wishes are known. This may be seen as 'hoping for the best, but planning for the worst'. For instance it may be important to discuss what may occur if there is limited or no discussion—studies have shown that ALS patients often undergo tracheostomy when there is no ACP and this may be without informed consent, as in the emergency situation when action is taken to support life (11,14).

The completion of ACP may be difficult, but often it gives the patient a sense of control over the future and can allow them to get on with living. This may help to maintain their QoL. However, for some people the discussion is very stressful and can be a negative experience. The approach needs to be individualized, with the provision of information about the positive and negative aspects. Moreover it is important to show that the AD can be changed, if the person still has capacity, and studies have shown that people do change their decision—in one study eight out of 26 people with ALS changed their decision on life sustaining measures over a 6 month period (15).

The decisions recorded in any ACP must be from the patient with ALS. However, the instigation of this process may be from the patient, their family or the professional team. Patients seem to want to start these discussions earlier, but they do feel that it should be the doctor who starts the discussion (16). There are times when this discussion may be particularly pertinent—at the diagnosis, during discussion of gastrostomy and when ventilatory support is discussed. In the UK the National Institute for Health and Care Excellence (NICE) has recommended that discussion of the future, including end of life issues and ACP, should start when respiratory function is monitored and certainly when non-invasive ventilation is being discussed and commenced (17). It is important to have these discussions earlier, as explained above, rather than waiting for an emergency, when there may be insufficient time to discuss carefully, or at the end of life, when the patient may find the discussion very tiring or difficult, due to communication issues.

The views of the professional do seem to alter how these discussions may take place. Although professionals may talk of supporting the autonomy of the person in decision making—ensuring that the person is able to make an informed preference or consent to whatever they do or what is done to them—they may find it difficult to accept patient and family decisions to refuse treatment (18). In Japan it was found that doctors would not wish tracheostomy if they had ALS, but they were suggesting this option to their patients (19,20). These issues need to be discussed more widely and the education of neurologists and other team members may allow a greater awareness of the issues (21, 22).

There is a need for the ACP to be specific if it is to be really applicable at the end of life. This may be easier for ALS patients as the issues that may be faced are relatively uniform—respiratory failure, swallowing difficulties, secretions, and death from respiratory failure (23). The use of specific ALS ADs may be useful as they will avoid any ambiguity as they should relate to specific issues seen in ALS (23). The use of online computer based systems has also been suggested, as this allows patients and families to complete these at their own pace and they encourage further discussion with professionals (24,25). This may avoid the difficulty of initiation of the discussion, with a computer seen as more objective, thus easing the consideration of the issues and allowing the patient more control over their actions.

Although there is little evidence that ACP leads to specific benefits, there does seem to be the benefit of facilitating discussion and allowing the views of the patient to be known. The patients completing the computer generated AD did feel more in control and were positive about the interaction with the computer programme, which completed a disease specific AD for them (25). This would seem to be supportive to all concerned and allow the person to feel more in control and that their views will be heard, even if they cannot express them themselves.

Respiratory interventions

As ALS progresses there will usually be increasing weakness of the respiratory muscles and diaphragm, leading to respiratory failure. This is the commonest cause of death (26) and there is increasing use of ventilatory support to reduce both the symptoms of respiratory failure—poor sleep, breathlessness, morning headache, daytime sleepiness, anorexia, fatigue, depression, personality change—as well as increasing length of life.

Non-invasive ventilation (NIV) has been shown to improve symptoms, improve QoL and extend life, in one RCT, by 11 months (27). However, although the symptoms of respiratory failure are eased the disease continue to progress and there is increased muscle weakness and increased disability. Initially NIV may be needed only at night, but as the respiratory muscle weakness progresses there may be increasing use, and this may cause distress to the patient and they may become totally dependent on NIV (28). The patient may become 'locked in' with very limited, or even no means of, communication.

These issues need to be discussed before the NIV is commenced and the NICE Guidelines on MND / ALS suggest that these issues should be discussed when monitoring respiratory function, when considering NIV, when starting NIV and throughout the use of NIV (17). This may allow the completion of ACP so that the patient can feel that their wishes are clear, including the time when they would wish to stop NIV, even though this could lead to their death. In many jurisdictions the stopping of NIV at the request of a patient with capacity is clear both ethically and legally and if there is a clear and specific AD the NIV could be stopped when the conditions set by the patient are reached, even if they have lost capacity (28). However, in many countries there may be a lack of clarity and in some, such as Japan, withdrawal of treatment may not be possible.

Although there is clarity regarding the legality and ethical nature of stopping NIV in many countries, the actual procedure can be very difficult for all involved. On a scale of 0 (not at all challenging) to 10 (very challenging), experienced Palliative Medicine physicians rated the discussions about withdrawal of NIV as 5.81/10 for practical issues, 6.22 /10 for emotional issues, and 5.08/10 for ethical issues, with more than half providing a score of greater than 7/10 for these discussions (29). As the patient may be dependent of NIV the withdrawal may cause severe symptoms of respiratory distress and anxiety. Therefore it is usually necessary to provide medication to prevent these symptoms before withdrawal, to ensure symptoms are managed. This may seem like assisting dying, although ethically it is seen as providing symptom management in anticipation of distress and that any doubt about the use of medication is covered under the doctrine of 'double effect'—the aim of the treatment is to minimize distress and not to cause death (7). As a result there has been further discussion and the production of guidelines in the UK (28) with the aim of supporting the professionals involved in these discussions and also providing the possibility of a mentor to support the professionals involved.

There is a variability across countries and cultures as to the acceptability of withdrawal of treatment. In some countries this is not legal and thus there is an even greater need to ensure that patients realize the implications of starting treatment, so that they can make an informed decision. There are implications for both patients and families with studies showing that the stresses for families can be great, and the effect of reduced QoL greater for family carers than the disabled patient (14).

Although NIV is widely used the use of invasive ventilation with a tracheostomy is more limited, but varies from country to country. In some cultures tracheostomy is common, for instance in Japan about 33% of all people with ALS have a tracheostomy and many survive for many years, even decades (30). However, many of these patients become more dependent and may lose the ability to communicate and up to 15–20% may become 'locked in' without any form of communication (31). This obviously has many implications for QoL and psychological issues for both patient and family. Moreover in many areas, such as Japan and Italy, the withdrawal of invasive ventilation is not legally possible.

The discussion regarding starting tracheostomy is more complex, as there are issues of prolongation of life, the extra stress on family and carers and the need to discuss possible later withdrawal. There is evidence that family members find tracheostomy particularly stressful and one study showed that 30% of carers rated their QoL lower than very disabled patients with tracheostomy and mechanical ventilation (14). These issues may need to be emphasized to all involved, although there is evidence that some patients do lack empathy and may not see this as an issue (6). If patients are to maintain their QoL they will need support—both physically and emotionally—to cope with the transition to tracheostomy. They may feel better physically as the issues of ventilation are relieved and any problems with coping with secretions, such as feelings of choking at times, will also lessen (28). However, the fears of dependency and increasing disease progression may cause added psychological concerns.

It is important to discuss ACP when a tracheostomy is being considered, as there is a greater likelihood that with disease progression the patient may lose capacity and / or communication ability to make decisions later. Their views as to further action is very helpful—such as their views on the use of antibiotics for infections if the disease has progressed, cardiopulmonary resuscitation, whether they would want active treatment if there were problems with the tracheostomy, and how they feel about withdrawal of ventilation. These could be recorded in a specific ALS AD (23) and the patient reassured that their wishes are known and would be adhered to.

Although ventilatory support may improve symptoms and QoL, at least initially, there are longer term issues. Patients with tracheostomy and mechanical ventilation have been found to rate their QoL similarly to ALS patients without ventilator support, despite their greater disability and dependency (32). Careful discussion throughout the disease is important so that any fears or concerns of the patient and /or family can be addressed. There may also be issues within the wider multidisciplinary team, as there are often different views across the team on the ethics of the use and withdrawal of these measures. For instance in a study of Palliative Medicine senior doctors, several spoke of the difficulties of managing conflicts within the multidisciplinary team and the need for recurrent discussions and explanations of the ethical aspects of care for these patients (29). Awareness of these team issues is also important if the care offered to the patient and family is to be as effective and supportive as possible (33).

End of life issues in ALS

The diagnosis of ALS is unknown to many people when they are first diagnosed. This may lead to apprehension about the disease and this can be worsened when they look at some of the media writings of ALS, There is often discussion of how 'distressing' ALS is and of 'choking to death' and there are concerns about how the disease will progress and how the person may die. At the same time there is also much written about some personalities with ALS, such as Professor Stephen Hawking, and the discussion of his survival for more than 40 years, which may give unrealistic optimism to patients.

The issues of the future need to be openly discussed—at the request of the patients and / or family and when there are certain management decisions made—such as gastrostomy or ventilatory support (14). Explanation of the probable progression of the disease may be helpful, emphasizing the individuality of every patient and that the possible issues to be faced are what *may* happen and are not necessarily what *will* happen for every individual. This discussion is difficult as some patients feel that they should know all information whereas others may be upset at being given information, which they feel is distressing.

There is the need to ascertain how people want to be told of their diagnosis and its progression. A Patient Preference Questionnaire (9) can be useful in allowing the person's preferences to be discussed. There is also evidence that some people with ALS want to know all information, others prefer to have information given to family or close carers, who then will moderate the information for them and some do not want any information (34). Many families may be concerned that discussion of end of life issues may be distressing for the patient, but this may reflect their own anxieties and reluctance to discuss these issues. If the patient has capacity to make a decision, their views are paramount, and the responsibility of the professional is to the patient, taking into consideration the views of families. These issues can cause professionals to be reluctant to start such discussions, but if the patient's needs are to be addressed and their psychological wellbeing maintained it is important to take on these discussions.

Many patients and families fear the end of life, as they have read or heard of a 'distressing death'. However, several studies have shown that distress is rare –a study of the first 100 patients with ALS at St Christopher's' hospice showed that distress was rare at the end of life and symptoms were managed effectively (35); a later study there of 124 patients again showed that distress was rare and one patient was suspected of choking to death, but a post mortem showed no airway obstruction and the cause of death was a myocardial infarction (2); in a UK and German study of 121 patients none died choking and 98% were reported as dying peacefully (3). Thus with good palliative care distress is rare and is certainly no greater than experienced with other patient groups. However, there are still fears and many of the people with ALS requesting assisted dying are fearful of the future and may choose to die before they face the last stages of life (36)—see Chapter 14 on Assisted Dying.

It is important to ensure that the issues are brought out into the open and patients given the opportunity to talk of their fears. This is often facilitated by the involvement of hospice or specialist palliative care services. These vary from country to country, but all aim to facilitate open discussion and the holistic assessment of the patient and family. Often the care can be continued at home—where many people wish to be—but admission to a hospice or specialist palliative care unit may be necessary if the care needs are too great for the family / carers to manage at home. If possible the decision should be made in a controlled way, without the pressure of a crisis or emergency situation. If discussion has not occurred a crisis may be reached and admission to emergency service occurs, without full consideration of the wishes of the patient and family. If there is the possibility of forward planning the crisis can be anticipated and extra care provided at home (17) and thus allowing care to continue at home.

The recognition of the end of life phase is important to allow the patient, family, and professionals to be prepared. It has been suggested that triggers to consider as indicating the end of life phase for all progressive neurological disease include swallowing problems, recurring infection, marked decline in functional status, first episode of aspiration pneumonia, cognitive difficulties, weight loss, and significant complex symptoms and for ALS in particular include breathlessness / respiratory failure, swallowing issues, cognitive change, and weakness (37). These triggers have been found to increase as death approaches in a retrospective study and further studies are being undertaken (38). This recognition is important so that preparations can be made:

- Discussion of the place of care and place of death—these may be different and need to be differentiated (39).
- Consideration of the completion of a DNACPR order.

- Provision of anticipatory medication—this may include morphine for pain / dyspnoea, midazolam for agitation / distress and an anticholinergic, such as glycopyrronium bromide, for chest secretions—as suggested in the UK MND Association's 'Just in case' kit (40). These medications are then readily available if the patient does become distressed and can be given by a visiting nurse or doctor without delay. Moreover before they are arranged this is an opportunity for discussion about what may happen at the end of life and ways of managing an episode of pain, breathlessness, or distress (40).
- Ensuring equipment is available to allow care at home—including an adjustable bed, hoist, or syringe driver for the administration of parenteral medication subcutaneously (17).
- Providing extra care if required, so that family members can be with the patient without having to continuously provide personal care (17).

The discussion and provision of these aspects of care can be reassuring to patient and family, as they show that the professionals are aware of the issues and are ensuring that any problems can be managed effectively.

Although the main aim of care should be of the person with ALS it is important to support the psychological, social, and spiritual concerns of the family / close carers (41, 42). They may need to be assessed separately from the patient, so that they are able to express their concerns and fears without being anxious of upsetting the patient. This care may need to be continued after death in bereavement, as carers who have been involved in close and personal care for a long period of time as the disease progresses may often have the need to express their feelings and concerns. Often they may feel ambivalent—feeling relieved that the caring has ended and the person is no longer 'suffering', but at the same time shocked that they should have such a reaction when their loved one has died (41).

The support of carers may be important for the professional caring team. Team members may have been involved in care for long periods of time and feel the loss following the death. This may be particularly true if there have been complex issues during the final days or weeks, such as severe cognitive change, feeding or swallowing problems, ventilator withdrawal, or a sudden death. An opportunity for team members to discuss the issues may be very helpful, so that they are able to return to their roles in the future (33).

Conclusion

The care of a patient with ALS at the end of life is often complex and challenging, but the aim of healthcare professionals should be to ensure that patients maintain their autonomy and QoL as much as possible, and are cared for as they would wish, whilst also supporting family and carers—both informal and professional. These latter individuals may face increasing burden of care, and often a poorer QoL. The challenge is to enable both the person with ALS and that person's family and carers to maintain as good QoL as possible, so that they may derive maximal benefit from their time together.

References

1. **World Health Organization**. (2002). Palliative care. Available at: www.who.int/cancer/palliative/definition/en/ (accessed 23 March 2017).

2. **O'Brien, T., Kelly, M.**, and **Saunders, C.** (1992) Motor neurone disease: A hospice perspective. *British Medical Journal*, **304**(6825), 471–3.

3. **Neudert, C., Oliver, D., Wasner, M.**, and **Borasio, G.D.** (2001) The course of the terminal phase in patients with amyotrophic lateral sclerosis. *Journal of Neurology*, **248**, 612–16.

4. **Renton, A.E., Chio, A.**, and **Traynor, B.J.** (2013) State of play in amyotrophic lateral sclerosis genetics. *Nature Neuroscience*, **17**, 17–23.

5. **Scott, A.** and **McPhee, M.** (2014) Multidiscplinary care: speech and language therapy. In: Oliver, D., Borasio, G.D., and Johnston, W. (eds) *Palliative Care in Amyotrophic Lateral Sclerosis—From Diagnosis to Bereavement*, 3rd edn, pp. 215–32. Oxford: Oxford University Press.

6. **Goldstein, L.H.** (2014) Control of symptoms: Cognitive dysfunction. In: Oliver, D., Borasio, G., and Johnston, W. (eds) *Palliative Care in Amyotrophic Lateral Sclerosis- From Diagnosis to Bereavement*, 3rd edn, pp. 107–25. Oxford. Oxford University Press.

7. **Chapman, S.** (2012) Advance care planning. In: Oliver, D. (ed.) *End of Life Care in Neurological Disease*, pp. 132–42. London: Springer.

8. **National End of Life Programme**. (2011) *Capacity, Care Planning and Advance Care Planning in Life Limiting Illness: a Guide for Health and Social Care Staff.* London: National End of Life Care programme.

9. **Murtagh, F.E.M.** and **Thorns, A.** (2006) Evaluation and ethical review of a tool to explore patient preferences for information and involvement in decision making. *Journal of Medical Ethics*, **32**, 311–15.

10. **Physical Orders for Life-Sustaining Treatment**. (2017) POLST and Advance Care Planning. Available at: http://polst.org/polst-advance-care-planning/.—(accessed 23 March 2017).

11. **Veronese, S., Valle, A., Chio, A., Calvo, A.**, and **Oliver, D.** (2014) The last months of life of people with amyotrophic lateral sclerosis in mechanical invasive ventilation: A qualitative study. *Amyotrophic Lateral Sclerosis and Frontotemporal Degeneration*, **15**, 499–504.

12. **Tsoh, J., Peisah, C., Narumoto, J.**, and **Wongpakaran, N.** (2015) Comparisons of guardianship laws and surrogate decision-making practices in China, Japan, Thailand and Australia: A review by the Asia Consortium, International Psychogeriatric Association (IPA) capacity taskforce. *International Psychogeriatrics*, **27** 1029–37.

13. **Creutzfelt, C.J., Robinson, M.T.**, and **Holloway, R.G.** (2016) Neurologists as primary palliative care providers. Communication and practice approaches. *Neurology Clinical Practice*, **6**, 1–9.

14. **Kaub-Wittemer, D., von Steinbuchel, N., Wasner, M., Laier-Groeneveld, G.**, and **Borasio, G.D.** (2003) Quality of life and psychosocial issues in ventilated patients with amyotrophic lateral sclerosis and their caregivers. *Journal of Pain and Symptom Management*, **26**, 890–6.

15. **Silverstein, M.D., Stocking, C.B., Antel, J.P., Beckwith, J., Roos, R.P.**, and **Siegler, M.** (1991) Amyotrophic lateral sclerosis and life-sustaining therapy: patients' desires for information, participation in decision making, and life sustaining treatment. *Mayo Clinic Proceedings*, **66**, 906–13.

16. **Johnston, S.C., Pfeifer, M.P., McNutt, R.**, et al (1995) The discussion about advance directives: Patient and physician opinions regarding when and how it should be conducted. *Archives of International Medicine*, **155**, 1025–30.

17. **National Institute for Health and Care Excellence**. (2016) *Motor Neurone Disease: Assessment and Management*, NICE Guideline NG42. www.nice.org.uk/guidance/NG42 (accessed 26 July 2017).

18. **Connolly, S., Galvin, M.,** and **Hardiman, O.** (2015) End–of-life management in patients with amyotrophic lateral sclerosis. *Lancet Neurology*, **14**, 435–42.

19. **Rabkin, J., Ogino, M., Goetz, R.,** et al. (2014) Japanese and American ALS patient preferences regarding TIV(tracheostomy with invasive ventilation): A cross-national survey. *Amyotrophic Lateral Sclerosis and Frontotemporal Degeneration*, **15**, 185–91.

20. **Veronese, S., Gallo, G., Valle, A.,** et al. (2017) Specialist palliative care improves the quality of life in advanced neurodegenerative disorders: Ne-PAL, a pilot randomized controlled study. *BMJ Supportive and Palliative Care*, **7**, 164–72.

21. **Carver, A.C., Vickrey, B.G, Bernat, J.L.,**et al. (1999) End-of-life care: A survey of US neurologists' attitudes, behavior and knowledge. *Neurology*, **53**(2), p. 284–93.

22. **Oliver, D., Borasio, G.D., Caraceni, A.,** et al. (2015) Consensus review on the development of palliative care for patients with chronic and progressive neurological disease. *European Journal of Neurology*, **23**(1), 30–8.

23. **Benditt, J.O., Smith, T.S.,** and **Tonelli, M.R.** (2001) Empowering the individual with ALS at the end-of-life: disease-specific advance care planning. *Muscle & Nerve*, **24**, 1706–9.

24. **Hossler, C., Levi, B.H., Simmons, Z.,** and **Green, M.J.** (2011) Advance care planning for patients with ALS: feasibility of an interactive computer program. *Amyotrophic Lateral Sclerosis*, **12**, 172–7.

25. **Levi, B.H., Simmons, Z., Hanna, C.,** et al. (2017) Advance care planning for patients with amyotrophic lateral sclerosis. *Amyotrophic Lateral Sclerosis and Frontotemporal Degeneration*. Available at: http://www.tandfonline.com/doi/full/10.1080/21678421.2017.1285317 (accessed 26 July 2017).

26. **Gelinas D.** (2014) Respiratory complications. In: **Oliver, D., Borasio, G., & Johnston W.** (eds) *Palliative Care in Amyotrophic Lateral Sclerosis: From Diagnosis to Bereavement*, 3rd edn, pp. 65–90. Oxford: Oxford University Press.

27. **Bourke, S.C., Tomlinson, M., Williams, T.L., Bullock, R.E., Shaw, P.J.,** and **Gibson, G.J.** (2006) Effects of non-invasive ventilation on survival and quality of life in patients with amyotrophic lateral sclerosis: a randomised controlled trial. *Lancet Neurology*, **5**, 140–7.

28. **Association for Palliative Medicine.** (2015) *Withdrawal of Assisted Ventilation at the Request of a Patient with Motor Neurone Disease: Guidance for Professionals.* Fareham: Association for Palliative Medicine of Great Britain and Ireland.

29. **Faull, C., Rowe Haynes, C.,** and **Oliver, D.** (2014) Issues for palliative medicine doctors surrounding the withdrawal of non-invasive ventilation at the request of a patient with motor neurone disease: a scoping study. *BMJ Supportive and Palliative Care*, **4**, 43–9.

30. **Rabkin, J., Ogino, M., Goetz, R.,** et al. (2013) Tracheostomy with invasive ventilation for ALS patients: Neurologists' roles in the US and Japan. *Amyotrophic Lateral Sclerosis and Frontotemporal Degeneration*, **14**, 116–23.

31. **Hayashi, H.** and **Oppenheimer, E.A.** (2003) ALS patients on TPPV. Totally locked-in satte, eurologic findings and ethical implications. *Neurology*, **61**, 135–7.

32. **Vianello, A., Acaro, G.,** and **Palmieri. A.** et al. (2011) Survival and quality of life after tracheostomy for acute repiratory failure in patients with amyotrophic lateral sclerosis. *Journal of Critical Care*, **26**(3), p329.e7–e14.

33. **Oliver, D.** and **Watson, S.** (2012) Multidisciplinary Care. In: Oliver, D. (ed.) *End of Life Care in Neurological Disease*, pp. 113–27. London: Springer.

34. **O'Brien, M.R.** (2004) Information-seeking behaviour among people with motor neurone disease. *British Journal of Nursing,* **13**, 964–68.

35. **Saunders, C., Walsh, T.D.,** and **Smith, S.** (1981) Hospice care in motor neurone disease. In: Saunders, C., Summers, D.H., and Teller, N. (eds) *Hospice: The Living Idea,* pp 126–55. London: Edward Arnold.

36. **Maessen, M., Veldink, J.H., Onwuteaka-Philipsen, B.D.,** et al. (2014) Euthanasia and physician assisted suicide in amyotrophic lateral sclerosis: A prospective study. *Journal of Neurology,* **261,** 1894–901.

37. **National End of Life Care Programme** (2010) End of life care in long term neurological conditions: A framework for implementation. London: National End of Life Care Programme. Available at: https://www.mssociety.org.uk/sites/default/files/Documents/ Professionals/End%20life%20care%20long%20term%20neuro%20conditions.pdf

38. **Hussain, J., Adams, D., Allgar, V.,** and **Campbell, C.** (2014) Triggers in advanced neurological conditions: prediction and management of the terminal phase. *BMJ Supportive and Palliative Care,* **4,** 30–7

39. **Agar, M., Currow, D.C., Shelby-James, T.M., Sanderson, C.,** and **Abernethy, A.P.** (2008) Preference for place of care and place of death in palliative care: are these different questions? *Palliative Medicine,* **22,** 787–95.

40. **Motor Neurone Disease Association.** Just in case Kit https://www.mndassociation.org/ life-with-mnd/treatment-and-care/mnd-just-in-case-kit/ (accessed 23 March 2017).

41. **Smith, S.** and **Wasner, M.** (2014) Psychosocial care. In: Oliver, D., Borasio, G.D., and Johnston, W. (eds) *Palliative Care in Amyotrophic Lateral Sclerosis: From Diagnosis to Bereavement,* 3rd edn, pp. 145–70. Oxford: Oxford University Press.

42. **Lambert, R.** (2014) Spiritual care In: Oliver, D., Borasio, G.D., and Johnston, W. (eds) *Palliative Care in Amyotrophic Lateral Sclerosis: From Diagnosis to Bereavement,* 3rd edn, pp. 171–86. Oxford: Oxford University Press.

Chapter 14

Hastened death: Physician-assisted suicide and euthanasia in ALS

James A. Russell and Zachary Simmons

Introduction

Deliberations regarding the role of the physician in hastened death date to early medical writings.(1) The preponderance of historical medical, legal, religious, and societal opinion has eschewed any role for the physician not intended to protect and maintain a patient's health. This perspective may be changing. The evolution of medical technology intended to restore health may not always do so, and may result in unintended prolongation of suffering. In addition, societal attitudes appear to be shifting away from deference to paternalistic medical opinion, toward patient autonomy, self-determination, and the quality, rather than duration of life. Physician-assisted suicide became lawful in the US for the first time in 1997 with the enactment of the Oregon Death with Dignity Act. This legislation allowed for the legal and carefully regulated prescription of lethal doses of medications by physicians at the request of their terminally ill adult patients. Annual reports are published and openly available. For some, but not all, of those who have followed this experience of nearly 20 years duration, concerns have been mollified that physician participation in hastened death will inevitably prey on the most vulnerable members of society and will escalate into less morally acceptable practices.

Considerations of hastened death are particularly germane to those with amyotrophic lateral sclerosis (ALS) and their caregivers.(2) Although there are many diseases that inflict suffering, ALS is arguably the worst. In support of this belief, ALS patients in Oregon have been repeatedly demonstrated to have an interest in hastened death that is higher than that of patients with any other disease, (3–9) being 4–10 times that found in terminally ill patients with cancer and 25 times that of patients with end-stage lung disease 10,11. A similar disproportionate interest in hastened death exists in ALS patients in the Netherlands. Twenty per cent of this population chooses hastened death, a rate two to four times that reported in cancer patients. (7,9)

This chapter addresses considerations of physician-hastened death relevant to the care of ALS patients. We recognize that this is an emotionally charged issue, where reasonable and thoughtful individuals disagree, and we have attempted to carefully consider the merits of all points of view in drawing our conclusions.

Definitions

Physician-assisted suicide (PAS)

PAS refers to the prescription of a lethal dose of a medication by a clinician, at the request of a terminally ill patient, administered by the patient with the intent of relieving their suffering by hastening their death. As the use of the word 'suicide' is considered by many to be both inaccurate and distasteful, physician-assisted dying, physician aid in dying, or physician-hastened death have been promoted as PAS surrogates (12). These euphemisms however, pose the threat of ambiguity, as they may not adequately distinguish between PAS and euthanasia, an ethically important distinction in the minds of many (13,14). In the USA, where euthanasia remains illegal in all jurisdictions, the term *lawful physician-hastened death* (LPHD) has been proposed. Although LPHD will have different meanings in different jurisdictions, it will be the primary acronym used within this document.

Euthanasia differs from PAS because the clinician both prescribes and administers a lethal dose of medication. It is currently legal only in a few European countries and Canada. Euthanasia may be considered either as a voluntary or non-voluntary act, depending on the decision-making capacity (DMC) of the patient. With non-voluntary euthanasia, the presumption exists that a surrogate decision maker utilizes substituted judgment, applying insight into a patient's premorbid wishes, based on the patient's prior statements or on an interpretation of the patient's historical value system.

Physician hastened-death (PHD) will be used as an inclusive term in this chapter to refer to PAS and euthanasia collectively, in order to efficiently facilitate understanding whenever the distinction between PAS and euthanasia is irrelevant.

Legal status of PHD

PAS, but not euthanasia, is legally sanctioned in five states in the USA—Oregon, Washington, Vermont, Montana, and most recently, California (15). In Canada, the Netherlands, and Luxembourg, both forms of PHD are lawful. In Belgium and Colombia, only euthanasia is legally sanctioned (16).

In 1997, the United States Supreme Court unanimously denied the existence of a constitutionally protected right to assisted suicide (17). Their opinion was based on two focal points:

- the absence of a liberty right as provided by the 14th amendment;
- the Court's opinion that withholding or withdrawing life-sustaining treatment and PAS were neither conceptually or legally synonymous.

As a consequence of these rulings, states were now free to either legally prohibit (or permit) PHD (18).

Ballot Measure 16, otherwise known as the Oregon Death with Dignity Act (ODDA) was passed into law with the support of 60% of the residents of Oregon in 1997 (2). Subsequently PAS has been legalized by statute in Washington (2008) and Vermont (2013) (1,16–20). In 2009, a local court in Montana exonerated a physician who had participated in PAS, a decision subsequently supported by the Montana Supreme Court (9). In 2014, the Second Judicial District Court in New Mexico endorsed PAS, but the ruling was subsequently challenged and overturned by the New Mexico Court of Appeals in August of 2015 (21). In October 2015, the End of Life Option Act was signed into law in California, effectively placing one in six US citizens into LPHD jurisdictions in the US (22). Further indication of public interest in hastened-death is provided by the recognition that 23 other states and the District of Columbia considered LPHD legislation in 2015 (16).

LPHD remains a prosecutable offence in most jurisdictions if specific legal requirements are not followed. In the USA, state regulations largely follow the ODDA template as summarized in Box 14.1, specifying both patient eligibility criteria and physician conduct (1,15,16,21). The prescribing physician is not required to be in attendance during ingestion of the prescribed agent or at the time of death in the US or Canada. Of note, the ODDA, unlike Bill C-14 in Canada (see later), is silent on the role of non-physicians with licensed prescription authority. Some of the requirements of the ODDA pose particular challenges to ALS patients, as will be addressed in the last section of this chapter.

In June 2014, 'The Act Respecting End of Life Care' providing 'medical aid in dying' was legalized in Quebec (16). It requires that patients be:

- at the end of life;
- in an advanced state of irreversible decline in capability;
- experiencing constant and unbearable physical or psychological suffering, which cannot be relieved in a manner the patient deems tolerable, as a consequence of a serious and incurable illness.

Box 14.1 Summary of eligibility requirements for Oregon Death With Dignity Act

- The patient is 18 years of age or older.
- The patient is a legal resident of the jurisdiction.
- The request originates from the patient and not from a lawful surrogate.
- The patient has a terminal illness with a life expectancy of 6 months or less.
- The patient possesses decision-making capacity and the ability to communicate, including the ability to sign their name in the presence of two witnesses.
- The patient's diagnosis, prognosis, and decision-making capacity are confirmed by a consulting physician.
- Mandatory psychiatric or psychological assessment must take place if either physician believes that the patient's judgment is impaired by a psychiatric or psychological condition.
- The patient is capable of self-administration.
- The request is durable over a period of at least 15 days.
- Notification of next of kin is recommended.
- The patient is counselled regarding feasible alternatives.

It does not mandate a specific life expectancy.

In February 2015, the Supreme Court of Canada reversed its historical position of 1993 and unanimously ruled in favour of medical assistance in dying (12,16,23,24). This occurred in response to a petition brought by ALS patient Gloria Taylor, holding for a constitutional right to hastened death for the terminally ill (23,25). The Court's position was heavily influenced by two considerations of ethical consequence:

♦ regulated, rather than unregulated hastened death was preferable from a societal perspective;

♦ arguments attempting to logically distinguish acts of commission causing hastened death from acts of omission causing hastened death such as withholding food and water were specious.12,23-26.

In early 2016, the Canadian House of Commons passed Bill C-14 providing lawful access to both PAS and euthanasia prescribed and/or administered by physicians or nurse practitioners. As in the US, implementation and regulation are the responsibilities of individual provinces.

LHPD laws in Europe differ from those in the US (16,25). In the Netherlands, both voluntary euthanasia and PAS have been historically illegal, yet largely condoned and unprosecuted practices (27). The Royal Dutch Medical Association (KDMA) first published guidelines in 1987 to assist physicians and patients in PHD practices (28). These have been updated on five subsequent occasions, most recently in 2012. Since 2002, the practice has been lawful, with the courts explicitly stating that physicians will not be prosecuted if compliant with statutory, 'due care' criteria, which include determination of patient decision making capacity (16). In Belgium, voluntary euthanasia, but not assisted suicide was legalized in 2002 (16,24,29). In Luxembourg, both euthanasia and assisted suicide have been legal since 2009 (16). All three countries maintain a federal registry and require documentation that a patient's condition is incurable, but only Luxembourg requires terminal illness (16). Refractory mental illness does not preclude eligibility in the Netherlands or Belgium. Documentation of mental capacity and confirmation of patient eligibility by a second physician are required in all three countries. Dementia does not preclude participation if an advance directive indicating a patient's premorbid choice is available. Euthanasia in Switzerland is not legal, but the penal code permits assisted suicide as long as the assisting individual does so for 'unselfish reasons' (16,30). Terminal illness, citizenship, physician participation, and mandated reporting are not required. The only other country where PHD is currently legal is Colombia, where euthanasia was sanctioned as of April 2015 (16).

Patient perspectives on PHD

A significant number of terminally ill patients consider, discuss, and in some cases implement PHD. The American Hospital Association estimates that 6000 deaths/day in the U.S. are in some way planned by patients, families and physicians (31). Fifteen to twenty per cent of dying Oregonians seriously considered a hastened death for themselves (18,32). As for those with ALS, 44% of 100 in one study endorsed their willingness to request a prescription for a lethal dose of medication (2). In a second study of 50 ALS patients, one-third discussed their interest in LPHD (33). In Germany and

Switzerland, a survey of 66 ALS patients and their caregivers indicated that half could imagine requesting hastened death and 14% possessed the current desire to do so (34).

The characteristics of dying patients requesting LPHD have been studied. In a survey Oregon physicians conducted in 2000, loss of independence, control, and quality of life, readiness to die, and patient perception of a pointless existence were thought to be the most frequent reasons for an interest in hastened death (35). Current physical symptoms, lack of social support and depressed mood were rated as unimportant. Concerns about future physical symptoms (potentially responsive to palliative intervention) were considered relevant (36). A small 2009 study of Oregonians requesting LPHD suggested that the most important underlying reasons were the desire to control the circumstances of death and die at home, and concerns about loss of independence, future pain, poor quality of life, and the ability to care for one's self, including the fear of becoming a burden (36). These studies emphasize the prevalence of existential reasons, in contrast to more tangible sources of suffering, such as pain, as the motivating influences on patient interest in hastened death. This, in turn, may explain in part physician and societal reluctance to endorse hastened death practices.

Societal perspectives on PHD

Societal support for hastened death appears to be increasing in North America. One of six individuals in the US now reside in states with LPHD, undoubtedly a consequence of public opinion (22). Between 1990 and 2003, the percentage of survey respondents who endorsed a moral right to suicide for an individual with great pain with no hope of improvement increased from 55 to 62% (37). In 2015, Gallup reported that 68% of Americans endorsed physicians assisting patients in hastening their deaths in the presence of incurable disease and severe pain, a 15% increase in 2 years (38). In Canada, 78% of respondents agreed with the Quebec law and only 9% strongly opposed it (24). In two separate Canadian polls, 84% of respondents supported physician-assisted dying and 78% agreed with the position taken by their Supreme Court (16). In Europe, there is a high acceptance of euthanasia in a small cluster of western European countries (Netherlands, Belgium, Luxembourg, Sweden, France, and Denmark) (39). In 1998, 90% of the Dutch population considered euthanasia to be an acceptable practice (40).

Physician and professional organization perspectives on hastened death

The American Public Health Association (APHA), the American Women's Medical Association, the American Medical Student Association, the Canadian Medical Association (CMA) and the Royal Dutch Medical Association (KNMG) are among the small group of professional medical associations that have endorsed member participation in PHD (22,41). The Oregon Medical Association neither endorsed nor opposed the legalization of PAS during the development of the ODDA (42). The California Medical Association recently became the first state medical society that dropped its opposition to physician-hastened dying, maintaining a neutral stance (16). Both the American Medical Association (AMA) (2016) and the American Academy of Neurology (AAN) (1998) remain resolutely opposed to member participation in hastened death (43,44).

Physician's attitudes regarding LPHD in the US appear to be more ambivalent than those of their parent organizations. In a 1998 USA survey of 1902 physicians, 239 of whom were neurologists, 36% said they would prescribe a lethal medication to a competent patient if they were legally permitted to do so (45). Forty-five per cent of 540 surveyed non-delegate members of the AMA endorsed LPHD as a concept in 2001, in contrast to the position of the parent organization (46). Similarly, a 1999 survey of AAN members found that 50% of respondents endorsed LPHD in concept, and 44% expressed a willingness to participate (3). Although smaller in size, a more recent, 2014 AAN-sponsored survey conducted by its Ethics, Law and Humanities Committee (a joint committee of the AAN, the American Neurological Association, and the Child Neurology Society), discovered that 73% of the 146 responding AAN member in LPAD states, and 54% of the 96 responding members in non-lawful states, viewed physician participation in LPHD as an ethically permissible act.

In their 2014 Update on Euthanasia and Assisted Death, the CMA stated its support for 'the rights of all physicians, within the bounds of existing legislation, to follow their conscience in deciding whether to provide medical aid in dying' as defined in their policy (47). Its member's attitudes however, are less clear, with only a significant minority being willing to participate (48). It has been suggested that CMA endorsement was driven more by an acceptance of legal inevitably rather than member support (24).

In the Netherlands, the KNMG guidelines largely address methodology primarily intended to ensure the safe and effective practice of hastened death in the Netherlands (28). Surveys indicate that 54–57% of Dutch physicians have performed euthanasia and an additional 13–27% have expressed a willingness to do so (49).

Ethical analysis of hastened death

Before embarking on an ethical analysis of physician participation in hastened death, it may be relevant identify two groups of individuals with philosophical perspectives that may preclude their acceptance of any ethical analysis. Individuals characterized as theists believe that life and death considerations fall exclusively within the purview of a deity. The belief system of vitalists holds that life is worthy of preservation under any circumstance.

There are, we believe, morally unassailable components of hastened death consideration. They include a physician's professional duty to exhaust all reasonable palliative efforts on behalf of their dying patients. Additionally there is an obligation to ensure that the patient's request is durable and based on satisfaction of all elements of informed consent including absence of coercion (26). Also in our view, a physician has a professional obligation to engage in a measured discussion regarding PHD when requested, regardless of their personal values and comfort level. To avoid this would represent an unwarranted abrogation of the patient's autonomy and a form of coercion. An unwillingness on the part of a physician to discuss hastened death could, at the same time, erect a barrier to a discussion that might change the patient's interest in PHD. This obligation to discuss, however, does not extend to a moral mandate to endorse or participate in LPHD, or even to identify another physician who is willing to do so, when a physician's conscience prohibits it (26,50).

Ethical analysis of the moral boundaries regarding physician participation in hastened death can be dichotomized. One consideration pertains to the morality of the action itself in the individual doctor–patient relationship. The other relates to the societal consequences that the legal endorsement of hastened death would pose if adopted as public policy.

There are many separate, but overlapping ethical aspects of the first consideration. In many cultures, autonomy may be viewed as the most influential of ethical principles, protected in the USA through the legal protections of liberty and self-determination. Autonomy should strongly influence medical decision making, but it does not by itself provide absolute moral authority (51).

The second ethical consideration relevant to the morality of hastened death as a concept pertains to the debate as to whether hastened death can provide any medical benefit. An answer of no would remove any authority of autonomy, as the authority of autonomy does not extend to futile treatment devoid of achievable medical goals (51). Furthermore, if LPHD has no medical benefit, it places it outside of a physician's professional purview, a perspective frequently emphasized by LPHD opponents. In consideration of harm, those opposed to LPHD express concern regarding the risk of misdiagnosis. The potential for misdiagnosis likely would be negligible in a terminally ill ALS patient who has undergone a mandated second evaluation.

LPHD advocates agree that when medical goals are to preserve and restore health, LPHD has no medical benefit and, therefore, no moral justification. Many would contend, however, that 'when death becomes unavoidable, medical care should allow (and provide) for the patient to die in a setting of his or her own choosing, as free as possible from pain and other burdensome symptoms, and with the optimal psychological and spiritual support of family and friends' (52). In contrast to the Hippocratic era, technology may lead to undesired prolongation of existence and postponement of inevitable death. In this context, PHD can be considered as a medical benefit when palliative measures fail (53).

The third issue focuses on the moral congruence or disparity related to acts of omission vs. acts of commission. Here, there is legal disagreement between the Supreme Courts of the United States and Canada. The former considers the two acts as conceptually different, whereas the latter considers them morally synonymous (15,24). Discourse regarding moral differences between acts of commission vs. acts of omission is not new to clinical medicine. (53,54). Within the professional lifetimes of the authors, it was common to encounter physician reluctance to initiate intubation for fear of unwanted ventilator dependency if treatment goals could not be realized. In such instances, extubation and resultant death was perceived as a homicidal act. Accordingly, the act of omission (not to intubate) seemed more acceptable to some than the act of commission (extubation) (31). Eventually, professional mores evolved from a physician-centric perspective focused on the perceived risks of extubation to an accepted state of moral equipoise when viewed from a patient-centric, goal-orientated perspective. Accordingly, using mechanical ventilation to achieve the patient's goal of restoring health, rather than sustaining existence is fulfilled in both cases (50).

These same considerations have been applied to the PHD debate. Using this morally defensible, patient-centric analysis, many would view withholding life-sustaining treatments (an act of omission) and the provision of a lethal dose of medication (an act of commission) as morally equivalent (53,54). Both accomplish the desired patient goal of alleviating suffering when requested by a terminally ill patient who both maintains decision-making capacity and who remains refractory to palliative intervention. The fourth and pivotal consideration is the potential harm that would occur if a physician's participation in hastened death compromised patient and societal trust in a physician's ability to maintain the primacy of an individual patient's welfare. PHD opponents support this contention (55–57). Supporters suggest the opposite, noting that a physician's willingness to offer aid, rather than abandon the patient in his or her time of need has the opposite effect (31,52–54,58–60). Compliance with a dying patient's request suggests physician empathy, and his or her desire to support the patient's need for control (7,58). Ironically, one reason for a patient's interest in PHD may be the dogmatic and coercive beliefs of physicians who maintain that hastened death is never acceptable. Expression of these beliefs to patients may incite the fear that whatever semblance of control they have over their lives will be hijacked by the very individual they have entrusted with their care (54). The willingness to restore patient control and engage in shared decision making contrasts with the historical and increasingly unpopular parentalistic approach of the medical profession. This attempt to preserve autonomy and control has been identified as a primary motivating factor in PHD interest in the ALS population (2,7,9,33,60–62).

Another potential benefit of patient empowerment provided by LPHD is that it may paradoxically influence patients to postpone or avoid hastened death. ODDA data reveals that since its inception, lethal prescriptions issued under this act have been used annually by only two-thirds of the patients who have received them (63). Presumably, those who acquired, but did not ingest these pills are seeking autonomy, not a hastened death. This same conclusion was reached from a prospective study of ALS patients when the reasons for their 'wish-to-die' were explored (60).

Support for the ethical permissibility of LPHD can also be derived from a comparative ethical analysis of the four interventions that may advertently or inadvertently hasten death:

- LPHD;
- euthanasia;
- withholding, withdrawing, or limiting life-sustaining treatment (WWLLST);
- palliative sedation (PS) (13,53,6).

In our minds, there are reasons to consider LPHD as morally equivalent if not superior to the other interventions from a patient-centric perspective (53). Unlike the others, LPHD requires that the patient both request and administer the medication (14,53). Accordingly, LPHD becomes insulated from concerns that the decision to implement the action may be made by someone other than the patient. Unlike PS, with its potential to be utilized as covert euthanasia, the intent of LPHD is never ambiguous (53,62).

Unlike WWLLST and PS, LPHD provides some reassurance afforded by required regulation and monitoring practices (54).

In the minds of many, ambivalence toward PHD originates more from its adoption as a public policy than from concerns pertaining to the morality of the act itself. This ambivalence is derived largely from the potential harm to vulnerable populations (the 'slippery slope'). Many, even PHD advocates, predict that hastened death practices will inevitably expand (65–67). Available US data is reassuring, but of course does not preclude the possibility of future abuse (18,54). Adoption of LPHD as a public policy has two other potential benefits. LPHD avoids criminalizing a behaviour that patients may pursue through clandestine means if necessary, as occurred with the prohibition of alcohol. It can be cogently argued that PHD is best practiced by those trained to do so in a controlled and regulated fashion (40,54,68,69). This consideration was emphasized by the Supreme Court of Canada as a contributory factor in their decision (24). Additionally, LPHD likely diminishes more stigmatizing and less socially acceptable means of hastened death that are sometimes sought prematurely by the terminally ill (14,18,53,68–70).

The major concern in adopting LPHD as a public policy is the potential for unacceptable coercive influence on vulnerable populations. Particularly concerning is the potential self-inflicted coercion of patients not to impose a burden on their caregivers, 'a duty to die' (70). There are also broader societal concerns that patients seeking PHD will be those who are disproportionately disadvantaged by a lack of decision making capacity (such as children and demented or depressed individuals), poverty, low levels of education, or the inability to receive appropriate palliative care. Realistic concerns also exist that the financial burdens of medical care will provide a coercive mechanism through political channels that influence future PHD policy decisions (67,70).

In fairness to PHD opponents, the European experience has been disconcerting. In the Netherlands, between 2003 and 2012, the incidence of euthanasia rose from approximately 10 to 30 per 1000 deaths annually (71). Between 2009 and 2013, the incidence of PHD (primarily euthanasia) in the Netherlands increased by 81% (16). In comparison, the incidence of LPHD in Oregon has remained relatively unchanged at 2.3 per 1000 deaths over the same interval (71). Additionally, attitudes in the Netherlands regarding PHD appear more permissive than in the US, allowing for both voluntary and non-voluntary euthanasia (7,16,40). In 1996, prior to the more careful reporting requirements for PHD that now exist, 1000 of 3300 euthanasia deaths in the Netherlands occurred in individuals lacking DMC (27). The Dutch Supreme Court has endorsed PHD on the basis of 'unbearable mental suffering', even if there is no concurrent medical disease. The stated philosophy of the Dutch courts is that the degree of suffering rather than its cause is the decisive factor (72). The majority of Dutch psychiatrists would considered PHD acceptable for psychiatric patients under certain circumstances (66). A review of Dutch euthanasia and assisted suicide cases from 2011 to 2014 revealed 66 who received PHD for psychiatric disorders (73). Although depression, anxiety, and post-traumatic stress disorder were the most common, the list included psychosis, substance abuse, eating disorders, neurocognitive impairment (including mental retardation), and autism spectrum. In 2002, in the Netherlands, the Groningen protocol was developed to provide guidelines to facilitate

PHD in severely and permanently injured newborns with refractory suffering, requiring consent of both parents and the medical team. It is estimated that there are 15–20 annual cases of PHD in neonates in the Netherlands (74,75). Additional behaviours of potential concern include the increased incidence of reported PS in the Netherlands. This promotes speculation that this trend may represent, at least in some cases, disguised PHD in which the need for monitoring and reporting is purposefully circumvented (65). Also concerning is the reported development of mobile end-of-life clinics in the Netherlands whose intent may be in part to provide PHD services to patients wishing to circumvent the judgment of their own physicians who have denied their request for PHD (73,75).

Similar concerns exist regarding the experience in Belgium (29,76,77). It has been estimated that 2–3% of patients who receive euthanasia in that country do so without their explicit request (76). In 2011, unbearable mental suffering was the sole justification in 3.5% of individuals requesting PHD (77). In 2014, legalization of euthanasia was extended to include chronically ill children with 'constant and unbearable suffering' that required an explicit request by the child, parenteral consent, and multidisciplinary assessment of decision-making capacity (29). The incidence of PS appears to be on the rise in Belgium as well, increasing from approximately 3 to 10 per 1000 deaths between 2003 and 2012 (71,76). In Belgium, 40 euthanized individuals have served as organ donors, raising concerns over potential associated coercive financial incentives (78–80). Although organ donation in ALS patients is a rare consideration, it has occurred (81).

These 'slippery slope' risks can never be dismissed, but fears have been ameliorated by the Oregon experience of the last 18 years (18,54,63). Although the absolute number of LPHD deaths in Oregon has grown gradually since its inception, its peak in 2014 remains at 105 of 33,931 (0.3%) deaths (63,71). This same detailed and publicly available data, in contrast with the lack of such data for WWLLST or PS, provides additional reassurance that LPAD is not disproportionately utilized in any of the disadvantaged populations listed above (18,54). Ninety-three per cent of patients who chose LPAD did so despite being enrolled in hospice and receiving palliative care (18). Furthermore, there has been no relaxation of LPAD procedural requirements or any movement toward euthanasia. LPAD, when scrupulously regulated and monitored, does not inevitably result in adverse consequences to patients or society.

ALS and PHD

In comparison to individuals with other terminal illnesses, ALS patients are disproportionately interested in PHD, both in the US and in Europe. In general, ALS patients seeking PHD, when compared with those not seeking such a course, are more likely to be men, and are generally more educated and less religious. They are likely to be distressed by what they perceive as a loss of autonomy and control, the inability to participate in pleasurable activities, and their increasing dependence on, and burden to, others. They also are more likely to experience insomnia, pain, and other forms of discomfort, and to have lower scores on hopelessness and quality of life assessments

(2,33,35,82). Financial status, culture, and disease severity do not appear to impact PHD decision making.

In the Netherlands, ALS patients choosing PHD were those for whom religion was less important (7,61). Interest in PHD appears dissociated from any particular disease characteristics, quality of care, income, or educational level (7). In another study, interest in PHD correlated with higher education and with an interest in dying at home, but not with quality of care, depression, or loss of function (61). A third European study involving German and Swiss patients reported that the wish to hasten death correlated with depression, loneliness, the perception of being a burden to others, a low quality of life, and the diminished personal importance of religion (34).

Both PHD opponents and advocates concur that once a patient's interest in PHD is identified, there is a professional obligation both to explore the underlying reasons for this interest and to provide palliative intervention in an attempt to alter that interest before PHD is implemented (18,53,54,69). The importance of this belief is emphasized by a report indicating that 46% of patients who expressed initial interest in PAS changed their minds after receiving some form of palliative care intervention as opposed to only 15% for whom no such interventions were provided (35).

We have posed six questions relevant to palliative care, PHD and ALS in Box 14.2. The initial four questions relate to the causes of suffering in ALS, considerations as to whether palliative care availability and efficacy would sufficiently diminish this morbidity, and what effect this would have on a patient's interest in PHD (4,6,9,61,83–86). Conceptually, the causes of suffering may be divided into those that are physical (e.g. pain, choking on secretions, suffocation) and those that are existential, social, and psychological (e.g. sense of burden, loss of dignity, hopelessness, loss of autonomy, and control) (4). It appears that these latter non-physical domains, notably prevalent in ALS, are less amenable to effective palliation with currently available interventions (2,4,33,65,86). Opponents of LPHD contend that patient interest would diminish with the adequate

---

Box 14.2 Six questions relevant to palliative care, physician-hastened death, and ALS

- What are the causes of suffering in ALS?
- Are these causes amenable to palliative care intervention?
- Is adequate palliative care available to all ALS patients in need?
- Does the implementation of palliative care affect an ALS patient's interest in PHD?
- Do depression and FTD, frequent comorbidities in ALS, affect decision-making capacity and interest in hastened death, and can they be influenced by treatment?
- What common characteristics of ALS impede implementation of lawful hastened death?

availability of effective palliative care services (6,7,35,53,54,59,68,69,83). Both ODDA data and the Dutch experience however, indicate that patients pursue LPHD despite palliative services (9,18,54,62,63,66). Also, as noted previously, interest in hastened death in ALS patients appears resolute (6,36). Thus, the limited evidence available does not support the hypothesis that addressing unmet palliative care needs, however beneficial to many patients, would eliminate requests for PDH by all patients with ALS (6,66,86).

The last two questions pertain to the impact of ALS comorbidities on patient decision-making capacity and ALS specific issues that may impact LPHD implementation. PHD requires informed consent, which in turn requires the capacity to understand the consequence of a decision and to communicate thought processes and reasons for decisions effectively (87). Decision-making capacity in ALS is jeopardized by a number of potential influences, including frontotemporal dementia (FTD), depression, and hypoventilation with resultant hypercarbia. The latter can be addressed through adequate ventilatory support, either non-invasive or invasive. The former two merit further consideration.

FTD is a prevalent comorbidity in ALS for which there are currently no effective medical treatments. Its effects may be overt or subtle, and its potential effects on decision-making capacity must be considered in any discussion of LPHD with ALS patients. The specific deficits encountered in FTD are addressed elsewhere (See Chapters 8 and 9). In a recent study of 274 ALS patients, 7% were identified as demented, with an additional 54% suffering from mild cognitive impairment (88). The salient concern that follows is the potential for these cognitive deficits to influence patient decision-making capacity and judgment when requesting LPHD. To that point, a recent study of 253 ALS patients from the same cohort, 58% of whom had some degree of cognitive impairment, failed to demonstrate any correlation between cognitive impairment, depression and interest in PHD (89).

Depression is the other major potential influence on decision-making capacity when assessing interest in PHD in the ALS population. It may be of even greater importance because it is potentially treatable. The reported incidence of depression in ALS varies widely from zero to 75%, with 20% appearing to be a common estimate (4,34,35,62,90–92). Even when ALS-specific assessments are used, estimates of the frequency of depression in ALS are still fairly broad, ranging from 28 to 48% (90), and do not appear to correlate with disease severity (90,91). The relationship between depression and interest in PHD remains uncertain. In terminally ill patients, the data appears to support a correlation (93–99), but this does not necessarily extrapolate to ALS, where the data is more ambiguous. One study supports the association (34), whereas others have failed to identify any relationship (2,9,33,61,89,92). Assessment of decision-making capacity and the wish for PHD must distinguish between depression and hopelessness. Further discussion of these related, but distinct concepts, and the relationships between the two, are discussed in more detail in Chapter 3.

Arguably, the major importance of identifying depression as a contributor to ALS patient interest in hastened death relates to treatment efficacy in mitigating both depression and the interest in hastened death. A review of 40 trials addressing the efficacy of treatment of depression in patients receiving palliative care arrived at no definitive conclusion (100). Reports from Oregon indicate that 'successful treatment of a major depressive disorder increases the desire for life-sustaining therapy in only a minority of terminally ill patients' (35,101,102). There are limited studies specifically addressing ALS that do not allow for any conclusions to be drawn regarding the efficacy of antidepressant treatment in treating the mood disorder (90). Confounding interpretation of these studies is that antidepressant use in ALS patients may be intended for symptom management, such as pseudobulbar affect or sialorrhoea, not for the treatment of depression (103,104). In a study of 204 Dutch ALS patients, no correlation was found between the use of antidepressant medication, symptoms of depression, or utilization of PHD (61).

LPHD implementation in ALS patients in the USA pose particular challenges. Patient eligibility may be precluded by impaired verbal and written communication necessary to request, swallowing difficulties necessary to ingest, and muscle weakness necessary for self-administration (4). It is not clear where the law stands in regard to the use of technology to circumvent these disease-related impediments to LPHD implementation (2). For example, the ODDA precludes injection, but is silent on infusion, potentially allowing for a parenteral barbiturate delivered by a pump activated by a quadriplegic and mute ALS patient through an eye gaze system.

Conclusions

Until such time as a meaningful treatment exists that favourably alters the natural history of ALS, there will probably continue to be an interest in PHD by this patient population and their caregivers. Clinicians caring for ALS patients in jurisdictions that permit LPHD will have the opportunity to consider the increasing public acceptance and lawfulness of PHD. Those in the USA will need to take into account the ODDA experience of the past 18 years, whereas those in other countries with different systems and laws will also need to consider data such as that from the Netherlands and Belgium. Beyond the data are the many ethical, social, existential, medical, and psychiatric factors discussed here. The current environment requires clinicians in jurisdictions in which PHD is legal to follow their consciences in making decisions that they believe are ethically and morally justifiable in response to their autonomous patients' requests. There are no absolute rules for such decisions, but it is our hope that this monograph will provide helpful guidance for personal deliberation.

References

1. **Lachman V.** (2010) Physician-assisted suicide: Compassionate liberation or murder. *Medsurg Nursing*, **19**(2), 121–5.
2. **Ganzini, L., Johnston, W.S., McFarland, B.H., Tolle, S., Tolle, S.W.,** and **Lee, M.A.** (1998) Attitudes of patients with amyotrophic lateral sclerosis and their care givers toward assisted suicide. *New England Journal of Medicine*, **339**(14), 967–73.
3. **Carver, A.C., Vickrey, B.G., Bernat, J.L., Keran, C., Ringel, S.P.,** and **Foley, K.M.** (1999) End of life care: A survey of US neurologists' attitude, behavior and knowledge. *Neurology*, **53**, 284–93.
4. **Ganzini, L., Johnston, W.S.,** and **Hoffman, W.F.** (1999) Correlates of suffering in amyotrophic lateral sclerosis. *Neurology*, **52**, 1434–40.

5. **Neudert, C., Oliver, D., Wasner, M., and Borasio, G.D.** (2001) The course of the terminal phase in patients with amyotrophic lateral sclerosis. *Journal of Neurology*, **248**, 612–16.

6. **Ganzini, L. and Block, S.** (2002) Physician-assisted death—a last resort? *New England Journal of Medicine*, **346**(21), 1663–5.

7. **Veldink, J.H., Wokke, J.H.J., van der Wal, G., Vianney de Jong, J.M.B., and van den Berg, LH.** (2002) Euthanasia and physician-assisted suicide among patients with amyotrophic lateral sclerosis in the Netherlands. *New England Journal of Medicine*, **346**, 1638–44.

8. **Hedberg, K., Hopkins, D., Leman, R., and Kohn, M.** (2009) The 10-year experience of Oregon's Death with Dignity Act: 1998–2007. *Journal of Clinical Ethics*, **20**(2), 124–32.

9. **Maessen, M., Veldink, J.H., van den Berg, L.H., Schouten, H.J., van der Wal, G., and Onwuteaka-Philipsen, B.D.** (2010) Requests for euthanasia: origin of suffering in ALS, heart failure and cancer. *Journal of Neurology*, **257**, 1192–8.

10. **Sullivan, A.D., Hedberg, K., and Hopkins, D.** (2001) Legalized physician-assisted suicide in Oregon, 1998–2000. *New England Journal of Medicine*, **344**, 605–7.

11. **Niemeyer, D.** (2016) Sixth annual report on Oregon's Death with Dignity Act. 2003, Portland OR: Department of Human Services. Available at: https://public.health.oregon. gov/ProviderPartnerResources/EvaluationResearch/DeathwithDignityAct/Documents/ year6.pdf (accessed 14 June 2016).

12. **Chochinov, H.M.** (2016) Physician-assisted death in Canada. *Journal of the American Medical Association*, **315**(3), 253–4.

13. **Fins, J.J. and Bacchetta, M.D.** (1995) Framing the physician-assisted suicide and voluntary active euthanasia debate: The role of deontology, consequentialism, and clinical pragmatism. *Journal of the American Geriatric Society*, **43**, 563–8.

14. **Angell, M.** (1997) The Supreme Court and physician-assisted suicide, the ultimate right. *New England Journal of Medicine*, **336**(1), 50–3.

15. **Gostin, L.O. and Roberts, A.E.** (2016) Physician-assisted dying: A turning point. *Journal of the American Medical Association*, **315**(3), 249–50.

16. **Dyer, O., White, C., and Rada, A.G.** (2015) Assisted dying: Law and practice around the world. *British Medical Journal*, **351**, h4481

17. **Burt, R.A.** (1997) The Supreme Court speaks: Not assisted but a constitutional right to palliative care. *New England Journal of Medicine*, **337**(17), 234–1236.

18. **Lindsay, R.A.** (2009) Oregon's experience: Evaluating the record. *American Journal of Bioethics*, **9**(3), 19–27.

19. **Steinbrook R.** (2008) Physician-assisted death—from Oregon to Washington State. *New England Journal of Medicine*, **359**(24), 2513–5.

20. **Jecker N.** (2009) Physician-assisted death in the Pacific Northwest. *American Journal of Bioethics*, **9**(3), 1–2.

21. **Harkness, K.** (2015) New Mexico Appeals Court Rules 'Assisted Suicide "is Not a Fundamental Liberty"'. *The Daily Signal*, 12 Aug. Available at http://dailysignal.com/2015/ 08/12/new-mexico-appeals-court-rules-assisted-suicide-is-not-a-fundamental-liberty/ (accessed 14 June 2016).

22. **Clodfelter, R.P.** (2016) The liberty to die: California enacts physician aid-in-dying law. *Journal of the American Medical Association*, **315**(3), 251–2.

23. **Webster, P.C.** (2015) Canada to legalise physician-assisted dying. *Lancet*, **385**(9969), 678.

24. **Attaran, A.** (2015) Unanimity on death with dignity—legalizing physician-assisted death with dying in Canada. *New England Journal of Medicine*, **372**(22), 2080–2.

25. **Schaefer, A.** (2013) Physician-assisted suicide; The great Canadian euthanasia debate. *International Journal of Law and Psychiatry*, **36**, 522–31.

26. **Wanzer, S.H., Federman, D.D., Adelstein, S.J.,** et al. (1989) The physician's responsibility toward hopelessly ill patients: A second look. *New England Journal of Medicine*, **320**(13), 844–9.

27. **Angell, M.** (1996) Euthanasia in the Netherlands-good news or bad. *New England Journal of Medicine*, **335**(22), 1676–8.

28. **The Royal Dutch Medical Association (KNMG)** (2016). Nieuw afweginskader scherpt aanpak kindermishandeling aan. Available at: www.knmg.nl (accessed 14 June 2016).

29. **Siegel, A.M., Sisti, D.A.,** and **Caplan, A.L.** (2013). Pediatric euthanasia in Belgium: Disturbing developments. *Journal of the American Medical Association*, **311**(19), 1963–4.

30. **Bosshard, G., Zellweger, U., Bopp, M.,** et al. (2016). Medical end-of-life practices in Switzerland; A comparison of 2001 and 2013. *Journal of the American Medical Association International Medicine*, **176**(4), 555–6.

31. **Cassel, C.K.** (1990). Morals and moralism in the debate over euthanasia and assisted suicide and euthanasia. *New England Journal of Medicine*, **323**(11), 750–2.

32. **Tolle, S.W., Tilden, V.R., Drach, L.L., Fromme, E.K.,** and **Phedberg, K.** (2004). Characteristics and proportion of dying Oregonians who personally consider physician-assisted suicide. *Journal of Clinical Ethics*, **15**, 111–18.

33. **Ganzini, L., Silveira, M.J.,** and **Johnston, W.S.** (2002). Predictors and correlates of interest in physician-assisted suicide in the final month of life among ALS patients in Washington and Oregon. *Journal of Pain and Symptom Management*, **24**, 312–17.

34. **Stutzki, R., Weber, M., Reiter-Theil, S., Simmen, U.,** and **Borasio, G.D.** (2013) Attitudes towards hastened death in ALS: A prospective study of patients and family caregivers. *Amyotrophic Lateral Sclerosis*, E1–9.

35. **Ganzini, L., Nelson, H.D., Schmidt, T.A., Kraemer, D.F., Delorit, M.A.,** and **Lee, M.A.** (2000). Physician's experiences with the Oregon Death with Dignity Act. *New England Journal of Medicine*, **342**, 557–63.

36. **Ganzini, L., Goy, E.R.,** and **Dobscha, S.K.** (2009). Oregonians' reasons for requesting physician aid in dying. *Archives of Neurology*, **169**(5), 489–92.

37. **Pew Research Center**. (2016). *Views on End-of-life Medical Treatments, November 2013*. Available at: http://www.pewforum.org/2013/11/21/views-on-end-of-life-medical-treatments/. Accessed June 14, 2016

38. **Dugan, A.** (2015) In US, support up for doctor-assisted suicide. *Gallup, Politics*, **May 27, 2015**. Available at http://www.gallup.com/poll/183425/support-doctor-assisted-suicide.aspx (accessed 14 June 2016).

39. **Cohen, J., Van Landeghem, P., Carpentier, N.,** and **Deliens, L.** (2014) Public acceptance of euthanasia in Europe: A survey study in 47 countries. *International Journal of Public Health*, **59**(1), 143–56.

40. **van der Heide, A.** (2013) Assisted suicide and euthanasia. In: Bernat, J.L. and Beresford, H.R. (eds) *Ethical and Legal Issues in Neurology. Handbook of Clinical Neurology* (3rd series), **118**, pp. 181–9. Amsterdam: Elsevier.

41. **American Public Health Association**. (2014) Patients' rights to self-determination at the end of life. Available at: http://www.apha.org/policies-and-advocacy/

public-health-policy-statements/policy-database/2014/07/29/13/28/patients-rights-to-self-determination-at-the-end-of-life (accessed 14 June 2016).

42. **Lee, M.A.** and **Tolle, S.W.** (1996) Oregon's assisted suicide vote: The silver lining. *Annals of Internal Medicine*, **124**(2), 267–9.

43. **American Medical Association.** (2015) Opinion 2.211—physician-assisted suicide. Available at http://www.ama-assn.org/ama/pub/physician-resources/medical-ethics/code-medical-ethics/opinion2211.page (accessed 14 June 2016).

44. **Pellegrino, T.R., Beresford, R., Bernat, J.L.,** et al. (1998) Assisted-suicide, euthanasia, and the neurologist. *Neurology*, **50**, 596–8.

45. **Meier, D.E., Emmons, C.A., Wallenstein, S., Quill, T., Morrison, R.S.,** and **Cassel, C.K.** (1998) A national survey of physician-assisted suicide and euthanasia in the United States. *New England Journal of Medicine*, **338**, 1193–201.

46. **Whitney, S.N., Brown, B.W.,** Jr, **Brody, H., Alcser, K.H., Bachman, J.G.,** and **Greely, H.T.** (2001) Views of United States physicians and members of the American Medical Associations House of Delegates regarding physician-assisted suicide. *Journal of General Internal Medicine*, **6**, 290–6.

47. **Canadian Medical Association** (2014) Euthanasia and assisted death (update 2014). Available at: http://policybase.cma.ca/dbtw-wpd/Policypdf/PD15-02.pdf. (accessed 14 June 2016).

48. **Canadian Medical Association** (2015) Canadian Medical Association members ready to lead principles-based discussion on end-of-life care. Available at: https://www.cma.ca/En/Lists/Medias/release-EOL-dialogue.pdf (accessed 14 June 2016).

49. **Onwuteaka-Philpsen, B.D., van der Heide, A., Koper, D.,** et al. (2003) Euthanasia and other end-of-life decisions in the Netherlands in 1990, 1995 and 2001. *Lancet*, **62**, 395–9.

50. **Miller, F.G.** and **Brody, H.** (1995) Professional integrity and physician-assisted death. *Hastings Central Reports*, **25**, 8–17.

51. **Gert, B.,** et al. (1994) Distinguishing between patient's refusals and requests. *Hastings Central Reports*, **24**, 13–15.

52. **Brody H.** (1992) Assisted death: A compassionate response to a medical failure. *New England Journal of Medicine*, **327**(19), 1384–8.

53. **Quill, T.E., Lo, B.,** and **Brock, D.W.** (1997) Palliative options of last resort: A comparison of voluntarily stopping eating and drinking, terminal sedation, physician-assisted suicide, and voluntary active euthanasia. *Journal of the American Medical Association*, **278**(23), 2099–104.

54. **Quill, T.E.** (2012) Physicians should 'assist in suicide' when it is appropriate. *Journal of Law and Medical Ethics*, **41**(1), 57–65.

55. **Yang, Y.T.** and **Curlin, F.A.** (2016) Why physicians should oppose assisted suicide. *Journal of the American Medical Association*, **315** (3), 247–8.

56. **Pellegrino, E.D.** (1993) Compassion needs reason too. *Journal of the American Medical Association*, **270**(7), 874–5.

57. **Davis, J.** and **Finlay, I.L.** (2015) Would judicial consent for assisted dying protect vulnerable people? *British Medical Journal*, **351**, h4437

58. **Quill, T.E., Back, A.L.,** and **Block, S.D.** (2016) Responding to patients requesting physician assisted death. *Journal of the American Medical Association*, **315**(3), 245–6.

59. **Quill, T.E.** (1991) Death and dignity. A case of individualized decision making. *New England Journal of Medicine*, **324**(10), 691–4.

60. **Albert, S.M., Rabkin, J.G., Del Bene, M.I.**, et al. (2005) Wish to die in end-stage ALS. *Neurology*, **65**, 68–74.

61. **Maessen, M., Vendink, J.H., Onwuteaka-Philipsen, B.D.**, et al. (2009) Trends and determinants of end-of-life practices in ALS in the Netherlands. *Neurology*, **73**, 954–61.

62. **Maessen, M., Vendink, J.H., Onwuteaka-Philipsen, B.D.**, et al. (2014) Euthanasia and physician-assisted suicide in amyotrophic lateral sclerosis: A prospective study. *Journal of Neurology*, **261**, 1894–901.

63. **Oregon Health Authority.** (2015) *Oregon Death With Dignity Act: 2015 Data Summary.* Available at https://public.health.oregon.gov/ProviderPartnerResources/ EvaluationResearch/DeathwithDignityAct/Documents/year18.pdf (accessed June 14, 2016).

64. **Papavasiliou, E., Payne, S.,** and **Brearley, S.** (2014) Current debates on end-of-life sedation: An international expert elicitation study. *Supportive Care Cancer*, **22**, 2141–9.

65. **van der Heide, A., Onwuteaka-Philipsen, D., Rurup, M.L.**, et al. (2007) End-of-life practices in the Netherlands under the euthanasia act. *New England Journal of Medicine*, **356**, 1957–63.

66. **Battin, M.P., Van der Heide, A., Ganzini, L., van der Wal, G.,** and **Onwuteaka-Philipsen, B.D.** (2007) Legal physician-assisted dying in Oregon and the Netherlands: Evidence concerning the impact on patients in 'vulnerable' groups. *Journal of Medical Ethics*, **33**, 591–7.

67. **Finlay, I.L.** and **George, R.** (2011) Legal physician-assisted suicide in Oregon and the Netherlands: Evidence concerning the impact on patients in vulnerable groups-another perspective on Oregon data. *Journal of Medical Ethics*, **37**, 171–4.

68. **Quill, T.E., Meier, D.E., Block, S.D.,** and **Billings, J.A.** (1998) The debate over physician-assisted suicide: Empirical data and convergent views. *Annals of Internal Medicine*, **128**, 552–8.

69. **Quill, T.E., Cassel, C.K.,** and **Meier, D.E.** (1992) Care of the hopelessly ill—proposed clinical criteria for physician-assisted suicide. *New England Journal of Medicine*, **327**, 1380–4.

70. **Misbin, R.I.** (1991) Physicians' aid in dying. *New England Journal of Medicine*, **325**(18), 1307–11.

71. **Gamondi, C., Borasio, G.D., Limoni, C., Preston, N.,** and **Payne, S.** (2014) Legalisation of assisted suicide: a safeguard to euthanasia. *Lancet*, **384**, 127.

72. **Groenewoud, J.H., van der Maas, P.J., van der Wal, G.,** et al. (1997) Physician-assisted death in psychiatric practice in the Netherlands. *New England Journal of Medicine*, **336**, 1795–801.

73. **Kim, S.Y.H., De Vries, R.G.,** and **Peteet, J.R.** (2016) Euthanasia and assisted suicide of patients with psychiatric disorders in the Netherlands 2011–2014, *Journal of the American Medical Association* Psychiatry, **73**, 362–8.

74. **Verhagen, E.** and **Sauer, P.J.J.** (2005) The Groningen protocol—euthanasia in severely ill newborns. *New England Journal of Medicine*, **352**(10), 959–62.

75. **Snijdewind, M.C., Willems, D.L., Diliens, L., Onwuteaka-Philipsen, B.D.,** and **Chambaere, K.** (2015) A study of the first year of the end-of-life clinic for physician-assisted dying in the Netherlands. *Journal of the American Medical Association Internal Medicine*, **175**, 1633–40.

76. **Bilsen, J., Cohen, J., Chambaere, K.,** et al. (2009) Medical end-of-life practices under the euthanasia law in Belgium. *New England Journal of Medicine*, **361**(11), 1119–20.

77. Deschepper, R., Distelmans, W., and Bilsen, J. (2014) Requests for euthanasia/physician assisted suicide on the basis of mental suffering: Vulnerable patients or vulnerable physicians. *Journal of the American Medical Association* Psychiatry, **71**(6), 617–18.

78. Bollen, J., Ten Hoopen, R. Ysebaert, D., van Mook, W., and van Heurn, E. (2016) Legal and ethical aspects of organ donation after euthanasia in Belgium and the Netherlands. *Journal of Medical Ethics*, **42**(8), 486–899.

79. Ysebaert, D., Van Beeumen, G., De Greef, K., et al. (2009) Organ procurement after euthanasia: Belgian experience. *Transplantation Proceedings*, **41**(2), 585–6.

80. Desschans, B. and Evrard, D. (2014) Organ donation and transplant statistics in Belgium for 2012 and 2013. *Transplantation Proceedings*, **46**, 3124–6.

81. Toossi, S., Lomen-Hoerth, C., Josephson, S.A., et al. (2012) Organ donation after cardiac death in amyotrophic lateral sclerosis. *Annals of Neurology*, **71**, 154–6.

82. Murphy, P.L., Albert, S.M., Weber, C.M., Del Bene, M.L., and Rowland, L.P. (2000) Impact of spirituality and religiousness on outcomes in patients with ALS. *Neurology*, **55**(10), 1581–4.

83. Borasio, G.D., Shaw, P.J., Hardiman, O., et al. (2002) Standards of palliative care for patients with amyotrophic lateral sclerosis: Results of a European survey. *Amyotrophic Lateral Sclerosis and Other Motor Neuron Disorders*, **2**, 159–64.

84. Simmons, Z. (2005) Management strategies for patients with amyotrophic lateral sclerosis from diagnosis through death. *Neurologist*, **11**, 257–70.

85. Blackhall, L.J. (2012) Amyotrophic lateral sclerosis and palliative care: where we are, and the road ahead. *Muscle & Nerve*, **45**, 311–18.

86. Connolly, S., Galvin, M., and Hardiman, O. (2015) End-of-life management in patients with amyotrophic lateral sclerosis. *Lancet Neurology*, **14**, 435–42.

87. Khin, E.K., Minor, D., Holloway, A., and Pelleg, A. (2015) Decisional capacity in amyotrophic lateral sclerosis. *Journal of the American Academy of Psychiatry Law*, **43**, 210–17.

88. Murphy, J., Factor-Litvak, P., Goetz, R., et al. (2016) Cognitive-behavioral screening reveals prevalent impairment in a large multicenter ALS cohort. *Neurology*, **86**, 813–20.

89. Rabkin, J.G., Goetz, R., Murphy, J., Factor Litvak, P., and Mitsumoto, H. (2016) Cognitive impairment, behavioral, depression, and wish to die in an ALS cohort. *Neurology* **87**(13), 1320–8.

90. Rabkin, J.G., Albert, S., Del Bene, M., O'Sullivan, I., Tider, T., and Rowland, L. (2005) Prevalence of depressive disorders and change over time in late-stage ALS. *Neurology*, **65**, 62–7.

91. McElhiney, M., Rabkin, J., Gordon, P., Goetz, R., and Mitsumoto, H. (2009) Prevalence of fatigue and depression in ALS patients and change over time. *Journal of Neurology, Neurosurgery, and Psychiatry*, **80**, 1146–9.

92. Rabkin, J.G., Goetz, R., Litvak-Factor, P., et al. (2015) Depression and wish to die in a multicenter cohort of ALS patients. *Amyotrophic Lateral Sclerosis and Frontotemporal Degeneration*, **16**, 265–73.

93. Breitbart, W., Rosenfeld, B., Pessin, H., et al. (2000) Depression, hopelessness, and desire for hastened death in terminally ill patients with cancer. *Journal of the American Medical Association*, **284**, 2907–11.

94. Chochinov, H.M., Wilson, K.G., Enns, M., and Mowchun, N. (1995) Desire for death in the terminally ill. *American Journal of Psychiatry*, **152**(8), 1185–91.

95. van der Lee, M.L., van der Bom, J.G., et al. Euthanasia and depression: A prospective cohort study among terminally ill cancer patients. *Journal of Clinical Oncology*, **23**, 6607–12.

96. Chochinov, H.M., Wilson, K.G., Enns, M., et al. (1995) Desire for death in the terminally ill. *American Journal of Psychiatry*, **152**(8), 1185–91.

97. Wilson, K.G., Scott, J.F., Graham, I.D., et al. (2000) Attitudes of terminally ill patients toward euthanasia and physician-assisted suicide. *Archives of Internal Medicine*, **160**(16), 2454–60.

98. Emanuel, E.J., Fairclough, D.L., and Emanuel, L.L. (2000) Attitudes and desires related to euthanasia and physician-assisted suicide among terminally ill patients and their caregivers. *Journal of the American Medical Association*, **284**, 2460–8.

99. Emanuel, E.J., Fairclough, D.L., Daniels, E.R., and Clarridge, B.R. (1996) Euthanasia and physician-assisted suicide: Attitudes and experiences of oncology patients, oncologists, and the public. *Lancet*, **347**(9018), 1805–10.

100. Ujeyl, M. and Müller-Oerlinghausen, B. (2012) Antidepressants for treatment of depression in palliative patients: A systematic literature review. *Schmerz*, **26**(5), 523–36.

101. Ganzini, L. and Lee, M.A. (1997) Psychiatry and assisted suicide in the United States. *New England Journal of Medicine*, **336**(25), 1824–6.

102. Ganzini, L., Lee, M.A., Heintz, R.T., Bloom, J.D., and Fenn DS. (1994) The effect of depression treatment on elderly patients' preferences for life-sustaining medical therapy. *American Journal of Psychiatry*, **151**, 1631–6.

103. Atassi, N., Cook, A., Pineda, C.M., et al. (2011) Depression in amyotrophic lateral sclerosis. *Amyotrophic Lateral Sclerosis*, **12**(2), 109–12.

104. Pisa, F.E., Logroscino, G., Casetta, A., et al. (2015) The use of antidepressant medication before and after the diagnosis of amyotrophic lateral sclerosis: A population-based cohort study. *Neuroepidemiology*, **44**(2), 91–8.

Chapter 15

Bulbar dysfunction in ALS: Psychological implications

Jashelle Caga and Matthew C. Kiernan

Bulbar dysfunction

Introduction

The most common manifestations of bulbar dysfunction in amyotrophic lateral sclerosis (ALS) are impairment of speech and swallowing. Among patients presenting with bulbar symptoms, 93% report problems with speech and 86% complain of trouble swallowing (1). While emotional lability, also referred to as pseudobulbar affect, may occur in association with a number of neurological disorders, it is most common among patients with ALS (2). The early identification of these changes in speech and swallowing is imperative given the negative prognostic implication of bulbar dysfunction (3).

Pathophysiology of bulbar symptoms

Approximately 25% of patients with ALS have bulbar-onset disease (4). For most patients, bulbar symptoms develop later in the disease course (5). Upper motor neuron degeneration manifests as pseudobulbar palsy, characterized by spasticity of the bulbar muscles, a brisk jaw jerk, and pseudobulbar affect. Lower motor neuron signs include tongue atrophy and fasciculations (bulbar palsy). Furthermore, degeneration of the motor neurons in the spinal cord contributes to respiratory muscle weakness, making communication and eating even more difficult (for reviews see (4,6,7)). The revised Amyotrophic Lateral Sclerosis Functional Rating Scale (ALSFRS-R) is one of the most frequently used scales to assess and track bulbar dysfunction (8,9).

Clinical features

Dysarthria

During the early course of the disease, changes in speech may be described as flaccid or spastic. Lower motor neuron involvement causes flaccid dysarthria while damage to the upper motor neurons results in spastic dysarthria (4). Flaccid dysarthria is characterized by a high-pitched voice (hypernasality), imprecise consonant production, and a soft (breathy) voice quality. Spastic dysarthria often manifests as imprecise consonant production and a harsh and monotonic voice quality (10). As ALS progresses, patients usually demonstrate a mixed spastic-flaccid dysarthria, characterized by difficulties saying certain vowels and consonants, slow and effortful speech, imprecise consonant production and hypernasality (for reviews see (9,11)).

Dysphagia

Involvement of the tongue, lips, palate, pharynx, larynx, and muscles of the upper thorax results in difficulties ingesting and transporting the food bolus (6,7,12,13). As a consequence, patients experience problems eating foods that are dry and tough and consuming thin liquids. This can lead to malnutrition, dehydration, chocking, prolonged eating times, and an increased risk of pulmonary infections due to aspiration (14–16). While the progression of dysphagia is extremely variable, problems swallowing saliva and drooling (sialorrhoea) as well as increased reliance on breathing through the mouth rather than through the nose causing dry lips and mouth are characteristic of advanced bulbar dysfunction (7).

Symptomatic and supportive treatment

Dysarthria

The clinical management of dysarthria focuses on preserving speech intelligibility and optimizing communicative interaction with a communication partner. When dysarthria is mild, patients may improve intelligibility by speaking more slowly, using repetition, and employing word substitution with an emphasis on short and simple words, preferably face-to-face (9). Speech and language therapy may be beneficial in improving speech intelligibility through breathing and relaxation exercises designed to optimize articulation and breathing rate (6). Well-developed verbal (e.g. confirming patients' answers to questions) and non-verbal (e.g. hand signals) communicative interaction with communication partners is crucial as dysarthria worsens (9).

Early intervention with augmentative and alternative communication (AAC) systems is recommended before speech intelligibility is severely compromised. Low-tech devices include pencil and paper (Fig. 15.1), an alphabet board, and tailored word or picture cards. High-tech devices such as electronic speech-generating and eye-gaze devices may be implemented, if desired, when patients are no longer able to use low-tech devices due to significant upper limb impairment (6,7,9,11,17).

Dysphagia

Mild dysphagia is usually managed with dietary changes and compensatory methods to ensure safe and effective swallowing (7,18). Foods that have a soft and moist consistency, thickened liquids, and postures that make swallowing safer may be tried initially (6,14–16).

Enteral nutrition is recommended when sufficient food and fluid intake cannot be maintained orally despite compensatory methods. In clinical practice, this is ideally discussed with patients and their caregivers well in advance of need. Percutaneous Endoscopic Gastrostomy (PEG) is the preferred method for administration of enteral tube feeding for most patients at most centres. Respiratory status must be carefully evaluated prior to PEG placement because of the need for sedation. A forced vital capacity of at least 50% of the predicted value is preferred at the time of the procedure (14–16,19).

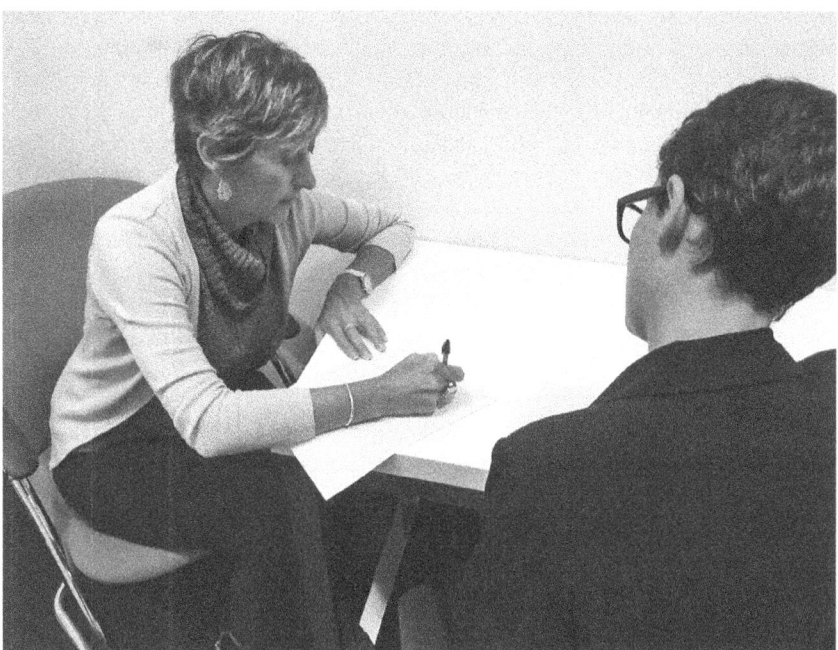

Fig. 15.1 In practice, a combination of communication methods may be used. For example, some patients with dysarthria may prefer to use pen and paper in one-on-one situations and more high-tech devices, such as smartphone voice output apps, in group settings.

Psychological consequences of speech impairment

The loss of the ability to speak can be one of the most distressing aspects of ALS for both patients and their caregivers (20,21). Speech impairment may affect patients' ability to interact effectively in personal, social, and occupational contexts and, consequently, may negatively impact their psychological well-being. Therefore, knowledge of the psychological consequences of speech impairment is fundamental to good clinical practice.

Problems with speech are a major source of psychological distress (22) and poor quality of life (QoL) in ALS (23,24). Early studies showed an association between more severe speech problems and greater anxiety. Interestingly, anxiety was specifically related to the impact of speech impairment on social interaction rather than communication (25). This is consistent with other studies, which suggest that QoL is not determined by physical function alone as psychosocial factors play an important role in maintaining QoL and psychological well-being (26,27). Patients with bulbar onset disease have also been found to present with higher levels of depression early in the course of the disease compared to those with limb-onset disease (28), which may reflect psychological distress related to the loss of ability to speak rather than clinical depression per se.

Being able to communicate enables patients to express their personal identity (7), which forms part of the self-concept and enables continued participation in usual activities and pastimes (29). Similar to that seen in other terminal conditions, being diagnosed with ALS and experiencing worsening disability may compromise the self-concept (how people think about and evaluate themselves) (30). Studies specifically examining the impact of speech impairment on the self-concept in ALS are limited, however, the importance of communication in preserving factors that contribute to beliefs about oneself such as personality (29) and self-efficacy (17,31) can be inferred from the literature.

A compromised self-concept may impact social interaction (30). For example, patients may be worried that their struggles to speak may cause distress for their family and friends. Furthermore, speech problems may make misunderstandings more common. As a consequence, patients and their families and friends may refrain from social interactions (30,32). This is likely to contribute to psychological distress, despair, and loneliness (17). Behavioural disengagement (giving up attempts to cope) has also been shown to be used more frequently by patients with bulbar onset disease (33), which undoubtedly reinforces feelings of hopelessness. Social withdrawal may also reflect the process of preparatory grief, whereby patients start to mourn future losses (30,34,35). For example, grief may be related to the loss of social roles and relationships (29,32) as communication becomes increasingly difficult. The inability to communicate makes the expression of grief even harder for patients (21).

Psychological consequences of swallowing impairment

Dysphagia can negatively affect mood and behaviour. Hillemacher and colleagues identified swallowing problems directly linked to symptoms of depression (36). The extent of dysphagia has also been found to contribute to poor QoL. ALS patients with limb onset disease who reported greater problems swallowing were more likely to perceive their QoL negatively than patients with mild dysphagia (37).

Various aspects of QoL are affected by swallowing problems. Compared to patients with intact swallowing function, patients with dysphagia reported worse QoL with respect to eating duration and desire as well as social life (38). Similarly, da Costa Franceschini and colleagues (37) demonstrated that eating duration and social function were the most affected areas of QoL among patients with limb onset disease. A more recent study showed that QoL was particularly low among ALS patients who aspirate (39). The idea that eating serves a social function may help explain these findings. Problems eating may decrease patients' chances of social interaction, adding to feelings of loneliness and isolation (37,40).

While it is widely acknowledged that the consequences of dysphagia can negatively affect psychosocial functioning in ALS (15,16,41), very few studies have systematically addressed this issue. Korner and colleagues (42) found that fatigue and a sense of demoralization accounted for poor QoL among ALS patients with weight loss, highlighting the importance of effectively managing weight via dietary modifications and/or PEG in this patient population. The psychological sequelae of dysphagia in other neurodegenerative diseases are well known. In Parkinson's disease, patients with swallowing problems reported more symptoms of anxiety and depression compared with those without swallowing problems (43). QoL is also reduced among Parkinson's disease patients with dysphagia, with those with more advanced disease reporting less desire to eat, food choice problems, and extended eating times (44). Perhaps not surprisingly, the swallowing-related QoL domain most affected among Parkinson's disease patients with dysphagia involve mental health and social functioning (45). As such, the psychological consequences of swallowing impairment in ALS warrant further investigation given its high prevalence and potential impact on psychosocial well-being, similar to that seen in other neurodegenerative diseases.

Psychological benefits of enhanced communication

The psychological benefits gained through the use of communication devices are well acknowledged. The use of a touch screen-tablet device early in the course of the disease has been shown to contribute to satisfactory QoL among patients, especially with regards to maintenance of existential and psychological well-being over time (46). High-tech devices, particularly eye tracking devices, also have a beneficial effect on QoL in the advanced stages of the disease (47). Intervention using these high-tech devices has been linked to lower levels of depression and enhanced QoL in ALS (48).

However, the exact mechanisms underlying the beneficial effects of communication devices are unclear. Social isolation and inability to participate in decision-making about clinical care have been proposed as reasons for poorer psychological well-being in patients not receiving a high-tech device intervention (48). This is perhaps related to a reduced sense of self-efficacy, self-esteem, and autonomy among patients not able to use these devices effectively (17,31). The need to feel connected to the community has also been shown to be an important factor that influences the acceptance of devices (49).

Social support is extremely important for coping among patients with bulbar dysfunction. As such, tailoring communication strategies and devices is imperative, especially since successful use of these devices is partly dependent on caregivers' (usually the main communication partner) support and perseverance (29). Indeed, family members' reluctance to assist patients with using communication devices has been associated with delayed AAC acceptance, which could have detrimental psychological consequences (49).

The introduction of communication devices early in the disease course has been shown to enhance caregiver QoL (46). Caregivers of patients using speech-generating devices described their usefulness in preserving patients' roles in the family (29). In more advanced stages of ALS, eye tracking devices alleviated caregiver burden by allowing caregivers to spend more time with other family members and to engage in their own hobbies and interests (47,48).

Having a means to communicate also allowed patients and caregivers to maintain social closeness. Being able to communicate strong emotions not only helped reduce stress, but also contributed towards a good marital relationship (29). The use of AAC devices also helped foster social closeness, preserving a healthy relationship (50). This is perhaps a case of positive benefit finding in the context of a devastating disease. This psychological phenomenon refers to the experience of positive outcomes as a result of adverse life events, such as greater resilience and stronger relationships (51).

Psychological well-being benefits of enhanced nutrition

The importance of interventions to preclude malnutrition and promote QoL is undeniable (15). Enteral nutrition is the most widely investigated intervention for maintaining adequate caloric and fluid intake in ALS (52). Early involvement of a gastroenterologist, speech pathologist, and dietitian regarding gastrostomy tube insertion has been associated with higher rate of use of gastrostomy tubes, perhaps because it provides these clinicians the opportunity to correct inaccurate illness perceptions about the value and implications of a gastrostomy tube (53). ALS patients with limited knowledge about the benefits of gastrostomy tubes for enteral nutrition have been shown to be more likely to defer tube insertion (54). Based on a survey of enteral nutrition practices among clinicians involved in treating patients with ALS, more than half of the clinicians reported that their patients were not adherent to enteral nutrition. Adverse effects such as diarrhoea and increased reliance on caregivers emerged as major factors affecting adherence. Depression and feelings of hopelessness were rarely mentioned as issues influencing adherence (55). This is perhaps not surprising as ALS patients experiencing depression may be reluctant to accept life-prolonging interventions such as gastrostomy in the first place. In another study, ALS patients who continued to find eating pleasurable were shown to be more likely to accept gastrostomy, although the reasons for this were not explored in detail (56).

This brings up the issue of considering patients' psychological status and the psychological and behavioural aspects of medical procedures as potential factors influencing uptake and adherence to interventions in ALS. Education about gastrostomy has been found to be helpful by ALS patients with respect to adjusting to artificial feeding. Furthermore, gastrostomy tube insertion was found to ease ALS patients concerns about eating and weight loss, offsetting gastrostomy-related anxieties that were affecting QoL (57). Indeed ALS patients have been shown to experience improved QoL rather than poorer QoL after feeding tube insertion, contrary to patient and caregiver expectations (42).

Considerations when assessing psychological morbidity in ALS patients with bulbar dysfunction

Cognitive and behavioural change

ALS patients with co-morbid frontotemporal dementia have been shown to be more likely to present with bulbar-onset rather than limb-onset disease. The cognitive profile of these patients was characterized by poor overall performance on tests of fluency (Fig. 15.2) (58), which are considered particularly sensitive to executive dysfunction in ALS (59). Markedly worse deficits on tests of verbal fluency among patients with pseudobulbar palsy compared to patients without pseudobulbar palsy and aged matched controls have also been identified (60). Other cognitive deficits more common in patients with bulbar onset compared to those with limb onset ALS extend to working memory, problem-solving, episodic memory, and visuospatial skills (61). Overall,

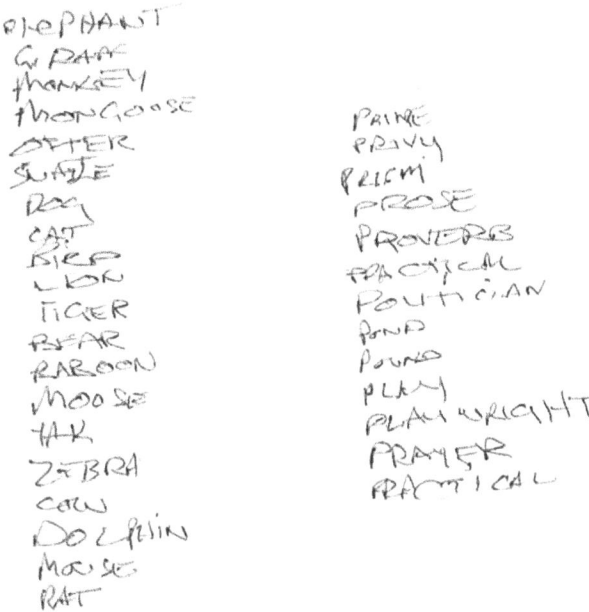

Fig. 15.2 For patients with severe dysarthria, written category (left) and letter (right) fluency tests are administered to assess executive function.

early occurrence and rapid progression of bulbar symptoms, particularly dysarthria are thought to be characteristic of ALS patients with co-morbid dementia (62–65).

Behavioural changes in ALS include lack of empathy, disinhibition, ritualistic behaviours, and apathy (66,67), which by themselves may be mistaken for 'normal' psychological responses to a diagnosis of a terminal illness and progressive disability, or vice versa (35). Changes in behaviour can manifest before classic motor symptoms (68), with marked changes significantly reducing survival time (69), highlighting the importance of assessing behaviour at the outset. Similar to cognitive impairment, behavioural changes may occur more frequently among patients with bulbar symptoms. Studies to date are limited, however, Chio and colleagues identified higher rates of behavioural symptoms, particularly apathy among patients with bulbar dysfunction rather than bulbar onset disease per se (70). Abnormal behaviours such as temper outbursts and delusions have also been observed among bulbar onset patients with cognitive impairment (71).

It seems likely that cognitive and behavioural symptoms among ALS patients with bulbar dysfunction would adversely affect their ability to provide accurate assessments of emotion and QoL and to manage symptomatic and supportive treatment for dysarthria and dysphagia. However, this is largely unexamined in the ALS literature. Indeed, emerging studies have shown that ALS patients with co-morbid frontotemporal dementia were more likely to be non-compliant with gastrostomy and non-invasive positive-pressure ventilation, but this finding was not specific to patients with bulbar dysfunction (65). In other neurodegenerative diseases such as Alzheimer's disease and Parkinson's disease, cognitive and behavioural impairment has been linked to poor treatment engagement and adherence (72–74). In addition to cognitive and behavioural impairment, other factors such as patient and caregiver perceptions about the disease and its treatment, symptom severity, depression, and caregiver burden were implicated in treatment uptake and adherence (72–74). Accordingly, assessment of cognitive and behavioural changes combined with provision of education and support strategies to caregivers regarding possible compliance issues may ultimately help reduce caregiver burden. For more information about cognitive and behavioural changes in ALS, see chapters 8 and 9.

Pseudobulbar affect

The clinical features of pseudobulbar affect are sudden and uncontrollable emotional outbursts, usually crying rather than laughter, occurring in association with spastic dysarthria (2,10). Synonyms for pseudobulbar affect include emotional or affective lability, emotional incontinence, excessive emotionality, pathological laughter, and crying (2).

It is important to differentiate pseudobulbar affect from psychological morbidity. Wicks and colleagues showed that patients and caregivers considered it important to be informed about pseudobulbar affect and cognitive impairment (75). Pseudobulbar affect may be mistaken for emotional distress by patients, caregivers, and also clinicians especially if it is less marked and not easily differentiated from commonly overlapping symptoms such as depression and changes in behaviour.

Pseudobulbar affect may contribute to difficulties with social interaction experienced by patients with bulbar dysfunction. There are increased risks of anxiety and depression with pseudobulbar affect (2). Indeed, patients have been found to experience high levels of psychological distress associated with pseudobulbar affect despite reporting satisfactory QoL (32,76). Pseudobulbar affect has also been associated with increased caregiver distress, which is perhaps related to social uneasiness (77).

Future directions

It is clear that bulbar dysfunction contributes to poor psychological well-being in ALS, however, the full extent of its psychological impact, especially dysphagia, is not yet well understood. Future directions for research include the need to investigate mediating and moderating psychological variables that affect emotional well-being and QoL in patients with dysarthria and dysphagia. This would also assist with identifying psychological factors that may complicate uptake and adherence to interventions for these symptoms. The severity of speaking and swallowing problems needs to be systematically taken into account when assessing the clinical relevance of findings as a certain level of psychological distress may be expected given the progressive nature and negative prognostic implication of bulbar dysfunction. Identification of protective factors such as self-efficacy beliefs and coping strategies associated with better adjustment to bulbar impairment may also contribute towards informing future approaches to psychological treatment.

Conclusions

Patients with ALS develop bulbar dysfunction almost universally, with significant impact on psychological well-being and QoL. The loss of speaking and swallowing ability is one of the most concerning and distressing features of ALS for both patients and their caregivers. Speech and swallowing problems may affect a patient's ability to interact effectively with others, maintain normal activities and interests, and participate in their own care. At the root of these issues is the desire to maintain social closeness, individuality and autonomy, which are factors important to patients' QoL. Interventions to manage problems communicating and swallowing can help patients live with dignity in spite of progressive loss of speech and ability to care for oneself.

References

1. **Chen, A.** and **Garrett, C.G.** (2005) Otolaryngologic presentations of amyotrophic lateral sclerosis. *Otolaryngology—Head And Neck Surgery*, **132**(3), 500–4.

2. **Miller, A., Pratt, H.,** and **Schiffer, R.B.** (2011) Pseudobulbar affect: the spectrum of clinical presentations, etiologies and treatments. *Expert Review of Neurotherapeutics*, **11**(7), 1077–88.

3. **Chio, A., Logroscino, G., Hardiman, O.,** et al. (2009) Prognostic factors in ALS: A critical review. *Amyotrophic Lateral Sclerosis*, **10**(5–6), 310–23.

4. **Kiernan, M.C., Vucic, S., Cheah, B.C.,** et al. (2011) Amyotrophic lateral sclerosis. *Lancet*, **377**(9769), 942–55.

5. **Fujimura-Kiyono, C., Kimura, F., Ishida, S.,** et al. (2011) Onset and spreading patterns of lower motor neuron involvements predict survival in sporadic amyotrophic lateral sclerosis. *Journal of Neurology, Neurosurgery, and Psychiatry*, **82**(11), 1244–9.

6. **Kuhnlein, P., Gdynia, H.J., Sperfeld, A.D.,** et al. (2008) Diagnosis and treatment of bulbar symptoms in amyotrophic lateral sclerosis. *Nature Clinical Practice Neurology*, **4**(7), 366–74.

7. **Hillel, A.D.** and **Miller, R.** (1989) Bulbar amyotrophic lateral sclerosis: Patterns of progression and clinical management. *Head & Neck*, **11**(1), 51–9.

8. **Cedarbaum, J.M., Stambler, N., Malta, E.,** et al. (1999) The ALSFRS-R: a revised ALS functional rating scale that incorporates assessments of respiratory function. BDNF ALS Study Group (Phase III). *Journal of the Neurological Sciences*, **169**(1–2), 13–21.

9. **Tomik, B.** and **Guiloff, R.J.** (2010) Dysarthria in amyotrophic lateral sclerosis: A review. *Amyotrophic Lateral Sclerosis*, **11**(1–2), 4–15.

10. **Freed, D.** (2011) *Motor Speech Disorders: Diagnosis & Treatment*, 2 edn. New York, NY: Cengage Learning.

11. **Hanson, E.K.Y.K.** and **Britton, D.** (2011) Dysarthria in amyotrophic lateral sclerosis: A systematic review of characteristics, speech treatment, and augmentative and alternative communication options. *Journal of Medical Speech-Language Pathology*, **19**(3), 12–30.

12. **Higo, R., Tayama, N.,** and **Nito, T.** (2004) Longitudinal analysis of progression of dysphagia in amyotrophic lateral sclerosis. *Auris, Nasus, Larynx*, **31**(3), 247–54.

13. **Kawai, S., Tsukuda, M., Mochimatsu, I.,** et al. (2003) A study of the early stage of Dysphagia in amyotrophic lateral sclerosis. *Dysphagia*, **18**(1), 1–8.

14. **Stavroulakis, T., Walsh, T., Shaw, P.J., McDermott, C.J.,** and **Progas, S.** (2013) Gastrostomy use in motor neurone disease (MND): A review, meta-analysis and survey

of current practice. *Amyotrophic Lateral Sclerosis & Frontotemporal Degeneration*, **14**(2), 96–104.

15. **Greenwood, D.I.** (2013) Nutrition management of amyotrophic lateral sclerosis. *Nutrition in Clinical Practice*, **28**(3), 392–9.

16. **Muscaritoli, M., Kushta, I., Molfino, A., Inghilleri, M., Sabatelli, M., and Rossi Fanelli, F.** (2012) Nutritional and metabolic support in patients with amyotrophic lateral sclerosis. *Nutrition*, **28**(10), 959–66.

17. **Brownlee, A. and Palovcak, M.** (2007) The role of augmentative communication devices in the medical management of ALS. *NeuroRehabilitation*, **22**(6), 445–50.

18. **Hardiman, O., van den Berg, L.H., and Kiernan, M.C.** (2011) Clinical diagnosis and management of amyotrophic lateral sclerosis. *Nature Reviews Neurology*, **7**(11), 639–49.

19. **Miller, R.G., Rosenberg, J.A., Gelinas, D.F.,** et al. (1999) Practice parameter: The care of the patient with amyotrophic lateral sclerosis (an evidence-based review): report of the Quality Standards Subcommittee of the American Academy of Neurology: ALS Practice Parameters Task Force. *Neurology*, **52**(7), 1311–23.

20. **Hecht, M., Hillemacher, T., Grasel, E.,** et al. (2002) Subjective experience and coping in ALS. *Amyotrophic Lateral Sclerosis and Other Motor Neuron Disorders*, **3**(4), 225–31.

21. **Centers L.** (2001) Beyond denial and despair: ALS and our heroic potential for hope. *Journal of Palliative Care*, **17**(4)259–64.

22. **Goldstein, L.H., Atkins, L., Landau, S., Brown, R.G., and Leigh, P.N.** (2006) Longitudinal predictors of psychological distress and self-esteem in people with ALS. *Neurology*, **67**(9), 1652–8.

23. **Lule, D., Hacker, S., Ludolph, A., Birbaumer, N., and Kubler, A.** (2008) Depression and quality of life in patients with amyotrophic lateral sclerosis. *Deutsches Arzteblatt International*, **105**(23), 397–403.

24. **Felgoise, S.H., Zaccheo, V., Duff, J., and Simmons, Z.** (2016) Verbal communication impacts quality of life in patients with amyotrophic lateral sclerosis. *Amyotrophic Lateral Sclerosis & Frontotemporal Degeneration*, **17**(3–4), 179–83.

25. **Hogg, K.E., Goldstein, L.H., and Leigh, P.N.** (1994) The psychological impact of motor neurone disease. *Psychological Medicine*, **24**(3), 625–32.

26. **Simmons, Z., Bremer, B.A., Robbins, R.A., Walsh, S.M., and Fischer, S.** (2000) Quality of life in ALS depends on factors other than strength and physical function. *Neurology*, **55**(3), 388–92.

27. **Ganzini, L., Johnston, W.S., and Hoffman, W.F.** (2006) Correlates of suffering in amyotrophic lateral sclerosis. *Neurology*, **52**(7), 1434–40.

28. **Rodriguez de Rivera, F.J., Oreja Guevara, C., Sanz Gallego, I.,** et al. (2011) Outcome of patients with amyotrophic lateral sclerosis attending in a multidisciplinary care unit. *Neurologia*, **26**(8), 455–60.

29. **McKelvey, M., Evans, D.L., Kawai, N, and Beukelman, D.** (2012) Communication styles of persons with ALS as recounted by surviving partners. *Augmentative and Alternative Communication*, **28**(4), 232–42.

30. **Taylor, S.E.** (ed.) (2006) Psychological Issues in Advancing and Terminal Illness, 6th edn. New York, NY: McGraw-Hill Higher Education.

31. **Nijboer, F., Sellers, E.W., Mellinger, J.,** et al. (2008) A P300-based brain-computer interface for people with amyotrophic lateral sclerosis. *Clinical Neurophysiology*, **119**(8), 1909–16.

32. Nelson, N.D., Trail, M., Van, J.N., Appel, S.H., and Lai, E.C. (2003) Quality of life in patients with amyotrophic lateral sclerosis: Perceptions, coping resources, and illness characteristics. *Journal of Palliative Medicine*, **6**(3), 417–24.

33. Montel, S., Albertini, L., and Spitz, E. (2012) Coping strategies in relation to quality of life in amyotrophic lateral sclerosis. *Muscle & Nerve*, **45**(1), 131–4.

34. Kubler-Ross E. (1969) *On Death and Dying*. New York, NY: Macmillan.

35. Caga, J., Ramsey, E., Hogden, A., Mioshi, E., and Kiernan, M.C. (2015) A longer diagnostic interval is a risk for depression in amyotrophic lateral sclerosis. *Palliative & Supportive Care*, **13**(4), 1019–24.

36. Hillemacher, T., Grassel, E., Tigges, S., et al. (2004) Depression and bulbar involvement in amyotrophic lateral sclerosis. *Amyotrophic Lateral Sclerosis and Other Motor Neuron Disorders*, **5**(4), 245–9.

37. da Costa Franceschini, A. and Mourao, L.F. (2015) Dysarthria and dysphagia in Amyotrophic Lateral Sclerosis with spinal onset: A study of quality of life related to swallowing. *NeuroRehabilitation*, **36**(1), 127–34.

38. Paris, G., Martinaud, O., Petit, A., et al. (2013) Oropharyngeal dysphagia in amyotrophic lateral sclerosis alters quality of life. *Journal of Oral Rehabilitation*, **40**(3), 199–204.

39. Tabor, L., Gaziano, J., Watts, S., Robison, R., and Plowman, E.K. (2016) Defining Swallowing-Related Quality of Life Profiles in Individuals with Amyotrophic Lateral Sclerosis. *Dysphagia*, **31**(3), 376–82.

40. Ekberg, O., Hamdy, S., Woisard, V., Wuttge-Hannig, A., and Ortega, P. (2002) Social and psychological burden of dysphagia: Its impact on diagnosis and treatment. *Dysphagia*, **17**(2), 139–46.

41. Rosenfeld, J. and Ellis, A. (2008) Nutrition and dietary supplements in motor neuron disease. *Physical Medicine and Rehabilitation Clinics of North America*, **19**(3), 573–89.

42. Korner S, Hendricks M, Kollewe K, et al. (2013) Weight loss, dysphagia and supplement intake in patients with amyotrophic lateral sclerosis (ALS): Impact on quality of life and therapeutic options. *BMC Neurology*, **13**, 84.

43. Manor, Y., Balas, M., Giladi, N., Mootanah, R., and Cohen, J.T. (2009) Anxiety, depression and swallowing disorders in patients with Parkinson's disease. *Parkinsonism & Related Disorders*, **15**(6), 453–6.

44. Leow, L.P., Huckabee, M.L., Anderson, T., and Beckert, L. (2010) The impact of dysphagia on quality of life in ageing and Parkinson's disease as measured by the swallowing quality of life (SWAL-QOL) questionnaire. *Dysphagia*, **25**(3), 216–20.

45. Plowman-Prine, E.K., Sapienza, C.M., Okun, M.S., et al. (2009) The relationship between quality of life and swallowing in Parkinson's disease. *Movement Disorders*, **24**(9), 1352–8.

46. Londral, A., Pinto, A., Pinto, S., Azevedo, L., and De Carvalho, M. (2015) Quality of life in amyotrophic lateral sclerosis patients and caregivers: Impact of assistive communication from early stages. *Muscle & Nerve*, **52**(6), 933–41.

47. Caligari, M., Godi, M., Guglielmetti, S., Franchignoni, F., and Nardone, A. (2013) Eye tracking communication devices in amyotrophic lateral sclerosis: Impact on disability and quality of life. *Amyotrophic Lateral Sclerosis & Frontotemporal Degeneration*, **14**(7–8), 546–52.

48. Hwang, C.S., Weng, H.H., Wang, L.F., Tsai, C.H., and Chang, H.T. (2014) An eye-tracking assistive device improves the quality of life for ALS patients and reduces the caregivers' burden. *Journal of Motor Behavior*, **46**(4), 233–8.

49. **Ball, L.J.B.D.** and **Pattee, G.L.** (2004) Acceptance of augmentative and alternative communication technology by persons with amyotrophic lateral sclerosis. *Augmentative and Alternative Communication*, **20**(2), 113–22.

50. **Fried-Oken, M., Fox, L., Rau, M.T.,** et al. (2006) Purposes of AAC device use for persons with ALS as reported by caregivers. *Augmentative and Alternative Communication*, **22**(3), 209–21.

51. **Tennen, H.** and **Affleck, G.** (2002) Benefit-finding and benefit-reminding. In: Snyder, C.R. and Lopez, S.J. (ed.) *Handbook of Positive Psychology*, pp. 584–97. New York, NY, Oxford University Press.

52. **Katzberg, H.D.** and **Benatar, M.** (2011) Enteral tube feeding for amyotrophic lateral sclerosis/motor neuron disease. *Cochrane Database of Systematic Reviews*, (1), CD004030.

53. **Zhang, L., Sanders, L.,** and **Fraser, R.J.** (2012) Nutritional support teams increase percutaneous endoscopic gastrostomy uptake in motor neuron disease. *World Journal of Gastroenterology*, **18**(44), 6461–7; discussion, p. 6.

54. **Stavroulakis, T., Baird, W.O., Baxter, S.K., Walsh, T., Shaw, P.J.,** and **McDermott, C.J.** (2014) Factors influencing decision-making in relation to timing of gastrostomy insertion in patients with motor neurone disease. *BMJ Supportive & Palliative Care*, **4**(1), 57–63.

55. **Zhang, M., Hubbard, J., Rudnicki, S.A.,** et al. (2013) Survey of current enteral nutrition practices in treatment of amyotrophic lateral sclerosis. *e-SPEN Journal*, **8**(1), e25–e8.

56. **Johnson, J., Leigh, P.N., Shaw, C.E., Ellis, C., Burman, R.,** and **Al-Chalabi, A.** (2012) Eating-derived pleasure in amyotrophic lateral sclerosis as a predictor of non-oral feeding. *Amyotrophic Lateral Sclerosis*, **13**(6), 555–9.

57. **Stavroulakis, T., Baird, W.O., Baxter, S.K., Walsh, T., Shaw, P.J.,** and **McDermott, C.J.** (2016) The impact of gastrostomy in motor neurone disease: Challenges and benefits from a patient and carer perspective. *BMJ Supportive & Palliative Care*, **6**(1), 52–9.

58. **Lomen-Hoerth, C., Murphy, J., Langmore, S., Kramer, J.H., Olney, R.K.,** and **Miller B.** (2003) Are amyotrophic lateral sclerosis patients cognitively normal? *Neurology*, **60**(7), 1094–7.

59. **Abrahams, S., Leigh, P.N., Harvey, A., Vythelingum, G.N., Grise, D.,** and **Goldstein, L.H.** (2000) Verbal fluency and executive dysfunction in amyotrophic lateral sclerosis (ALS). *Neuropsychologia*, **38**(6), 734–47.

60. **Abrahams, S, Goldstein, L.H., Al-Chalabi, A.,** et al. (1997) Relation between cognitive dysfunction and pseudobulbar palsy in amyotrophic lateral sclerosis. *Journal of Neurology, Neurosurgery, and Psychiatry*, **62**(5), 464–72.

61. **Strong, M.J., Grace, G.M., Orange, J.B., Leeper, H.A., Menon, R.S.,** and **Aere, C.** (1999) A prospective study of cognitive impairment in ALS. *Neurology*, **53**(8), 1665–70.

62. **Cavalleri, F.** and **De Renzi, E.** (1994) Amyotrophic lateral sclerosis with dementia. *Acta Neurologica Scandinavica*, **89**(5), 391–4.

63. **Caselli, R.J., Windebank, A.J., Petersen, R.C.,** et al. (1993) Rapidly progressive aphasic dementia and motor neuron disease. *Annals of Neurology*, **33**(2), 200–7.

64. **Ishihara, K., Araki, S., Ihori, N.,** et al. (2013) Pseudobulbar dysarthria in the initial stage of motor neuron disease with dementia: a clinicopathological report of two autopsied cases. *European Neurology*, **69**(5), 270–4.

65. **Olney RK, Murphy J, Forshew D,** et al. (2005) The effects of executive and behavioral dysfunction on the course of ALS. *Neurology*, **65**(11), 1774–7.

66. Raaphorst, J., Beeldman, E., De Visser, M., De Haan, R.J., and Schmand, B. (2012) A systematic review of behavioural changes in motor neuron disease. *Amyotrophic Lateral Sclerosis*, **13**(6), 493–501.

67. Mioshi, E., Hsieh, S., Caga, J., et al. (2014) A novel tool to detect behavioural symptoms in ALS. *Amyotrophic Lateral Sclerosis & Frontotemporal Degeneration*, **15**(3–4), 298–304.

68. Mioshi, E., Caga, J., Lillo, P., et al. (2014) Neuropsychiatric changes precede classic motor symptoms in ALS and do not affect survival. *Neurology*, **82**(2), 149–55.

69. Caga, J., Turner, M.R., Hsieh, S., et al. (2016) Apathy is associated with poor prognosis in amyotrophic lateral sclerosis. *European Journal of Neurology*, **23**(5), 891–7.

70. Chio, A., Vignola, A., Mastro, E., et al. (2010) Neurobehavioral symptoms in ALS are negatively related to caregivers' burden and quality of life. *European Journal of Neurology*, **17**(10), 1298–303.

71. Portet, F., Cadilhac, C., Touchon, J., and Camu, W. (2001) Cognitive impairment in motor neuron disease with bulbar onset. *Amyotrophic Lateral Sclerosis and Other Motor Neuron Disorders*, **2**(1), 23–9.

72. Brady, R. and Weinman, J. (2013) Adherence to cholinesterase inhibitors in Alzheimer's disease: a review. *Dementia and Geriatric Cognitive Disorders*, **35**(5–6), 351–63.

73. Choi, J. and Twamley, E.W. (2013) Cognitive rehabilitation therapies for Alzheimer's disease: a review of methods to improve treatment engagement and self-efficacy. *Neuropsychology Review*, **23**(1), 48–62.

74. Daley, D.J., Myint, P.K., Gray, R.J., and Deane, K.H. (2012) Systematic review on factors associated with medication non-adherence in Parkinson's disease. *Parkinsonism & Related Disorders*, **18**(10), 1053–61.

75. Wicks, P. and Frost, J. (2008) ALS patients request more information about cognitive symptoms. *European Journal of Neurology*, **15**(5), 497–500.

76. Palmieri, A., Abrahams, S., Soraru, G., et al. (2009) Emotional Lability in MND: Relationship to cognition and psychopathology and impact on caregivers. *Journal of the Neurological Sciences*, **278**(1–2), 16–20.

77. Goldstein, L.H., Atkins, L., Landau, S., Brown, R., and Leigh, P.N. (2006) Predictors of psychological distress in carers of people with amyotrophic lateral sclerosis: A longitudinal study. *Psychological Medicine*, **36**(6), 865–75.

Chapter 16

ALS caregiver quality of life and psychological implications

Peggy Z. Shipley

Introduction

Caregiver general characteristics

Caregiving for someone with a terminal disease can include formal care, which is commonly done by health care professionals, and informal care, which is performed by unpaid non-professionals (1,2). In patients with amyotrophic lateral sclerosis (ALS) this informal care is most commonly performed by a family member (3–5).

The majority of informal family caregivers are women, but demographic and health-trends research has predicted an increased number of male caregivers in the future (6). The overall number of adult family caregivers actively providing care is expected to increase due to the ageing of the US population and improved survivorship rates for advanced chronic conditions (5–8) yet these caregiving duties can come at significant physical and mental cost for family caregivers. For example, spousal family caregivers are 63% more likely to die within a 4-year time frame than non-caregivers (9).

ALS family caregiver features

Informal family caregiving often extends over months or years, beginning with the ALS diagnosis and continuing through the disease progression until the death of their loved one (2,10,11). During this time, family caregivers must perform many activities that encompass both physical and emotional care (5,7), and that commonly increase as the disease progresses (12–14).

Informal caregivers may experience physical, financial, psychological, and spiritual distress (15–19). This distress often leads to increased mortality rates among informal caregivers (20). Because of these risks, informal caregivers should not be seen by health care providers as solely co-providers of care to their loved one, but should be examined for their unique needs as care recipients as well (21).

Many ALS family caregivers tend to focus solely on the needs of their dying loved one to the exclusion of their own physical or mental needs (22,23). This is due to the caregiver's own perception of not seeing themselves as being a recipient of care and typically interactions with health care providers fail to change this caregiver perception (24).

The care of a family member living with ALS is often associated with a particularly intensive caregiving experience and recognition that the toll on these family caregivers has increased (25,26). With ALS, as the disease progresses, the amount and intensity of the family caregiving experience increases as well. It is estimated that ALS caregivers spend an average of 11 hours per day in caregiving, but this time increases as the final stages of the disease approach (27).

As ALS progresses, family caregivers assume more complex caregiving roles and a need for round the clock care often develops toward the end of the illness trajectory (28). This caregiving occurs largely away from a formal medical setting, instead taking place in the community, where family members assume most of the responsibility for the care of these ALS patients (29).

Financial concerns for ALS caregivers are great due to the many out-of-pocket costs associated with caring for their loved ones (30). The cost of maintaining the patient's QoL and autonomy in the home setting for as long as possible often demands expensive equipment and home renovation. Although the exact financial cost is debated and some of these items can be covered by insurance, out of pocket expenses to caregivers and patients can climb to thousands of dollars per year (31). Even with financial help from support and advocacy organizations, this can contribute to overwhelming financial burdens for both caregiver and the ALS patient they care for (32). Often, this financial strain can result from the remodelling of homes to meet the physical demands of the illness, and the selling or downsizing of family homes can occur, especially if the ALS patient was the main breadwinner for the family (30). Also, many family caregivers need to dramatically reduce their job hours or stop working outside the home entirely as their caregiving duties increase during the progression of the disease (30). In addition, ALS family caregivers provide the majority of support and play a pivotal role in clinical decision-making for their loved one with ALS (33).

ALS caregiving, quality of life, and mental health

By far, the largest category of research in ALS caregiving has been QoL for ALS family caregivers, either as the sole focus of the research, or compared with QoL in the patients for whom they care. It has also been shown that there is a strong concordance between patient and caregiver distress, and that providing attention to the ALS caregiver's mental health may well decrease the patient's distress (30). In other words, the well-being of caregivers can impact the well-being of their loved one with ALS.

The health status of an ALS patient can have a significant impact on the health of the family caregiver, and it has been shown that ALS family caregivers have a poorer health status than the general population (34). Specifically, ALS family caregiver physical health status is negatively impacted by the ALS patients' physical limitations as the disease progresses. This is due to the increased physical demands placed upon the family caregiver as the physical limitations of the ALS patients increase. Greater negative emotional reactions in patients also corresponded with greater emotional demands being placed on the caregivers. In addition, caregiver burden, anxiety, and somatic expressions of depression are positively related to the ALS patient's loss of physical function (34).

Anxiety has a very powerful negative impact on a family caregiver's QoL because as the ALS disease progresses, the family caregiver has less time to adjust to the multitude of caregiving changes demanded by the disease progression. This causes psychological, physical, and emotional changes in the caregivers. In addition, the increasing financial, emotional, and physical caregiving strains (35), and the ongoing need to continuously adapt to the ALS disease presentation in their loved one, can lead to increased anxiety. In addition, these demands can result in increased caregiver burden and depression (36).

Researchers have examined caregiver reactions to the process of caregiving. Many experience symptoms of severe depression and substantial drop in self-esteem. To examine this phenomenon, stress process models have been utilized (37–39). This research has focused on identifying risk factors for caregivers, as well as exploring theoretical frameworks to provide targeted caregiving interventions. These stress process models have examined both primary stressors for caregivers and stressors that arise directly from caregiving for the patient, as well as secondary stressors, such as lack of social support/interaction and declining caregiver health. The Stress Process Model has been applied to research on caregiver of cancer patients at the end of life (18) and researchers have developed a theoretical model based on their findings. Depression has also been shown to be more likely in caregivers who feel less satisfied in their caregiving role, and in those who find little meaning in the experience of caregiving (40–42).

The use of complementary and alternative therapies (as discussed in Chapter 5 by Pagnini and Palmieri) to treat anxiety and depression has shown to be very helpful, especially in those individuals who experience panic attacks and severe depression (43). This could have implications for ALS family caregivers as most, at some point, say depression and anxiety over their loved one are concerns. In addition, most patients who receive treatment from a mental health professional also practice complementary and alternative therapies in addition to therapeutic medication administration (43). Inquiries by health care professionals to ALS family caregivers about the utilization of complementary and alternative therapies could maximize the usefulness of therapeutic measures directed to relieve the anxiety and depression commonly seen in this caregiving population.

Quality of life research has also focused on separating the needs of patients from those of family caregivers. One of the few qualitative inquiries comparing perception and experiences of ALS patients and their caregivers found that both should be viewed as having their own needs and preferences as related to the disease (44). Perceptions of needs, as well as how the ALS disease is viewed, judged, evaluated, and processed, greatly differ between patients and their caregivers. Also, the need for caregivers to have someone to confide in and give them support is important.

Passage of time does not appear to impact QoL in ALS patients, but caregivers' overall psychological well-being and QoL decline with the progression of the ALS disease (36). This could be due to the accumulation of stress and fatigue that results as the disease progresses and the caregiving demands increase. An additional contributing factor may be the caregiver's perception of a lack of leisure time as a result of their caregiving duties. This lack of being able to participate in activities with friends, family, or even the ability to leave the home can have significant impact on the caregiver (46,47). Even though most ALS caregivers do not believe their loved one's requests are unreasonable, some caregivers are very much challenged by their caregiving duties and never truly reach a successful level of adaptation to their caregiving role (47). Lastly, negative social support and caregiver satisfaction with family and social relationships can be related to psychological distress in ALS caregivers (48).

ALS caregiving and burden

The concept of burden has also been explored in the ALS caregiving literature due to the unique demands the disease places on both patients and caregivers. The two components that appear to impact ALS caregiver burden are physical and emotional health, and personal and social restrictions (48). Some research has shown that the burden of care on the ALS family caregiver increases as the functional impairment of the ALS patient increases (49). Somewhat surprisingly, the addition of formal paid caregivers to the home does not always decrease the burden of care of the family caregiver. This is most probably because the home care given by paid caregivers is often inadequate and occurs too late in the ALS disease trajectory to relieve the amount of burden in caring for their loved one by the family caregiver (44).

ALS patients appear to recognize the burden that ALS places on their family caregivers, however this perception appears to be different from what is experienced by their family caregivers (50,51). Also, the ALS patient's degree of decline is directly related to caregiver burden, anxiety, and depression, and the increased caregiver burden is exhibited through a higher level of anxiety and depressive symptoms (26). Other research has revealed that caregiver burden is positively correlated with that family caregiver's level of depression and their own perception of their QoL, and that, in contrast to some other chronic diseases, caregiver burden increases as the patient's disability worsens (46).

With caregivers, perceived burden of caregiving is significantly associated with finding positive meaning in the caregiving experience. For some, caregiver burden can be perceived as being excessive (47). A significant relationship was found between caregiver and patient distress, which suggests the importance of paying attention to the mental health needs of the caregiver and how it might impact patient distress (36).

ALS caregiving experience

Delayed diagnosis and knowing something is wrong

A delay in the diagnosis of ALS can be common especially if a family physician or neurologist does not recognize the symptoms presented as indicative of ALS (52). Delay in diagnosis can also occur if the neurologist does not make a prompt referral to a neurologist who specializes in ALS diagnosis and treatment. One study showed that 75% of the ALS family caregivers experienced delays in the diagnosis of ALS in their loved one, even though the affected individuals were showing symptoms that something was physically wrong an average 2 years prior to their ALS diagnosis (53). This was due to the patients and their caregivers dismissing commonly overlooked motor difficulties, such as tripping, hand weakness, or dropping of common objects such as pens or pencils, which in turn led to delays in seeking medical evaluations for these issues. In addition, unnecessary surgeries were performed based on a misdiagnosis of their loved one's symptoms. This ALS diagnosis delay substantiates other research findings that an ALS diagnosis occurs an average of 9–11 months after symptoms first appear (32).

Caregiver role adaptation

Caring for a loved one with ALS requires many adaptations from their family caregivers. Changing roles in the family, uncertainty about being alone after the death of their loved one, uncertainty about treatment plans, and financial concerns imposed on the family have been identified as important to the ALS family caregiver (55). Financial concerns are particularly difficult as most ALS family caregivers need to decrease their working hours as the ALS disease progresses or even relocate to more affordable housing as the financial burdens of caregiving increase. The loss of privacy due to the need for outside support as caregiving demands increase, as well as changes in the marital partnership role, and the sexual relationship between ALS patient and spouse are also adaptations many family caregivers face (53).

Future planning

From the initial diagnosis of ALS, all family caregivers know that the disease is fatal. In addition, ALS family caregivers are aware that plans, such as advanced directives and living wills for their loved one need to be made, if not now, then in the future (53). Planning for the future is often an important caregiving role and family caregivers deal with planning in different ways. Some prefer to plan ahead for the anticipated future manifestations of the disease in their loved ones, while others like to deal with things as they happen. Regardless of how they preferred to plan for the future, ALS family caregivers are aware of the end point of their loved one's ALS diagnosis (53). In addition, these family caregivers try to 'seek normal' (i.e. dependable patterns in everyday life) in the midst of whatever challenges they face as caregivers for their loved ones (55,56).

Caregiver main challenges

Caregiver obstacles have been described as situations that make it more difficult for ALS family caregivers to perform their caregiving role. These can be 'speed bumps' (i.e. each new symptom experienced in the ALS disease trajectory) or can be caused by the ALS patient him/herself (53). For many ALS caregivers, homes need to be transformed into hospital-like settings and this change often stresses the entire family system in that household. If the patient has been the primary wage earner for that family, financial concerns and anxiety levels may be high (30). As care levels increase, family caregivers experience frequent mental and physical exhaustion. These factors create considerable stress on the caregiver and patient alike. In fact, this stress can be so great that patients may actually start to wish they were dead, and family caregivers may wish that the patient were dead as well. These feelings can lead to guilt-ridden behaviour and feelings of hostility by both patients and family caregivers toward one another (57).

Family caregivers show multiple ways of dealing with these obstacles, including relying on written materials from ALS support and advocacy organizations or the ALS clinical care team, support from friends and family, prayer, respite, and hospice resources. Regardless of the strategy they choose, ALS family caregivers utilize varying forms of family or social support depending on where their loved one is in relation to the expected death trajectory and the current symptoms present (56).

Caregiver support, benefits, and burdens

Although social and family support is necessary for the caregiving role, support can have a negative impact and produce increased stress on the family caregiver (58). This is due mainly to the fear of becoming indebted to the supporter, having their freedom restricted, or perceiving the support as a blow to their self-esteem because of perceived inability to independently care for their loved one (58,59). Many caregivers struggle, at least when their loved one is first diagnosed with ALS, to ask for help and many try to do as much of the caregiving on their own as possible before asking for additional support (53).

Respite for the caregiver

Caregiver respite time is essential because it provides the ALS caregiver with the opportunity to devise a plan of care for themselves, a need which is commonly overlooked (60). This interval of rest or relief provides the ALS caregiver with a much-needed break from the physical, emotional, or mental caregiving role, and can involve just a few hours a day or days at a time. By experiencing respite self-care time, many caregivers find that quality of life can be improved for themselves and ALS patients alike by presenting a respite or break from the normal everyday responsibilities of ALS disease care, which can take a deep toll on the ALS family caregiver (61). In order for caregiver respite to take place, ALS family caregivers usually need to arrange for support in providing care for their loved one while the respite takes place. Knowing that their loved one is safe while they take respite time is a primary concern for the ALS family caregiver (53). Commonly described respite activities include going shopping, spending time reading or listening to/performing music, being out in nature, participating in hobbies, being with friends, and spending time with family members other than their ALS loved one. Regardless of the type of respite chosen, having 'downtime' from their caregiving role is important to the physical and emotional health of the ALS family caregiver.

Role of family, friends, and health care professionals in support

ALS family caregivers receive support in their caregiving roles from family, friends, community, church, and health care professionals (53). The amount of support varies depending on the progression of their loved one's ALS and the caregiver's willingness to seek and accept support, but support from others helps ALS family caregivers in learning about the disease, planning for the future, and performing their daily caregiving roles. The resources and support systems that a family caregiver has in place can dramatically decrease their burden (62). If a family caregiver does not have access to support systems, they can experience loneliness and decreased QoL. It is essential, especially with the growing dependent older population and the rise in chronic illnesses, that social and personal resources are more readily accessible for family caregivers (63). In addition, it is important for the health care provider to remember that targeting the health of the caregiver also offers the health care provider another mechanism to optimize the quality of life for their patient.

Predictors of caregiver distress

One predictor of caregiver distress involves the focus of others, including the health care professional, which commonly is directed toward the ALS patient and not the ALS family caregiver. Many ALS family caregivers found that when their loved one was initially diagnosed with ALS, friends and family would ask about their loved one, as well as the family caregiver, but as the disease progressed, the focus shifted to only the ALS patient (53). The physical and emotional strain to the family caregiver of providing care to an ALS loved one has been documented (25,27), and the importance for family caregivers to be seen not only as co-providers of care to their loved one, but also co-recipients of care, due to the equal importance of the family caregiver's physical/mental needs, has been demonstrated (56). In particular, the environment of care, including a focus of care on the family caregiver, can have a dramatic effect on the caregiving experiences of family caregivers of loved ones with life-limiting illnesses.

Another predictor of caregiver distress involves the descendants of an ALS patient. Familial forms of ALS (i.e. those in which the patient has a history of ALS in the family) account for only about 10% of all ALS cases (61). However, in those families, the distress and anxiety for a son or daughter of a familial ALS patient can be significant (61). The person they are caring for is faced with a decision about whether to undergo genetic testing, the family caregiver (who is at risk for inheriting the deleterious mutation) must have a discussion with the affected individual about whether such information would be shared with them, and the family caregiver must also decide whether they do or do not want to know whether they are carrying a genetic mutation for a disease for which there is no effective treatment. Beyond this, even when ALS is known to be familial, the causal mutation can be identified only 60–70% of the time (61,64,65). Adding to the distress over FALS, the cost of genetic testing may not be covered by health insurance (61).

Interventions to support caregivers

Caregiver assessment as intervention

Because most ALS family caregivers willingly assume the role of being a caregiver to their loved one, and this choice is undertaken out of love and commitment, assessing caregiver physical and mental health should be a primary concern for health care professionals (61). This is especially important because over time, caregiving will exert an enormous emotional toll, and will commonly impact the caregiver's own psychological and physical health, which will then compromise their ability to provide care to their loved one with ALS. Because ALS family caregivers will overlook their own basic needs of adequate food, rest, exercise, and respite, it is important for health care providers to make sure that the family caregiver's basic needs are met.

Assessing these basic needs can be done when the family caregivers accompany their loved one to the ALS multidisciplinary clinic. In addition, it is essential that family caregivers receive regular health check-ups through their primary care health provider, although many family caregivers are reluctant to make their own health a priority when providing care to their loved one (66). In fact, health professional's lack of attention to family caregivers has proved to be a serious gap in health care delivery even though researchers for the past 20 years have documented the potential hazards that accompany family caregiving (66,67). Often family caregivers are the 'hidden figures' in the room, where focus is primarily on the patient alone. Furthermore, assessing family caregivers for signs of depression, role strain, powerlessness, guilt, or grief can be useful in initiating care plans, assessments, and interventions that will help meet the need of these lay caregivers (66,67).

One study (68) administered a Caregiver Needs Assessment questionnaire to 27 ALS caregivers during their loved ones' disease trajectory over the course of the illness and showed that ALS family caregivers need to be assessed by health care providers with respect to preparing for their futures. This study found that ALS family caregivers needs are high, and that family caregivers expressed the need to be educated and kept up to date on treatments, and involved in any decision making that involves their loved one. In addition, health care professionals need to plan psychological support for each caregiver based on his/her individual needs by completing a careful evaluation based on that caregiver's own capacity to meet the difficult needs of their caregiving role. This family caregiver assessment should be done on an ongoing basis with each ALS clinical visit or primary care contact throughout the disease trajectory.

The assessment of family caregivers can be complicated by the fact that they will rarely ask for any personal help or assistance in providing support for their loved one; instead they will be commonly focused on how to perform the demanding physical aspects of their caregiving, as well as how to improve the sharing of information with health care providers. Another factor for health care providers to consider is that especially during the first year of caregiving, family caregivers expressed the need for more emotional and social support (68), a need that primary care providers and members of the ALS multidisciplinary team can support.

Providing education and resources

The primary resources for ALS family caregivers in the USA are the ALS multidisciplinary clinical team, the ALS association (61), and the Muscular Dystrophy Association (69). These three resources provide written, verbal, digital, and taped resources for family caregivers and patients covering the entire disease trajectory. In the UK, in addition to multidisciplinary clinics, the Motor Neurone Disease Association (70) plays a large role, and other countries have a variety of organizations serving similar functions, many of whom are members of the International Alliance of ALS/MND Associations (71).

Seeking a new normal

As ALS family caregivers journey with their loved ones through the disease trajectory, they encounter many challenges through phases and transitions in their caregiving as the disease progresses. This causes family caregivers to experience many phases where the 'steady state' of their caregiving is no longer present and some new aspect of the disease causes the caregivers to adapt their caregiving activities to meet the latest challenge. This basic social process has been called 'seeking normal' as family caregivers try to maintain everyday activities in the midst of their changing and often challenging new or modified caregiving experiences (56). In other words, these caregivers try to establish reliable patterns in their everyday life, while their caregiving duties evolve to meet the deteriorating health and function of their loved one.

As family caregivers interpret the changes in their loved ones' condition, their focus can be directed at current symptoms or toward the future while they interpret the present situation and accompanying caregiving duties (56). The family caregivers attempt to process the information at hand and then try to recreate a new state of normal in the midst of the chaos presented by the different stages of the ALS disease. Often, this involves changing the pattern of their way of life. When family caregivers successfully 'seek this normal', they state they are more confident, more certain, and feel more in control in their caregiving duties, which is congruent with the conceptualization of QoL explored by other researchers (72).

Connection with other ALS caregivers

Local and regional support groups are of great value to many family caregivers. The use of online as well as written resources, can be very valuable as well, and is explored in depth in Chapter 11. Stories of courage (44) is a website that profiles ALS patients and their family caregivers, telling their own stories of courage and dedication to maintaining an optimal QoL, as well as encouraging others living the ALS disease journey. The MDA (69) also provides a link for Share the Care that provides a model for organizing a volunteer caregiving group for family caregivers that are interested. MDA offers an online caregiver discussion forum and support groups, and an online mentoring programme under Today's Caregiver and Well Spouse Association (https://www.mda.org/). In addition to these online sources, the ALS clinics routinely supply lists of local in-person support groups that are available to family caregivers. ALS Chat (http://www.alsforums.com) is a free volunteer resource that can provide support, discussion and information for any ALS family caregiver. Also, Daily Strength (http://www.dailystrength.org) offers free support for ALS family caregivers where a caregiver can post his/her feelings, emotions, and thoughts, as well as respond to other caregiver postings or read through other family caregivers experiences that are shared in the chat room. Finally, Facebook ALS groups have provided support for family caregivers (http://www.facebook.com). Postings are shared to read or family caregivers can post their own thoughts to be shared with others.

ALS caregiver assessment instrument

One research team conducted a study to better understand ALS caregiver perceptions during the trajectory of the disease. A caregiver questionnaire (73) was developed using an evidence-based approach, including literature reviews, medical providers' input, and caregiver feedback. A total of 297 caregivers completed a caregiver survey prior to each ALS clinical visit, usually once every 3 months. All questionnaires were reviewed at each clinical visit by members of the ALS multidisciplinary team. Results (unpublished data) indicated that taking time (by the ALS multidisciplinary team) to review the impact of caregiving on the primary caregiver did not interfere with the busy clinic process, and the information provided was useful to medical and social service providers in meeting the needs of the patient and caregiver. Caregivers' confidence in their own problem-solving abilities was significantly related to their QoL, and meeting the patient's social and emotional needs was more challenging than providing the physical assistance needed by the patient. In addition, lack of time for social activities had a negative relationship with quality of life for the family member caring for the patient. Between 14 and 25% of the caregivers appeared to be at risk for clinical depression. Caregivers became more concerned about their ability to provide caregiving activities over time, with a decrease of the initial advantage of women over men. Caregivers who were women engaged in more support activities than did those who were men, but this decreased over time. Importantly, caregiving in motor neuron disease appears to be a dynamic process. Ongoing monitoring and re-assessment of caregivers is necessary to identify appropriate interventions throughout the disease trajectory.

Summary

ALS impacts every family member, but most heavily the family caregivers who provide the majority of care for their loved ones with ALS. Making health care providers more aware of the many challenges an ALS family caregiver faces throughout the disease trajectory is the first step in a process that can and should lead to more effective communication between health care providers and ALS family caregivers. This has the potential to result in interventions to target each caregivers' specific needs, thus optimizing their psychological well-being and physical health, and enabling those caregivers to become better able to serve in their highly challenging, but invaluable role in caring for their loved one with ALS. Targeting the health of the caregiver also offers the health care provider another mechanism to optimize the quality of life for their patient.

References

1. Navaie-Waliser, M., Feldman, P.H., Gould, D.A., Levine, C., Kuerbis, A.N., and Donelan, K. (2002) When the caregiver needs care: The plight of vulnerable caregivers. *American Journal of Public Health*, **92**, 409–13.

2. Waldrop, D.P., Kramer, B.J., Skretny, J.A., Milch, R.A., and Finn, W. (2005) Final transitions: Family caregiving at the end of life. *Journal of Palliative Medicine*, **8**, 623–38.

3. Aoun, S.M., Kristjanson, L.J., Currow, D.C., and Hudson, P.L. (2006) Caregiving for the terminally ill: At what cost? *Palliative Medicine*, **19**, 551–5.

4. Fromme, E.K., Drach, L.L., Tolle, S.W., et al. (2005) Men as caregivers at end of life. *Journal of Palliative Medicine*, **8**(6), 1167–75.

5. Hauser, J.M. and Kramer, B.J. (2004) Family caregivers in palliative care. *Clinics in Geriatric Medicine*, 2004; **20**:671–88.

6. **National Consensus Project** (2002) Clinical practice guidelines for quality palliative care. In: Kramer, B.J. and Thompson, B.H. (eds) *Men as Caregivers: Theory Research and Service Implications*, pp. 3–19. New York, NY: Springer.

7. **Rabow, M.W., Hauser, J.M.**, and **Adams, J.** (2004) Supporting family caregivers at the end of life: 'They don't know what they don't know'. *Journal of the American Medical Association*, **291**, 483–91.

8. **Sorrell, J.M.** (2007) Caring for the caregivers. *Journal of Psychosocial Nursing*, **45**, 17–20.

9. **Schultz, R.** and **Beach, S.** (1999) Caregiving as a risk factor for mortality: The caregiver health effects study. *Journal of the American Medical Association*, **282**, 2215–19.

10. **Lunney, J.R., Lynn, J.**, and **Hogan, C.** (2002) Profiles of older Medicare decedents. *Journal of the American Geriatric Society*, **50**, 1108–12.

11. **Lynn, J.** (2001) Perspectives on the care at the close of life: serving patients who may die soon and their families: the role of hospice and other services. *Journal of the American Medical Association*, **285**, 925–32.

12. **Hebert, R.S.** and **Schulz, R.** (2006) Caregiving at the end of life. *Journal of Palliative Medicine*, **9**, 1174–87.

13. **Schumacher, K.L., Stewart, B.J., Archbold, P.G., Dodd, M.J.**, and **Dibble, S.L.** (2000) Family caregiving skill: Development of the concept. *Research in Nursing & Health*, **23**, 191–203.

14. **Soothill, K., Morris, S.M., Harman, J., Francis, B.J., Thomas, C.**, and **McIllmurray, B.** (2001) Informal carers of cancer patients: what are their unmet social needs? *Health and Social Care in the Community*, **9**, 464–75.

15. **Emanuel, E.J., Fairclough, D.L., Slutsman, J.**, and **Emanuel, L.L.** (2000) Understanding economic and other burdens of terminal illness: The experience of patients and their caregivers. *Annals of Internal Medicine*, **132**, 451–59.

16. **Hanratty, B., Holland, P., Jacoby, A.**, and **Whitehead, M.** (2007) Financial stress and strain associated with terminal cancer: A review of the evidence. *Palliative Medicine*, **21**, 595–607.

17. **Levesque, L., Ducharme, F., Zarit, S., Lachance, L.**, and **Giroux, F.** (2008) Predicting longitudinal patterns of psychological distress in older husband caregivers: Further analysis of existing data. *Aging and Mental Health*, **12**, 333–42.

18. **Weitzner, M.A., Haley, W.E.**, and **Chen, H.** (2000) The family caregiver of the older cancer patient. *Hematology and Oncology Clinics of North America*, **14**, 269–81.

19. **Zivin, K.** and **Christakis, N.A.** (2007) The emotional toll of spousal morbidity and mortality. *American Journal of Geriatric Psychiatry*, **15**, 772–9.

20. **Rhee, Y., Degenholtz, H., Lo Sasso, A.T.**, and **Emanuel, L.L.** (2009) Estimating the quantity and economic value of family caregiving for community-dwelling older persons in the last year of life. *Journal of the American Geriatric Society*, **57**, 1654–59.

21. **Harding, R.** and **Higginson, I.J.** (2003) What is the best way to help caregivers in cancer and palliative care? A systematic literature review of interventions and their effectiveness. *Palliative Medicine*, **17**, 63–74.

22. **Lowder, J.L., Buzney, S.J.**, and **Buzo, A.M.** (2005) The caregiver balancing act: giving too much or not enough. *Care Management Journals*, **6**, 159–65.

23. **Schulz, R.** and **Martire, L.M.** (2004) Family caregiving of persons with dementia: Prevalence, health effects, and support strategies. *American Journal of Geriatric Psychiatry*, **12**, 240–9.

24. **Stajduhar, K.I.** (2003) Examining the perspectives of family members involved in the delivery of palliative care at home. *Journal of Palliative Care*, **19**, 27–35.

25. **Armon, C.** (2006) Who cares for the carers? *Amyotrophic Lateral Sclerosis*, **7**(3), 131.

26. **Pagnini, F., Rossi, G., Lunetta, C.,** et al. Burden, depression, and anxiety in caregivers of people with amyotrophic lateral sclerosis. *Psychology, Health & Medicine*, **15**(6), 685–93.

27. **Murphy, V., Felgoise, S.H., Walsh, S.M.,** and **Simmons, Z.** (2009) Problem solving skills predict quality of life and psychological morbidity in ALS caregivers. *Amyotrophic Lateral Sclerosis*, **10**(3), 147–53.

28. **MDA/ALS** (2008) *Caregiver's Guide.* Tucson, AZ: Muscular Dystrophy Association, Inc.

29. **Mockford, C., Jenkinson, C.,** and **Fitzpatrick, R.** (2006) A review: Carers, MND and service provision. *Amyotrophic Lateral Sclerosis*, **7**, 132–41.

30. **Rabkin, J.G., Wagner, G.J.,** and **Del Bene, M.** (2000) Resilience and distress among amyotrophic lateral sclerosis patients and caregivers. *Psychosomatic Medicine*, **62**, 271–9.

31. **Obermann, M.** and **Lyon, M.** (2015) Financial cost of amyotrophic lateral sclerosis: A case study. *Amyotrophic Lateral Sclerosis and Frontotemporal Degeneration*, **16**(1–2), 54–7.

32. **Mitsumoto H.** and **Rabkin, J.G.** (2006) Palliative care for patients with amyotrophic lateral sclerosis: Prepare for the worst and hope for the best. *Journal of American Medicine*, **298**(2), 207–16.

33. **Emanuel, E.J., Fairclough, D.L.,** and **Slutsman, J.** (1999) Assistance from family members, friends, paid caregivers, and volunteers in the care of terminally ill patients. *New England Journal of Medicine*, **34**(13), 956–63.

34. **Jenkinson, C., Fitzpatrick, R., Swash, M., Peto, V,** and **the ALS-HPS Steering Group** (2000) The ALS health profile study: quality of life of amyotrophic lateral sclerosis patients and carers in Europe. *Journal of Neurology*, **415**, 835–40.

35. **Clark, M.** and **Standard, P.L.** (1996) Caregivers burden and the structural family model. *Family and Community Health*, **18**, 58–68.

36. **Gauthier, A., Vignola, A., Calvo, A.,** et al. (2007) A longitudinal study on quality of life and depression in ALS patient-caregiver couples. *Neurology*, **68**, 923–6.

37. **Haley, W.E., Levine, E.G., Brown, S.L.,** and **Bartolucci, A.A.** (1987) Stress, appraisal, coping, and social support as predictors of adaptational outcome among dementia caregivers. *Psychology and Aging*, **2**, 323–30.

38. **Lazarus, R.S.** and **Folkman, S.** (1984) *Stress Appraisal and Coping.* New York, NY: Springer.

39. **Pearlin, L.I., Mullan, J.T., Semple, S.J.,** and **Skaff, M.M.** (1990) Caregiving and the stress process: An overview of concepts and their measures. *Gerontologist*, **30**, 583–94.

40. **Folkman, S.** and **Moskowitz, J.T.** (2000) Positive affect and the other side of coping. *American Psychologist*, **55**, 647–54.

41. **Haley, W.E.** and **Bailey, S.** (1999) Research on family caregiving in Alzheimer's disease: Implications for practice and policy. In: Vellas, B. and Fitten, J.L. (eds) *Research and Practice in Alzheimer's Disease*, **vol. 2**, pp. 321–32. Paris: Serdi Publisher.

42. **Oberst, M.T., Gass, K.A.,** and **Ward, S.E.** (1989) Caregiving demands and appraisal of stress among family caregivers. *Cancer Nursing*, **12**, 209–15.

43. **Kessler, R.C., Davis, R.B., Foster, D.F.,** et al. (2001) Long-term trends in the use of complementary and alternative medical therapies in the United States. *Annals of Internal Medicine*, **135**(4), 262–8.

44. **ALS Association** (2016) *Family Caregiving.* London: ALS Association. Available at: http://www.alsa.org (accessed 26 July 2017).

45. **Bolmsjo, I.** and **Hermeren, G.** (2001) Interviews with patients, family, and caregivers in amyotrophic lateral sclerosis: Comparing needs. *Journal of Palliative Care*, **17**, 236–40.

46. Chio`, A., Gauthier, A., Calvo, A., Ghiglione, P., and **Mutani, R.** (2005) Caregiver burden and patients' perception of being a burden in ALS. *Neurology*, **64**, 1780–82.

47. Gelinas, D.F., O'Connor, P., and **Miller, R.G.** (1998) Quality of life for ventilator-dependent ALS patients and their caregivers. *Journal of Neurological Sciences*, **160**(Suppl. 1), 134–6.

48. Goldstein, L.H., Atkins, L., Landau, S., Brown, R., and **Leigh, N.P.** (2006) Predictors of psychological distress in carers of people with amyotrophic lateral sclerosis. *Psychology and Medicine*, **36**, 865–75.

49. Hecht, M.J., Graesel, E., Tiggers, S., et al. (2003) Burden of care in amyotrophic lateral sclerosis. *Palliative Medicine*, **17**, 327–33.

50. Trail, M., Nelson, N.D., Van, J.N., Appel, S.H., and **Lai, E.C.** (2004) Major stressors facing patients with amyotrophic lateral sclerosis (ALS): A survey to identify their concerns and to compare with those of their caregivers. *Amyotrophic Lateral Sclerosis*, **5**, 40–5.

51. Adelman, E.E., Albert, S.M., Rabkin, J.G., Del Bene, M.L., Tider, T., and **O'Sullivan, I.** (2004) Disparities in perception of distress and burden in ALS patients and family caregivers. *Neurology*, **62**, 1766–70.

52. **ALS Association.** Diagnosing ALS (2008) [Cited 2017 Jan 30]. Available at: http://www.alsa.org/2015-non-responsive-pages/about-als/diagnosing-als.html

53. Shipley, P.Z., Penrod, J., and **Falkenstern, S.** (2018) Life patterns of family caregivers of patients with amyotrophic lateral sclerosis. *Nursing Science Quarterly* [Under review].

54. Grbich, C., Parker, D., and **Maddocks, I.** (2001) The emotions and coping strategies of caregivers of family members with a terminal cancer. *Journal of Palliative Care*, **17**, 30–6.

55. Penrod, J., Hupcey, J., Baney, B., and **Loeb, S.** (2010) End-of-life caregiving trajectories. *Clinical Nursing Research*, **20**(7), 7–24.

56. Penrod, J., Hupcey, J., Shipley, P., Loeb, S., and **Baney, B.** (2011) A model of caregiving through the end-of-life: seeking normal. *Western Journal of Nursing Research*, **34**(2), 174–93.

57. **Mitsumoto, H.** (2002) Caregiver assessment: summary. *Amyotrophic Lateral Sclerosis and Other Motor Neuron Disorders*, **3**(Suppl. 1), S31–S34.

58. **Greenberg, M.S.** (1980) A theory of indebtedness. In: Gergen, K.J., Greenberg, M.S., and Willis, R.H. (eds), *Social Exchange: Advances in Theory and Research*, pp. 3–26. New York, NY: Plenum.

59. Brehm, J.W. and **Cole, A.H.** (1966) Effect of a favor which reduces freedom. *Journal of Personal and Social Psychology*, **3**, 420–6.

60. **ALS Association.** (2010) Family Caregiving. Why Respite? London: ALS Association. Available at: http://www.alsa.org/als-care/resources/publications-videos/factsheets/fyi-respite.html

61. **ALS Association.** (2014) Home page. [Internet]. 2014; Available from: www.alsa.org

62. Ekwall, A.K., Sivberg, B., and **Hallberg, I.R.** (2005) Loneliness as a predictor of quality of life among older caregivers. *Journal of Advanced Nursing*, **49**, 23–32.

63. **Greenberger, H.** and **Litwin, H.** (2003) Can burdened caregivers be effective facilitators of elder care-recipient health care? *Journal of Advanced Nursing*, **41**, 332–41.

64. Su, X.W., Broach, J.R., Connor, J.R., Gerhard, G.S., and **Simmons, Z.** (2014) Genetic heterogeneity of amyotrophic lateral sclerosis: Implications for clinical practice and research. *Muscle & Nerve*, **49**, 786–803.

65. **Family Caregiver Alliance** (2016) *What is ALS?* Available at: www.caregiver.org (accessed 26 July 2017).

66. **Reinhard, S., Given, B., Petlick, N.H.,** and **Bemis, A.** (2008) *Supporting Family Caregivers in Providing Care.* Available at: https://www.ncbi.nlm.nih.gov (accessed 26 July 2017).

67. **Ruppert, R.** (1996) Psychological aspects of lay caregiving. *Rehabilitation Nursing,* **21**(6), 315–20.

68. **Ferullo, C.M., Mascolo, M., Ferrandes, G.,** and **Caponnetto, C.** (2009) Amyotrophic lateral sclerosis: An assessment of the needs of patients and caregivers in the Liguria region of Italy. *Giornale Italiano Di Medicina Del Lavoro Ed Ergonomia,* **31**, A16–23.

69. **Muscular Dystrophy Association** (2017) *Home Page.* Available at: www.mdausa.org (accessed 26 July 2017).

70. **Motor Neurone Disease Association** (2016) Our Vision, Mission, Values. Available at: www.mndassociation.org (accessed 26 July 2017).

71. **International Alliance of ALS/MND Associations.** (2017) Home Page. Available at: www. alsmndalliance.org (accessed 26 July 2017).

72. **Ferrell, B.R.** (1999) The impact of pain on quality of life: A decade of research. *Nursing Clinics of North America,* **30**, 609–24.

73. **Bremer, B., Stephens, H.E., Reading, J., Fink, A., Walsh, S.,** and **Simmons, Z.** (2017) *Longitudinal Assessment of Caregivers of Patients with Motor Neuron Disease.* Available at: http://www.pennstatehershey.org/c/document_library/get_file?uuid=a4a986be-9b45-4589-a4df-16e4657b17f7&groupId=22147 (accessed 26 July 2017).

Chapter 17

Providing holistic care for the individual with ALS: Research gaps and future directions

Francesco Pagnini and Zachary Simmons

Despite recent progress by researchers on quality of life (QoL) and psychological well-being in ALS, many gaps remain in our understanding of these concepts and in our knowledge of how best to address them. Future efforts should not only build upon the solid foundation of knowledge and approaches described in this book, but should make full use of technologies and discoveries from other fields that have opened up new research opportunities.

Healthcare professionals caring for persons with ALS have largely re-defined the concept of QoL for those with the disease, moving from a narrow, physician-defined, physically centred medical definition to a broad construct of patient-defined well-being. One central element to this change in perception is the realization and acceptance by health care professionals that a person with profound physical impairment can have a high QoL, as his or her values, interests, and passions change and adapt to new situations (1). We have developed instruments and tools that seek to quantify QoL, and that have proven to be helpful in both clinical and research settings (2). Most of these assessments reflect current knowledge and thinking in psychometrics, using a 'traditional' approach to psychological testing. As such, they have their intrinsic limitations, and some may also be lengthy and exhausting for physically limited patients. As the field of psychometrics evolves, ALS researchers should consider applying new testing strategies and methods, such as item response theory and computer-adaptive tests, to further refine QoL assessments, optimizing patients' time and efforts (3). These techniques allow a reduction of the number of test questions by 'estimating' the answers to some questions, predicted through advanced algorithms (4).

Many studies have explored the psychological impact of the disease, often focusing on depressive and stressful reactions, which represent threats to overall QoL. A number of gaps exist. New research on coping skills and resilience has the potential to provide insightful and applicable clinical suggestions to reduce psychological distress. Furthermore, certain needs of ALS patients have been overlooked by most psychological and QoL studies, particularly sexuality and intimacy. Exploration of such 'embarrassing' and uncomfortable themes should be part of clinical practice, as well as research, because of the potential to improve psychological well-being. As additional studies are undertaken, emphasis should be placed on longitudinal studies, which are scarce in the psychologically-oriented ALS literature. Further studies about how psychological outcomes change over time are needed, as they may identify new predictors of QoL that can be addressed by specific interventions.

Another gap exists with regard to studies of the end-of-life in ALS. Most of the conventional literature focuses on symptom management (e.g. dyspnoea, pain, sialorrhoea), rather than the psychological aspects of facing imminent death.

Research on psychological intervention in ALS is a relatively recent and much-needed development (5), and it is providing promising and interesting results. Some psychological treatments appear to result in the reduction of distress and depressive features, leading to a higher QoL (6). Given the unique features of ALS, the simple replication of an intervention protocol that has been proven to be effective in a different field may not be optimal. The development of new psychological practices that can address specific needs of people with ALS (and, possibly, their caregivers) is desirable. Specific needs include coping with progressive physical impairment resulting in the need for assistive devices, bulbar dysfunction resulting in impaired swallowing and communication, and the inevitable terminal nature of the condition. Further studies are required to explore the potential benefits of such psychological treatments in promoting both psychological and physical benefits. Importantly, the impact of psychological treatments on physical disease progression warrants further research. This is an underexplored area for which there is some promising early data on the effects of mindfulness (7) and hypnosis (8).

Complementary and alternative medicines (CAMs) generally receive little attention in the world of conventional medicine. However, even if such treatments demonstrate limited efficacy in altering disease progression, physicians and researchers should be mindful of their psychological effects, particularly in providing patients with a way to increase their perceived control and self-efficacy. In this way, CAMs could represent a source of hope and, therefore, psychological well-being. This is an area that would benefit from rigorous scientific investigation.

During the past decade, it has become clear that behavioral and cognitive changes are an important part of the ALS disease spectrum. It is noteworthy that a major journal in the ALS world has changed its name from *Amyotrophic Lateral Sclerosis* to *Amyotrophic Lateral Sclerosis & Frontotemporal Degeneration*. Cognitive deterioration and behavioral change are aspects that have been extensively explored, but that require additional investigation, not only from the perspective of assessment ('what is happening'), but of intervention and management ('what can we do to reduce the impact of cognitive and behavioral change on the patient and caregiver?').

Recent advances in our scientific knowledge have made tools and opportunities available that were inconceivable in even the recent past. Genetic tests can now help identify the risk for developing ALS, and provide data to support the development of new drugs targeting genetic expression. Technological changes, ranging from inexpensive text-to-speech devices to eye-gaze systems to brain-computer interfaces are offering new opportunities for patients with marked physical impairments to communicate, not only with people in the same room, but long-distance, via the internet. New challenges for future researchers will include the increasing incorporation of these technologies into clinical practice. Specifically, the availability of new communication technologies, particularly complex ones such as brain-computer interfaces, does not directly translate into clinical usage. Studies that unite efforts and knowledge from basic science and engineering with those from clinical research are essential.

Technological innovations and new discoveries will have to be mindfully communicated and shared with patients and their families. As new scientific knowledge becomes available, an important role of scientists and physicians is to effectively communicate this knowledge to patients and to the general public. To be effective, science must be viewed, by both those who perform it and those who may potentially benefit from it, as not simply a series of isolated laboratory experiments, but as a field that can and will impact people's lives. The increasing interest by patients and families in genetic testing to predict the risk of developing ALS, or the explosion of discussion about physician-hastened death, highlights the importance of a social and cultural debate about the effects of new discoveries. These discussions are increasingly being conducted on the internet, from patient-to-patient, researcher-to-researcher, and patient-to-researcher. Via such mechanisms, the transition from research to practice is greatly facilitated.

Although most studies on QoL and psychological well-being in ALS focus on the person with the disease, it is becoming increasingly clear that the impact of the disease is not limited to that person alone, but extends to family, friends, and others who provide care or are close to that individual. Reducing caregiver stress and burden should be an integral part of ALS care. Interventions that focus on this warrant further research. Often overlooked is the impact on healthcare professionals of providing care to patients (9,10). This may be particularly relevant when the patients have a chronic, fatal diseases, such as ALS. Although healthcare providers caring for ALS patients have high job satisfaction, stress and burnout appear to be significant considerations (9). Further exploration of this, and of interventions to mitigate it, would improve the well-being not only of the healthcare professional, but potentially of the healthcare recipient (patient) as well.

In the Introduction, we noted, 'This book attempts to provide a solid scientific foundation for an approach to care that does not just treat the disease, but rather *takes care* of the person as a whole.' We believe that the chapters of this book individually and cumulatively support this goal. The classical medical paradigm that sees the patient in the same way that a mechanic sees a car, as something to be 'fixed' by a series of procedures, is doomed to failure for a disease such as ALS, in which there are no medical treatments that can reverse the widespread neurological damage. However, an inability to cure should never result in a failure to provide care and treatment for the person with ALS. The unifying theme of the book can be crystalized in one concept: the effective practice of medical care is directed not to the illness, but to the *person*. A healthcare professional should attend to as many of the individual characteristics of each patient as possible. No two patients with ALS are like one another, even if their physical disease courses are essentially identical. If the health care professional's approach to care and management of an individual with ALS is to be effective in optimizing QoL and psychological well-being, it must be individualized to the physical, psychological, social, existential, and other characteristics of each patient. In practicing conventional medicine, healthcare professionals may overlook this broad perspective, leading to a narrow focus on medical issues alone. Paying attention not only to the medical information that is being conveyed, but to non-medical information, including the feelings and emotions of the patient, can lead to the establishment of a connection that goes beyond the mechanics of 'fixing' the problem, and facilitates the creation of a strong patient-physician relationship. Such an approach may be the most effective 'medicine' of all (11).

References

1. **Simmons, Z., Bremer, B.A., Robbins, R.A., Walsh, S.M.,** and **Fischer, S.** (2000) Quality of life in ALS depends on factors other than strength and physical function. *Neurology,* **55**(3), 388–92.
2. **Simmons, Z.** (2015) Patient-perceived outcomes and quality of life in ALS. *Neurotherapeutics,* **12**(2), 394–402.
3. **Gibbons, C., Bower, P., Lovell, K., Valderas, J.,** and **Skevington, S.** (2016) Electronic quality of life assessment using computer-adaptive testing. *Journal of Medical Internet Research,* **18**(9), e240.
4. **Embretson, S.E.** and **Reise, S.P.** (2013) *Item Response Theory.* Hove: Psychology Press.
5. **Pagnini, F., Simmons, Z., Corbo, M.,** and **Molinari, E.** (2012) Amyotrophic lateral sclerosis: Time for research on psychological intervention? *Amyotrophic Lateral Sclerosis,* **13**(5), 416–17.
6. **Gould, R.L., Coulson, M.C., Brown, R.G., Goldstein, L.H., Al-Chalabi, A.,** and **Howard, R.J.** (2015) Psychotherapy and pharmacotherapy interventions to reduce distress or improve well-being in people with amyotrophic lateral sclerosis: A systematic review. *Amyotrophic Lateral Sclerosis and Frontotemporal Degeneration,* **16**(5–6), 293–302.
7. **Pagnini, F., Phillips, D., Bosma, C., Reece, A.,** and **Langer, E.** (2015) Mindfulness, physical impairment and psychological well-being in people with amyotrophic lateral sclerosis. *Psychology & Health,* **30**(5), 503–17.
8. **Kleinbub, J.R., Palmieri, A., Broggio, A.,** et al. (2015) Hypnosis-based psychodynamic treatment in ALS: A longitudinal study on patients and their caregivers. *Frontiers in Psychology,* **6,** 624.
9. **Bromberg, M.B., Schenkenberg, T.,** and **Brownell, A.A.** (2011) A survey of stress among amyotrophic lateral sclerosis care providers. *Amyotrophic Lateral Sclerosis,* **12**(3), 162–7.
10. **Kahn, M.W.** (2008) Etiquette-based medicine. *New England Journal of Medicine,* **358**(19), 1988–9.
11. **Larson, E.B.** and **Yao, X.** (2005) Clinical empathy as emotional labor in the patient-physician relationship. *Journal of the American medical Association,* **293**(9), 1100–6.

Index